Praise for *The Complete Mediterranean Diet*

This comprehensive book contains an easy-to-understand section on how the Mediterranean diet and lifestyle can lead to health and longevity. It also contains more than 500 delicious recipes that are easy to make. The ingredients for the recipes can be found in any supermarket and nutrition information is listed for each recipe including calories, carbohydrate counts, and fiber. The book can be used by calorie counters, diabetes patients using carbohydrate exchanges, Paleo folks who need veggie/protein ideas, and the rest of us mortals in need of inspiration.

—Maria A. Bella, MS, RD, CDN

Praise for Dr. Ozner and *The Miami Mediterranean Diet*

I strongly recommend Dr. Ozner's book, *The Miami Mediterranean Diet*, for anyone who is interested in living a long and healthy life. This book is a concise, no-nonsense approach for heart disease prevention. With so many fad diets that are here today and gone tomorrow, finally there is a clinically proven and sensible approach, as Dr. Ozner provides practical dietary and lifestyle guidelines for defeating heart disease.

—Barry T. Katzen, MD
Medical Director, Baptist Cardiac & Vascular Institute of Miami

---

The current medical literature is replete with articles confirming what Dr. Ozner has been advocating for many years—that prevention is the best treatment for heart disease. In his book, *The Miami Mediterranean Diet*, he outlines a strategy that, combined with an exercise program, has allowed me to reduce my weight, my blood pressure, and my cholesterol. I have a greater sense of well-being and I feel that I will live a longer and healthier life.

—Jerrold Young, MD

In *The Miami Mediterranean Diet*, Dr. Michael Ozner not only makes a compelling argument for the importance of the Mediterranean diet and lifestyle for overall health, but gives a comprehensive guide for ways to incorporate this diet into all of our lives. Research has clearly shown that those who follow a life-long Mediterranean diet and lifestyle are giving themselves the best insurance for a healthy life and now Dr. Ozner brings that to our shores.

—Randolph P. Martin, MD
Director of Noninvasive Cardiology, Emory University Hospital

A valuable resource from preventive cardiologist Michael Ozner providing heart-healthy dietary information, sample meal plans, and an exciting array of recipes.

—NANETTE K. WENGER, MD
Professor of Medicine (Cardiology),
Emory University School of Medicine

This book is a direct path to the visceral pleasure of well-prepared food and cardiovascular health. *The Miami Mediterranean Diet* provides a sane alternative to the faddist and extremist diets that lead to short-term weight loss and long-term weight gain.

—JOSEPH L. IZZO, JR., MD
Professor of Medicine & Pharmacology,
State University of New York at Buffalo, Clinical Director of Medicine,
Erie County Medical Center, Buffalo, New York

I wholeheartedly endorse the Mediterranean diet, a way of eating that has been in existence for thousands of years. *The Miami Mediterranean Diet* is based on this way of life, encouraging a balanced, well-nourished food plan including whole grains, fresh fruits and vegetables, and lower fat intake. Following Ozner's stated food plan, coupled with caloric control and daily exercise, can lead to both weight loss and a healthy heart. The recipes are easy to produce and generate delicious meals; no one would feel deprived adhering to the stated plan.

—KAREN LIEBERMAN, PhD, RD
Professor and Chair, the Hospitality College,
Johnson & Wales University, Florida Campus

I have bounced from one diet to another, including the "low-carb" diets. My weight would go up and down on these fad diets and I felt that I was mortgaging my long-term health in order to achieve weight loss. I adopted Dr. Ozner's dietary and lifestyle guidelines and I have achieved my goal—controlled and steady weight loss. In addition, my cholesterol has dropped, my blood pressure has normalized, and I have more energy. I highly endorse this book for anyone seeking to decrease their risk of heart disease and improve their overall health.

—PATIENT (CP)

EVERYTHING YOU NEED TO KNOW
TO LOSE WEIGHT AND LOWER
YOUR RISK OF HEART DISEASE...
WITH 500 DELICIOUS RECIPES

The Complete Mediterranean Diet

*Lifesaving Advice Based on the Clinically Proven
Mediterranean Diet and Lifestyle*

Michael Ozner, MD
MEDICAL DIRECTOR
Cardiovascular Prevention Institute of South Florida

BENBELLA BOOKS, INC.
Dallas, Texas

BenBella

BenBella Books, Inc.
10440 N. Central Expy., Suite 800
Dallas, TX 75231
Send feedback to feedback@benbellabooks.com • www.benbellabooks.com

Printed in the United States of America
10 9 8 7

Library of Congress Cataloging-in-Publication Data

Ozner, Michael D.
    The complete Mediterranean diet : everything you need to know to lose weight and lower your risk of heart disease . . . with 500 delicious recipes / Michael Ozner, M.D., Medical Director, Cardiovascular Prevention Institute of South Florida.
        pages cm
    Includes bibliographical references and index.
    ISBN 978-1-939529-95-4 (pbk.)—ISBN 978-1-939529-96-1 (electronic) 1. Reducing diets—Recipes. 2. Cooking, Mediterranean. 3. Heart—Diseases—Diet therapy—Recipes. I. Title.
    RM222.2.O959 2014
    641.59'1822—dc23
                                                                                                2013039368

Proofreading by Kimberly Marini, Amy Zarkos, and Cape Cod Compositors, Inc.
Full cover design by Faceout Studio
Text design and composition by John Reinhardt Book Design
Index by WordCo Indexing Services
Printed by Versa Press

Distributed by Perseus Distribution • perseusdistribution.com

To place orders through Perseus Distribution:
Tel: 800-343-4499
Fax: 800-351-5073
E-mail: orderentry@perseusbooks.com

Special discounts for bulk sales (minimum of 25 copies) are available.
Please contact Aida Herrera at aida@benbellabooks.com.

Acknowledgments

I would like to thank my patients and colleagues who gave me the inspiration and motivation to write *The Miami Mediterranean Diet* and this expanded edition, *The Complete Mediterranean Diet*.

I am especially grateful to the following individuals who took extensive time and effort to review and critique *The Miami Mediterranean Diet*: Barry T. Katzen, MD, a pioneer in interventional radiology and Medical Director of the Baptist Cardiac & Vascular Institute at Baptist Hospital of Miami; Randolph P. Martin, MD, Director of Noninvasive Cardiology at Emory University in Atlanta; and Karen Lieberman, PhD, RD, Professor and Chair of the Hospitality College at Johnson & Wales University, Florida Campus. I would also like to thank Nanette K. Wenger, MD, and Joseph L. Izzo, MD, for reviewing and commenting on *The Miami Mediterranean Diet*.

I would like to express my gratitude to all of the nurse educators who share my passion for cardiovascular disease prevention and who have helped me organize and promote the Wellness & Prevention Program at the Baptist Cardiac & Vascular Institute at Baptist Hospital of Miami. This program provides education and prevention strategies for patients who have heart disease or diabetes and for those with risk factors for cardiovascular disease.

I am also grateful to Glenn Yeffeth, Adrienne Lang, and Lindsay Marshall at BenBella Books for their steadfast guidance and advice.

Finally, and most importantly, I would like to thank my wife, Christine Ozner, RN, who has a special interest in nutrition and Mediterranean cooking and has contributed immensely to the writing and editing of this book.

To my wife, Christine, and my children, Jennifer and Jonathan:
You are my heart and soul.

Congratulations! By reading this book and following the principles of the Mediterranean diet and lifestyle, you will begin to take charge of your cardiovascular health.

This book is intended to provide information on cardiovascular disease prevention. However, it is *not* intended to replace the doctor-patient relationship. I recommend that you discuss all prevention and treatment options with your personal treating physician. Regular office visits between a patient and his or her doctor to discuss cardiovascular prevention strategies provide the optimum approach in the ongoing battle against heart disease.

Contents

Foreword   xi

PART ONE
The Mediterranean Diet and Lifestyle

How Your Diet and Lifestyle Are Affecting Your Health   3
The Mediterranean Diet and Lifestyle   9
Why Choose the Mediterranean Diet?   19
Putting the Pieces Together   27
It's Your Choice!   41

PART TWO
Recipes

A 14-Day Menu Plan   45
A Guide to Cooking Method Terminology   65
Salads   67
Soups   107
Pizza, Pizza Sauces, and Pizza Crusts   139
Omelets, Eggs, Frittatas, and Cereals   155
Pancakes   165
Main Dishes   169
Side Dishes   309
Wraps and Sandwiches   363
Breads   383
Desserts   395

Smoothies and Coolers 439
Appetizers, Dips, and Snack Foods 445
Spices, Sauces, Marinades, and Dressings 475

Appendices

APPENDIX A: The Atherogenic Metabolic Stew 503
APPENDIX B: Important Medications for
    Cardiovascular Disease Prevention 505
APPENDIX C: Tips on Purchasing, Preparing, and Eating
    Foods in the Mediterranean Diet 507
APPENDIX D: Eating Out on the Mediterranean Diet
    (The Restaurant Survival Guide) 521

Glossary 523
Recipe Index 529
Index 553
About the Author 561

Foreword

I hate the word "diet." Ask any girl over the age of thirteen for the definition of "diet," and she will undoubtedly tell you a story of denial and deprivation. The word "diet" has a negative connotation because we as a culture have given it just that. In all actuality, the *Oxford Dictionary* definition for diet is simply, "the kinds of food that a person, animal, or community habitually eats."

In America, I believe, we have a strange relationship with our food. Whether we overeat and feel a sense of guilt and shame, therefore starving ourselves the next day, or we subscribe to a very strict regimen of eating whatever fits one's definition of "health," we are constantly obsessing about the food that goes into our bodies. And truthfully, how can we not? Everything in our culture, it seems, revolves around food. Whether at breakfast meetings, lunch with the girls, dinners with friends, holidays, birthdays, even funerals, we are constantly eating. If we are not careful, we can easily fall into the vicious cycle of binging and depriving indefinitely.

Although I, too, fell prey to this food trap, I managed to make my way back to the diet of my ancestors, which today we call the "Mediterranean diet." I am the first person in my family to have been born in the United States. My parents immigrated to America from Greece in the early 1970s. Besides two suitcases and two children (my brother and sister), they brought along with them centuries of culture and tradition, most of which also revolves around food. However, my family's relationship with food was quite different than the American norm. Our diet was primarily based around whole natural foods straight from the earth. My mother's kitchen was filled with fresh, seasonal fruits and vegetables from our garden, extra-virgin olive oil, mint, oregano, parsley, lemons, all sorts of beans, and, of course, lamb—after all, we are Greek! I always ate to my heart's content, always feeling satiated. Whether she was conscious of it back then or not, my mother's cooking was way ahead of its time.

It was not until I moved to New York City to work at MTV and attend NYU that I realized how fortunate I was to have been raised in the traditional Greek way of eating. As a first-year college student and intern at MTV, I was constantly on the run, and my diet shifted dramatically. I began eating like college students do. It was all take-out and deli food. It was cheap and fast. I was eating less, never feeling satiated, and yet gaining weight. I couldn't believe it! How could food labeled *fat free* or *diet* cause me to gain weight? Well, it did. Although I thought I was eating in a healthy way, it turns out that I was consuming all processed foods loaded with sodium and empty calories.

Exasperated by my expanding waistline, splotchy skin, and general lethargy, I knew something needed to be done. While visiting home one weekend and eating my mom's cooking morning, noon, and night, I noticed my jeans fitting a little looser. Feeling excited and encouraged, I asked her what she was putting in the food and why I was no longer feeling bloated and sluggish. My mom was surprised by my question, and she responded, "Nothing, honey! Olive oil, vegetables, and meat!" Suddenly, a light bulb went off in my head and I realized the key to fixing my diet: If a food has ingredients in it that I cannot pronounce, then I should not be eating it.

Upon my return to New York City, I made a concerted effort to start eating the foods on which I was raised. The Greeks have an ancient life philosophy that basically states *everything in moderation*, and that is exactly how I began to live. I soon returned to my natural weight, my energy skyrocketed, and my skin cleared up. Needless to say, it was great for my self-esteem and my social calendar. I was healthy and vibrant and have stayed that way ever since.

More important, there are also unbeatable long-term health benefits to eating the way the Greeks do. Earlier this year, I had the pleasure of meeting Dr. Michael Ozner. He shared his book *The Complete Mediterranean Diet* with me and helped me understand some of the science behind the ancient traditions I had learned as a child. Dr. Ozner is an award-winning cardiologist and advocate for heart disease prevention, and his work has helped me identify why and how my switch back to a traditional Greek diet transformed my body, both inside and out.

In this revised edition of his popular book *The Miami Mediterranean Diet*, which has more than 100,000 copies, Dr. Ozner goes into depth regarding why and how eating whole, non-processed foods, rich in a wide variety of vitamins and nutrients, reduces the risk of heart disease, obesity, diabetes, cancer, and numerous other diseases. In addition to sound clinical advice and the latest scientific findings, Dr. Ozner also shares 200 new, healthy, and delicious recipes, making a total of 500 dishes, all built from the main ingredients of a Mediterranean diet—whole grains, fresh fruits and vegetables, nuts, beans, fish, olive oil, and even a little red wine.

The Complete Mediterranean Diet is a fantastic combination of nutrition text and cookbook. I am confident it will prove to be a useful resource for you as well, with its simple and delicious approach to regaining your health while trimming your waistline. So, here's to the well-being I've rediscovered through the food of my ancestors and to the hope that, with Dr. Ozner's help, you'll find that same vitality, too. *Kali orexei* and *Opa*! (Good appetite and Opa!)

—DEBBIE MATENOPOULOS
Actress, TV personality, and coauthor of *It's All Greek to Me*

PART ONE

THE MEDITERRANEAN DIET AND LIFESTYLE

How Your Diet and Lifestyle
Are Affecting Your Health

Ted and Giovanni

It was a typical day for Ted. He awoke at 6 A.M. and had his usual breakfast of bacon, eggs, and fried potatoes. He left home in a hurry after an argument with his wife and drove to his office to begin another stressful day as a real estate executive. At a 9:30 A.M. board meeting, he presented a proposal for purchasing a large office complex. During the meeting he had coffee and doughnuts and smoked several cigarettes. It was customary for Ted to argue with his partners, and today was no different. After several phone calls he was off to the airport to catch a noon flight. He had no time to sit down for lunch, so he went to his favorite fast-food drive-through for a burger and fries, which he ate quickly on the way to the airport. After parking his car and walking briskly to the terminal, he felt a crushing chest pain and broke into a sweat. He grabbed a roll of Tums from his pocket and chewed several tablets. The pain subsided briefly, only to return with a vengeance several minutes later. This time the pain was an intense sensation of pressure in his chest that radiated out to his arms and his jaw. He collapsed at the security gate and lost consciousness. When he awoke, he was in a nearby emergency room, having been resuscitated by paramedics. It was clear that Ted had suffered a massive heart attack and was lucky to be alive. Following an extensive hospital stay including heart catheterization and coronary bypass surgery, Ted's life would never be the same.

Giovanni awoke the same day in his small Italian village. He ate a light breakfast of whole grain bread with jam and fruit. He walked to his nearby office and passed a pleasant morning with his clients in his import/export business. At 2:00 P.M., he returned home, where he shared an enjoyable lunch with his family and friends. Lunch consisted of a salad with olive oil, whole wheat pasta, whole grain bread with garlic, goat cheese, red wine, and fresh fruit. Following lunch, he rested for an hour, and then returned to work.

Was Ted's heart attack preventable? Is Giovanni's good health a matter of luck? Or are both the consequences of diet and lifestyle?

The Toxic American Diet and Lifestyle

The American diet and lifestyle are toxic. Our food is contaminated with pesticides and preservatives and contains an excessive amount of dangerous fat, sugar, and salt. We no longer exercise, and our lives are plagued by chronic stress. In the last fifty years, there's been an explosive rise in heart disease, stroke, high blood pressure, diabetes, and obesity, diseases that have been directly linked to the food we eat and the lifestyle we lead.

We have been led to believe that the solution to this epidemic is to be found in medical or surgical intervention: in prescription medications and invasive surgeries. But despite the billions of dollars we spend on health care, we continue to suffer and die unnecessarily from diseases *that can be prevented*.

I have been practicing preventive cardiology for more than twenty-five years and have helped countless patients discover the real secret of long-term health: the optimal nutrition and healthy daily practices of the Mediterranean diet and lifestyle.

Heart Disease: Your First Symptom May Be Your Last

Why do I practice preventive cardiology? Because heart disease is the number one killer of men and women in America and in most developed countries around the world—and most people never see it coming.

It would be nice if we had a warning system that alerted us to heart disease. Many people think chest pain is that warning system. Unfortunately, for the majority of men and women, the first symptom you experience is a heart attack—or sudden death. By then, it's too late.

In many respects, coronary heart disease is a silent killer—we are completely unaware of its presence in our body until a plaque ruptures and a heart attack occurs. Recent data has revealed that small plaques (which cause no symptoms) are in fact *more* likely than large plaques to suddenly rupture and lead to a heart attack or sudden death. The only way to defeat this formidable enemy, cardiovascular disease, is to attack when the enemy is most easily defeated—prior to the onset of symptoms!

The Mediterranean diet has been shown to reduce the risk of:

- Allergies
- Alzheimer's disease
- Arthritis
- Asthma
- Cancer
- Cardiovascular disease
- Chronic obstructive lung disease
- Depression
- Diabetes
- High blood pressure
- High cholesterol
- Inflammatory bowel disease
- Metabolic syndrome

Believing in preventive cardiology doesn't mean I think surgery is never a necessary step. There are absolutely situations where surgical or cardiac catheterization procedures are not only needed but also may save lives, especially in the case of patients with "unstable" heart disease, meaning they have an impending heart attack or are actually experiencing one. However, the vast majority of patients a doctor sees in his or her office are not unstable. Rather, they are stable patients who either have risk factors for coronary heart disease or have "stable" blockages in their arteries. And too often, doctors rely on coronary artery bypass surgery and coronary stent placement when the best treatment for the patient is aggressive prevention, which can halt the progression of cardiovascular disease and potentially even reverse it.

Through my practice, I've learned that prevention is more important than medication or bypass surgery in achieving greater heart health. And together, diet and lifestyle can reduce or eliminate the need for expensive medications and risky surgical interventions.

Susan's Story

About four and a half years ago, I awoke at about 5 A.M. with the most horrible pain in my chest and extreme shortness of breath. In a panic and with an unbelievable sense of impending doom, I woke my husband, who immediately called 911. Forty thousand dollars later, through the grace of God, I had survived a major heart attack.

Seven months earlier, I had experienced a few minor symptoms that led me to see a group of doctors. They did some tests, performed a heart procedure to put a stent in one of my coronary arteries, and told me that I could go home and relax because they had "taken care" of my problem. After my heart attack, those same doctors told me that I was "stable" now that they had put in a second stent, but that I should return to the emergency room if I experienced any more chest pain. I realized that I needed to do more than just wait for the next heart attack to occur. I needed to take steps personally that would help me avoid another such experience, or worse. I have two grown children and three adorable grandkids. I desperately want to be around to enjoy them and to spend those coveted golden years with my husband. There had to be more that could be done. I felt it was just a matter of time before I once again found myself lying on an ER stretcher, praying that I would survive. The word "despondent" barely describes my anxiety.

I was determined to learn more about heart disease and what my options were. A few months later, my husband learned about a cardiologist in Miami who exclusively practiced cardiovascular prevention. We learned that Dr. Ozner gave lectures on heart disease prevention to other physicians as well as to the general public. After doing some research, I began to feel there was hope for me, so I made an appointment to see him.

Dr. Ozner started me on the Mediterranean diet and a regime of medical therapy to lower my cholesterol and blood pressure. He also started me on a walking program. When Dr. Ozner first mentioned lifestyle changes and diet, I became concerned; I had tried other diets, but after the initial weight loss I would eventually gain the weight back. I began to realize that those diets didn't make much sense. Dr. Ozner told me he had based the Mediterranean diet on a way of eating that has been in existence for thousands of years and has been proven over the last fifty years to reduce heart disease risk.

I've lost a lot of weight on the Mediterranean diet and now maintain a normal weight. This is a diet I can live with for the rest of my life! As a matter of fact, it's a way of life that my entire family can embrace; my entire family now follows the diet and exercise program.

As for me, I haven't needed any more cardiac procedures and I feel better than I have in years!

Beyond Heart Disease Prevention

But this isn't just about heart disease. The Mediterranean diet and lifestyle lowers the risk of a multitude of chronic diseases. You may very well wonder how a single eating plan can afford all these benefits. That's a fair question. The secret seems to lie in the fact that the Mediterranean diet is *synergistic*. This means that the components are not only nutritious in themselves, but when combined with one another, act together to provide added benefits as well. They are more powerful in combination than if they were eaten separately.

The Mediterranean diet is full of fruits and vegetables rich in antioxidants, which help prevent the damage to your body's cells that cause heart disease, cancer, and other diseases. The diet also features whole grain foods rich in fiber, which has been shown to help balance cholesterol and also prevent some forms of cancer. In addition, the diet decreases inflammation, which has been strongly linked to the development of heart disease, cancer, and other ailments such as arthritis.

In short, if you're looking for a diet that will benefit your entire body, you can do no better than to choose the Mediterranean diet.

The Mediterranean Diet
and Lifestyle

The Mediterranean Diet

The Mediterranean diet—a diet of whole non-processed foods, rich in a wide variety of health-promoting vitamins and nutrients—is the ideal dietary plan for long-term heart health and weight control; multiple clinical trials have demonstrated its beneficial impact. Indeed, a landmark study from Spain was recently reported in the prestigious *New England Journal of Medicine* (February 25, 2013), comparing a Mediterranean diet to a low-fat diet. The study was stopped after 4.8 years due to a highly significant 30 percent reduction in major cardiovascular events (heart attack, stroke, death) in those following the Mediterranean diet. As reported in the *New York Times* on March 2, 2013, medical experts stated, "This is a watershed moment in the field of nutrition. For the first time, a diet has been shown to have an effect as powerful as drugs in preventing what really matters to patients—heart attacks, strokes and death from cardiovascular disease."

Below is a brief summary of some of the other important clinical trials demonstrating a beneficial impact of the Mediterranean diet on cardiovascular health:

The Seven Countries Study
This landmark twenty-year study by Dr. Ancel Keys demonstrated that a diet low in saturated animal fat and processed food was associated with a low incidence of mortality from coronary heart disease and cancer. Beginning in the late 1950s, the study followed almost 13,000 men from seven different countries (Italy, Greece, Yugoslavia, Netherlands, Finland, United States, and Japan). Men living in the Mediterranean region had the lowest incidence of heart disease and

the longest life expectancy. And Greek men had a 90% lower likelihood of premature death from heart attack compared to American men!

The Lyon Diet Heart Study

This study compared a Mediterranean diet to a control diet resembling the American Heart Association Step 1 diet in heart attack survivors and found that, compared to the American Heart Association Step 1 diet, the Mediterranean diet afforded significantly better protection against recurrent heart attacks and death. The Mediterranean diet was associated with a 70% decreased risk of death and a 73% decreased risk of recurrent cardiac events.

The DART Study

This study of more than 2,000 men who had suffered heart attacks tested the hypothesis that fatty fish such as salmon and tuna, rich in omega-3 fatty acids, are protective against coronary heart disease. The results demonstrated that a modest intake of fatty fish twice per week (around 300 grams per week) reduced the risk of coronary heart disease death by 32% and overall death by 29%.

The Singh Indo-Mediterranean Diet Study

This study placed 499 patients with risk factors for coronary heart disease on an Indo-Mediterranean diet rich in fruits, vegetables, whole grains, walnuts, and almonds. The study found that the diet change resulted in a reduction in serum cholesterol and was associated with a significant reduction in heart attack and sudden cardiac death. Subjects were also found to have fewer cardiovascular events than those on a conventional diet.

The Alzheimer's Disease Study

This study by Dr. Nikolaos Scarmeas and colleagues from Columbia University Medical Center in New York demonstrated that a Mediterranean diet reduced the risk of developing Alzheimer's disease by 68%. Another study from this same group showed that patients with Alzheimer's disease who followed a Mediterranean diet had reduced mortality.

The Metabolic Syndrome Study

This study by Dr. Katherine Esposito and colleagues from Italy evaluated the effects of a Mediterranean diet on patients with metabolic syndrome (obesity, elevated blood sugar, elevated blood pressure, abnormal cholesterol profile, and markers of vascular inflammation). A Mediterranean diet was shown to improve all of the components of the metabolic syndrome.

Why does the Mediterranean diet lower the risk of death from heart disease and cancer compared to an American or Western diet? There are many theories. Scientific studies have linked the intake of saturated fat and trans fat to the development of heart disease and other diseases, including cancer. The consumption of saturated fat is limited in the Mediterranean diet, and trans fats are not present. This is in stark contrast with the typical Western or American diet, which contains an excessive amount of saturated fat and trans fat. Many of the foods present in the Mediterranean diet have been shown to decrease inflammation, and current research has demonstrated the pivotal role that inflammation plays in the development and progression of heart disease, cancer, diabetes, and an increasing list of other diseases. In contrast, the typical American (Western) diet, with its high levels of saturated fat, trans fat, and omega-6 fat, promotes inflammation and increases the incidence of heart disease and a multitude of other diseases initiated and aggravated by a state of chronic inflammation.

Whatever the reasons, I have witnessed the diet's success over and over again in my Miami cardiovascular disease prevention practice. And by adapting the traditional Mediterranean diet to our modern lifestyle, I have created a delicious and easy diet for long-term health.

How has the traditional Mediterranean diet been adapted? Nutritional science has introduced new and exciting ways to cook and prepare food. For instance, newly developed non-hydrogenated buttery spreads are a great, healthier replacement for butter or margarine in cooking and baking (they contain no trans fats and support heart health by providing omega-3 fat and plant sterols). Another example is the introduction of pomegranate juice, which has recently been shown to lower blood pressure and help reverse the build-up of fatty deposits (atherosclerosis) in our arteries. Nevertheless, the basics of a traditional Mediterranean diet remain unchanged: a wide variety of fresh whole non-processed foods, frequently enjoyed with a glass of wine in a relaxed setting with family and friends.

Let's take a look at the main components of the Mediterranean diet and their chief health benefits.

Whole grains

Whole (non-refined) grains are an integral part of the Mediterranean diet and have been shown to decrease the risk of heart disease, diabetes, and cancer. A whole grain kernel consists of an outer layer, the bran (fiber); a middle layer (complex carbohydrates and protein); and an inner layer (vitamins, minerals, and protein). The process of refining, common outside the Mediterranean region, destroys the outer and inner layer of the grain, resulting in grains that lack fiber and disease-fighting vitamins and phytochemicals. Examples of whole grains that are common to the Mediterranean diet are oatmeal, kasha, quinoa, and barley.

Fresh Fruits and Vegetables

Go to any market in the Mediterranean basin and you will find a bountiful supply of fresh, native fruits and vegetables. Fruits and vegetables contain an abundance of vitamins, minerals, fiber, and complex carbohydrates that lower the risk of heart disease and cancer. In particular, phytonutrients, concentrated in the skin of fruits and vegetables, are powerful plant-derived nutrients that help fight disease and improve our health. It is recommended that we eat a wide variety of colors (oranges, blueberries, red apples, spinach, yellow squash, etc.) in order to get all the nutritional benefits that fruits and vegetables can provide.

Nuts

Nuts, like olive oil, have been an essential part of the Mediterranean diet since antiquity. Nuts such as almonds and walnuts are rich in monounsaturated fat and omega-3 fatty acids, as well as good sources of protein, fiber, and vitamins. Nuts are an excellent snack that can assist with weight loss thanks to their high satiety. Several clinical trials have demonstrated that regular nut consumption leads to lower cholesterol, lower risk of coronary heart disease, and a significant reduction in the risk of heart attack.

Beans (Legumes)

Beans are also consumed on a regular basis in the Mediterranean region and are a rich source of soluble and insoluble fiber, which help curb appetite and reduce cholesterol. In addition, beans are an excellent source of protein and vitamins. Regular bean consumption lowers the risk of heart disease, cancer, and diabetes.

Fish

Oily fish, prevalent in the Mediterranean diet, provide us with a rich source of protein and omega-3 fatty acids. Omega-3 fatty acids have a favorable impact on cholesterol and triglyceride levels and reduce the risk of heart attack. They also help to reduce inflammation and, with regular consumption, decrease the risk of sudden death due to fatal cardiac arrhythmias.

A warning: Several species of fish may contain high levels of mercury and other contaminants, so pregnant women and young children should exercise caution. Nevertheless, for most adults, the cardiovascular benefits of fish consumption outweigh the risks, especially if you choose fish varieties that provide the highest amount of omega-3 fatty acids and tend to contain the lowest amount of mercury.

The best choices are salmon, albacore tuna, herring, sardines, shad, trout, flounder, and pollock. Avoid tilefish, swordfish, shark, and king mackerel, as these fish species tend to have the highest mercury content.

Olive Oil

Olive oil, made by crushing and then pressing olives, is the "soul" of the Mediterranean diet and provides the taste and flavor that is so much a part of Mediterranean dishes. It is rich in monounsaturated fat—the type of fat that is beneficial for heart health.

The regular use of olive oil instead of butter or margarine is associated with a reduced risk of heart disease, cancer, diabetes, and inflammatory disorders like asthma and arthritis. Olive oil also has a favorable impact on cholesterol. Besides decreasing total cholesterol, it also lowers bad (LDL) cholesterol and makes our bodies less susceptible to oxidative damage by free radicals. Olive oil also helps maintain or increase good (HDL) cholesterol, so the total cholesterol to HDL cholesterol ratio (an important key to cholesterol health) is improved.

In addition, olive oil can help you lose weight. A study in Boston showed that a diet that included olive oil and nuts resulted in sustained weight loss over eighteen months compared to a low-fat diet. People also stayed on the diet longer because they did not feel deprived.

Red Wine

Moderate alcohol consumption has been shown to lower the risk of coronary heart disease, and red wine, often part of a Mediterranean meal, is believed to have several advantages over other forms of alcohol. Red wine contains polyphenols and resveratrol, two substances that help to promote heart health. Resveratrol, a powerful antioxidant, is more abundant in red wine than white wine; it lowers the bad (LDL) cholesterol and raises the good (HDL) cholesterol, and it also has a beneficial impact on clotting.

Remember, alcohol should be consumed in moderation: wine consumption should not exceed one to two (5-ounce) glasses per day. For those individuals who do not wish to consume wine, grape juice is an excellent alternative: grape juice—specifically purple grape juice—also lowers the risk of heart attack. Since most heart attacks occur in the morning, many patients with cardiovascular risk factors often have a small glass of purple grape juice with breakfast.

The Mediterranean Diet Pyramid

Lean
Red Meat
(Limited)

Red Wine
(Moderation)

Poultry
(skinless)

Low Fat Dairy
(ex.yogurt)

Extra-Virgin Olive Oil

Fish
(ex.Salmon, Mackeral, Trout, Sardines)

Beans

Nuts
(ex.Almonds, Walnuts)

Fruits and Vegetables
(Wide variety of color)

Whole Grains
(ex.bread, cereal, pasta, rice, wheat)

Daily Exercise   Relaxation   Smoking Cessation

The Mediterranean Lifestyle

You'll notice that, in the anecdote I used to open the book, Giovanni's day differed from Ted's in more than just diet. The pace of Giovanni's day was more relaxed—yet more active!—with more room for enjoyment. It is important not just what you eat, but the circumstances in which you eat it, and the way you live between meals!

Stress: The Silent Killer

People living in Mediterranean countries tend to have less stress in their daily lives compared to their American counterparts. They spend more time enjoying their meals with family and friends. They often relax and take a short nap after lunch. A recent study showed that a regular midday nap reduced the risk of death from heart disease by 37%!

Often, doctors don't discuss the deleterious impact of chronic stress on long-term health with patients during routine office visits. This does not mean that stress is not an important risk factor—indeed, it may be the most important! The problem with stress is that it cannot be measured the way cholesterol or blood pressure can. In addition, what causes stress for one person may not cause stress for another. I am reminded of a story I once heard about two matadors from Spain. Pepe and Poncho were having lunch before a bullfight. Pepe said, "Poncho, isn't this great? I love bullfighting. I live to enter the stadium and fight the bull in front of all those people." Poncho replied, "That's great, Pepe, but I hate what I do for a living—I have constant nightmares of being gored by the bull, and my stomach is tied up in knots for days before each fight." Here are two men in the same profession with completely opposite views regarding the stress it causes.

Chronic stress increases stress hormones, such as cortisol and adrenaline, which in turn increase blood pressure, cause the heartbeat to become rapid, and increase the likelihood of forming blood clots. Studies have shown that chronic stress significantly increases the risk of heart attack. To make matters worse, those individuals who are "hot reactors"—who have a short fuse, are impatient, and have a high hostility index—are especially prone to cardiovascular calamities.

What, then, is the treatment for stress? First, let's be realistic—we all have periods of stress in our lives. Some of us, unfortunately, have more stress than others. Regardless, the first step in handling stress is to take a realistic view of the factors responsible for stress in our lives and try our best to modify them. Next, I recommend a physical exercise program—not because exercise eliminates stress, but rather because people who exercise are better able to handle stress. There is a physiological explanation for the beneficial effects of exercise on stress: people who engage in regular aerobic exercise have lower catecholamine levels—in other words, their adrenaline levels are lower and rise less dramatically with stressful situations. In addition to a regular exercise program, I encourage my patients to begin relaxation response training, yoga, self-hypnosis, or meditation. Finally, prayer offers significant stress reduction for some individuals. If these lifestyle changes do not result in a significant reduction in stress, then a consultation with a psychologist or psychiatrist may be appropriate.

10 Steps for Stress Reduction

- Exercise daily
- Meditate
- Pray
- Enjoy a close relationship with family and friends

- Set realistic goals in life
- Live within your means
- Try yoga
- Enjoy hobbies and interests outside of your work
- Have a positive outlook on life and never lose your sense of humor
- Laugh, smile, and enjoy your life!

Exercise Daily—Your Heart Will Thank You

Daily exercise is an integral part of the Mediterranean lifestyle, and it does more than just help you handle stress. Whether it's walking to the market or working in the garden, regular daily exercise is essential for good health. Exercise raises good (HDL) cholesterol, lowers blood pressure, and optimizes bone health, reducing the risk of osteoporosis. Regular exercise also provides a sense of well-being. Physical inactivity, along with poor dietary habits, has led to an epidemic of obesity in America. And several studies have shown that being unfit is even more deleterious to our health than being overweight. Unfortunately, we have become a nation of "couch potatoes." Getting people to exercise is difficult. We use the elevator instead of stairs; we ride in golf carts instead of walking; we park as close as possible to the store in order to walk the fewest number of steps.

The solution is to incorporate exercise into our daily activities. Exercise does not necessarily mean jogging five miles a day; simply walking for thirty minutes a day has been shown to decrease the risk of heart attack and cardiovascular death. The benefits of regular aerobic exercise are significant. Besides the benefits listed above, a regular exercise program will also reduce fatigue and improve lung function. And adding resistance training with light weights can improve bone health further and help maintain muscle tone.

5 Easy Exercise Tips

- Walk in place for thirty minutes while watching your favorite TV show—get off the couch!
- Park farther away from your destination (office, store, etc.) and enjoy a short walk
- Climb stairs instead of using the elevator
- Walk for the initial part of your lunch break, before eating lunch
- Use a pedometer—strive for 10,000 steps per day

The Ten Commandments of the Mediterranean Diet and Lifestyle

1. Eat a wide variety of fresh, non-processed food
2. Avoid saturated fat, trans fat, refined sugar, and excess sodium
3. Substitute olive oil or trans fat–free vegetable spreads for margarine or butter
4. Limit portion size
5. Drink an adequate amount of water
6. If you consume alcohol, do so in moderation
7. Exercise daily (minimum thirty minutes per day)
8. Abstain from smoking
9. Relax (especially after meals)
10. Never lose your sense of humor—laugh, smile, and enjoy life!

Why Choose the Mediterranean Diet?

What Is Wrong with the Popular Fad Diets?

Americans have always been enamored with "quick fix" diets that promise rapid, sustained weight loss. The problem with these diets is that they have no scientific basis, and there is no long-term data demonstrating their effectiveness regarding sustained weight loss or long-term health.

I consider these diets to be fad diets. Fad diets usually promise quick and easy weight loss, but the sad truth is that, although some of these diets may result in initial weight loss, the weight is quickly gained back. That initial weight loss is often not healthy weight loss, either. Starving yourself can also lead to weight loss, but it deprives you of the vitamins and nutrients you need to live and can do permanent damage to your body.

Here's a round-up of some popular diets and their drawbacks:

- *Low-fat diets (Ornish and Pritikin)*: These low-fat, high-carbohydrate, and mainly vegetarian diets are hard to follow and not palatable for most Americans.
- *AHA (American Heart Association) diet*: This low-fat diet can lead to decreased good (HDL) cholesterol, and heart disease may progress regardless. The AHA diet contains less monounsaturated fat and omega-3 fat than the Mediterranean diet and is associated with a higher risk of heart attack and death; the Lyon Heart Study demonstrated a 73% reduction in cardiovascular endpoints (heart attack or death) in patients following a Mediterranean diet rather than an AHA Step 1 diet.

- *Low-carbohydrate diets (Atkins)*: There is no long-term data demonstrating clinical benefit of following these diets, and concern about increasing the risk of heart disease and cancer make low-carbohydrate diets suspect according to many doctors. These diets are high in protein and saturated fat and restrict carbohydrates. They do often lead to a quick, early drop in weight due to water loss, but this process of water loss can result in fluid and electrolyte changes that may lead to serious cardiac arrhythmias (heart rhythm disturbances) and kidney malfunction. The impact of these diets on cholesterol levels is unpredictable. Eating an excessive amount of saturated fat while following these diets causes some people to experience a significant rise in their bad (LDL) cholesterol—especially if they absorb cholesterol at a higher-than-average rate.

Low-carbohydrate diets that achieve an "artificial" weight loss due to water loss from glycogen breakdown and ketosis (a condition that occurs when there is a lack of carbohydrates in the diet) are usually not effective in the long run. They are, however, potentially more dangerous, which is why many doctors do not recommend them. Some of the reported side effects and complications of these diets include a potential increased risk of:

- Cancer
- Cardiac arrhythmia (disorder of the heart rhythm)
- Coronary heart disease
- Deficiency of micronutrients
- Dehydration
- Diabetes
- Elevated cholesterol
- Elevated CRP (a marker of inflammation)
- Gout
- Halitosis (bad breath)
- Impaired cognitive (memory) function
- Kidney malfunction
- Kidney stones
- Optic neuropathy

Juan's Story

I have always been a quick-fix weight loss junkie and jumped from one fad diet to another. It's not that I didn't take these diets seriously; I did. I tried protein shakes, miracle pills, and low-carb diets. The Atkins and South Beach diets really sounded good to me because you could eat as much as you wanted and still have a few carbs and a variety of meat without having to worry about portion size or exercise. What could be better? At first I lost sixteen pounds. Fabulous! The only trouble was that I regained the weight. It became a vicious cycle. Sadly, I finally realized that these diets just didn't work.

I knew I had to do something that would actually work. I'm only thirty-eight, and even though I was overweight, I was otherwise healthy. But I have a strong family history of heart disease. My father had a heart attack early in life, and he died at the age of fifty-two from a second one. My uncle had a stroke and subsequently died of a heart attack when he was sixty-one. My aunt has diabetes, and my sister, who is overweight, was recently diagnosed with it as well.

Because of my family history, I went to see Dr. Ozner a year ago. He put me on the Mediterranean diet. I've been on it ever since, have lost twenty-eight pounds, and kept it off. I enjoy eating this way, and I find the diet quite easy to adhere to. I haven't just lost weight, I also have much more energy and feel healthier and stronger. I eat a wide variety of delicious, healthy foods, and I exercise daily by walking. Best of all, with this change in lifestyle and diet, I feel that I will live a longer and healthier life.

Why Choose the Mediterranean Diet Instead?

The Mediterranean diet—as a well-balanced diet including healthy fats and complex carbohydrates—offers the best alternative if you're looking to lose weight without sacrificing your health. There's a reason the Mediterranean diet has been around for thousands of years! By pairing the Mediterranean diet with increased exercise and lowered stress, you can not just lose weight, but also lower your cholesterol, blood sugar, and blood pressure—and as you've already seen, that's just the beginning of the benefits.

The Secret to Weight Loss

The secret to weight loss is simple: burn more calories than you consume. Americans consume too many calories! We eat large meals and then snack in the evening while we sit and watch TV. This excessive caloric intake combined with our sedentary lifestyle is the reason why obesity is a major public health threat.

We must learn to eat smart. First, we need to limit the portions of food we eat. Over the years, restaurant portions and packaged food portions have increased in size. The average bagel now weighs four to five ounces (equal to four or five slices of bread), cookies are the size of saucers, and an order of pasta in a restaurant would once have fed a family of four. To determine what an "average" serving of a packaged food is, check the nutrition label. You'll probably be surprised to learn that the "single" packaged food portion you assumed was for one is actually intended for two or more. You don't need to weigh and measure foods, but use common sense, and learn to eyeball correct portions. For instance, a medium-sized orange is about the size of a tennis ball, and a three-ounce piece of meat is the size and thickness of a deck of cards.

Second, we need to burn more calories by being physically active—there's no other way to do it!

Third, we must replace processed food, refined sugar, trans fats, and saturated fats with healthier, lower-calorie whole foods—as in the Mediterranean diet.

People who live in the Mediterranean region and follow a Mediterranean diet and lifestyle are leaner than their American counterparts for a number of reasons:

- Exercise is a part of everyday life.
- Consumption of food with high fiber content, like fruits, vegetables, beans, nuts, and whole grains, leads to high satiety: a feeling of being full.
- Trans fats, which are associated with weight gain and obesity, are avoided, whereas healthy fats, such as monounsaturated fat and omega-3 fat, are encouraged. Fat consumption, in the form of olive oil, nuts, and fish, also leads to satiety.
- Consumption of complex rather than simple carbohydrates, and avoidance of the refined sugars linked with obesity, makes the eater feel full longer.
- Food is not "super-sized" in Mediterranean countries like it is in America. It is the quality of food, not the quantity of food, that makes a good meal!

Lower Your Cholesterol—The Natural Way

In addition to weight loss, one of the chief benefits of the Mediterranean diet and lifestyle is its impact on cholesterol. The Mediterranean diet has been shown to lower the bad (LDL) cholesterol, raise the good (HDL) cholesterol, and lower triglycerides. I have had many patients reduce or eliminate their cholesterol-lowering medications after several months on the Mediterranean diet (but remember, any decision to adjust your medications should be made by your personal treating physician). This improvement in cholesterol helps explain the cardiovascular benefit of following a Mediterranean diet: it decreases the build-up of fatty deposits in artery walls.

The top foods responsible for the favorable impact on cholesterol are listed below—you may recognize many of them as the key nutritional components of the Mediterranean diet!

- Fruits and vegetables
- Whole grains (bread, cereal, etc.)
- Olive oil
- Nuts (especially almonds)
- Beans
- Soy protein
- Coldwater fish (and other foods rich in omega-3 fats)
- Red wine
- Cinnamon

There's a reason so many plants and plant products are included on this list. Whereas cholesterol is derived from animals, when we eat fruits, vegetables, and grains, we ingest plant sterols (or phytosterols), the plant equivalent. Plant sterols are beneficial because they interfere with the intestinal absorption of cholesterol, thereby lowering cholesterol levels. Certain vegetable spreads found in the grocery store also contain plant sterols and can lower cholesterol and benefit long-term health, especially when used to replace butter or margarine.

In addition, exercise, an integral part of a Mediterranean lifestyle, raises good (HDL) cholesterol, lowers triglycerides, and makes bad (LDL) cholesterol particles larger and less likely to cause heart attack and stroke.

Lower Your Blood Pressure with Diet and Lifestyle

Blood pressure is the term used to refer to the force of the blood against the artery walls, and it is measured in two numbers: systolic and diastolic. Systolic pressure is the level of force as the heart beats, and diastolic pressure is the level of force as the heart relaxes between beats. We used to think that only diastolic pressure was important, but both numbers matter in all individuals. Elevated systolic pressure is a key indicator of your risk for stroke, especially in the elderly population. Left uncontrolled, high blood pressure can also result in kidney disease, vascular disease, and increased risk of heart attack.

What is a normal reading? It used to be less than 140/90 millimeters of mercury (mmHg), with 120/80 mmHg being ideal. But according to recent changes in the guidelines, less than 120/80 mmHg is now considered optimal. The range between 120/80 mmHg and 140/90 mmHg is now called pre-hypertension.

This guideline change means more people are now considered hypertensive or pre-hypertensive.

It is healthy for your blood pressure to fluctuate during the day due to physical activities or stressful stimuli, as it should return to normal as your body adjusts to the situation. But if it does not, it becomes a chronic condition called hypertension (elevated blood pressure). The condition is unfortunately common, affecting more than 50 million Americans.

While there is a lifestyle component to hypertension, the most common cause is aging. As we age, blood vessels lose their elasticity, or the ability to expand and contract. When the heart contracts and then relaxes, this reduced elasticity may lead to a rise in systolic pressure and a decrease in diastolic pressure.

Another common cause is heredity predisposition, as hypertension has a neuro-hormonal component that is under genetic control. People with a strong family history of hypertension are at higher risk of developing hypertension later in life compared to someone with no family history of the condition.

Hypertension caused by certain treatable conditions is called secondary hypertension. Reversible nutritional causes are surprisingly common. I always ask patients who show signs of hypertension if they eat licorice, as it contains glycyrrhizin, a substance that may cause sodium retention and thus can lead to hypertension. Excessive salt, alcohol, and caffeine can also increase blood pressure, so it is prudent to decrease or eliminate their consumption.

Other secondary causes of hypertension can be reversible through surgery. These include constriction or coarctation of the aorta, adrenal gland tumor (pheochromocytoma), or a blocked renal artery. People who snore might have obstructive sleep apnea, a cause of hypertension that has several treatment options.

Looking at the possible causes of hypertension, you can see that even someone who is leading the right lifestyle could still have a problem. This is why a complete evaluation by your personal physician is necessary: diagnosing and eliminating any secondary causes can significantly reduce or eliminate hypertension.

If you have no secondary causes, however, you should follow appropriate lifestyle changes, even if you also need medications (see Appendix B for a list of common medications and what they do). I recommend a four-part program for all my patients with high blood pressure. The first three components, you'll notice, are also the cornerstones of the Mediterranean diet and lifestyle: good nutrition, exercise, and stress management. The fourth, when applicable, is smoking cessation.

Nutrition

Many foods contain nutrients derived from plants (phytonutrients) that help lower blood pressure, so it makes sense to eat a diet rich in such foods. As it happens, those foods are beneficial for weight control, which can also help to reduce blood pressure. The Mediterranean diet emphasizes the importance of eating heart-healthy fruits and vegetables, whole grains, olive oil, coldwater fish, low-fat dairy products, red wine, nuts, and beans—foods that can lower blood pressure. What the Mediterranean diet does not contain is also important: it is low in saturated fat, has no trans fat, and is low in sodium—all factors that can lower blood pressure.

We have long seen the evidence that a Mediterranean diet supports cardiovascular health and can lower blood pressure, and science has backed this theory. Fruits, vegetables, and nuts provide potassium, calcium, and magnesium for lowering blood pressure. Extra-virgin olive oil supports healthy blood pressure by causing blood vessels to dilate. Red wine in moderation (one 5-ounce glass per day for women and two for men) and red or purple grape juice may help relax arteries, which can lower blood pressure. Numerous studies have documented the blood pressure–regulating benefits of fresh garlic, abundant in a Mediterranean diet. And fish is rich in omega-3 fatty acids, which are beneficial for numerous disease states, including hypertension.

Exercise

We exercise far too little, which is unfortunate, since exercise lowers blood pressure in a couple of ways. One way is by supporting weight loss, particularly the reduction of abdominal fat. Fat in this area is associated with elevated levels of a protein called angiotensinogen, which can lead to hypertension. Exercise also strengthens the heart and makes the cardiovascular system more efficient by relaxing and dilating blood vessels. And if you exercise rather than raiding the refrigerator as an outlet for stress, you can both eliminate emotional eating and maintain a healthy weight.

Stress Management

Stress releases catecholamines, chemicals that prepare the body for physical activity and can therefore increase blood pressure. There is ample evidence that managing and reducing stress can significantly lower the risk of hypertension. We know this from the works of Dr. Herbert Benson of Harvard University, who popularized a stress-reduction technique in his book *The Relaxation Response*, and from cardiologist Dr. Robert S. Eliot, who coined the phrase "the hot reactor" for his patients who had an exaggerated rise in heart rate or blood pressure in response to stimuli that would only cause a small reaction in an average person.

There are many stress-reduction techniques to choose from: transcendental meditation, self-hypnosis, breathing techniques, Benson's relaxation response, yoga, prayer, and deep muscle relaxation. Find something that works for you and that you enjoy. Your exercise program may also reduce stress and make you better able to handle the stress you do encounter. Whatever method you choose, just stick with it!

Smoking Cessation

A word about smoking: Quit! This is a no-brainer. Cigarette smoking increases the risk of developing heart disease for a variety of reasons. The nicotine causes arteries to constrict, and the carbon monoxide from cigarette smoke decreases the amount of oxygenated blood reaching the heart muscle. No amount of smoking is safe, and it is counterproductive to an otherwise healthy lifestyle. There are many methods to help you quit, including nicotine patches or gum, acupuncture, and hypnosis, to name a few. Several new medications are also available to help "kick the habit." If you are unable to quit on your own, discuss smoking cessation with your doctor—don't let your good health go up in smoke!

Putting the Pieces Together

There are many important components to the Mediterranean diet, and although each component is responsible for conferring a certain degree of health, it is the combination of all the components that makes the Mediterranean diet so beneficial. The better you understand how each component contributes to your overall health, however, the better you'll be at understanding how everything works together.

This section goes more in depth on a few of the most important aspects of the Mediterranean diet. As a result, you'll be more capable than ever of making the best food choices for your health.

Fat: The Good, the Bad, and the Ugly

There are three types of fat in our diet: unsaturated fat, saturated fat, and trans fat...or the good, the bad, and the ugly.

The Good

Unsaturated fats, including polyunsaturated fats and monounsaturated fats, are good fats. Omega-3 and omega-6 fatty acids are polyunsaturated fats. Omega-3, which comes from oily fish, vegetables, and nuts, is cardioprotective (decreases the risk of heart disease). Monounsaturated fat, from nuts, seeds, and olive oil, is also cardioprotective, thought to be beneficial since it has a positive impact on our cholesterol ratio and helps to decrease inflammation. Vegetable oils (which include various amounts of both mono- and polyunsaturated fat) like soybean, sunflower, and corn oils, are neutral, meaning they have no effect, either good or bad, on heart health.

The Bad

Saturated fats, which raise the bad (LDL) cholesterol and increase the risk of heart disease and cancer, are bad fats. They're found in animal products, such as red meat, butter, milk, cheese, and lard, as well as tropical oils, like coconut and palm oils.

The Ugly

Then there are trans fatty acids, or trans fats. These fats are particularly harmful to our health, as they raise the bad (LDL) cholesterol, lower the good (HDL) cholesterol, increase inflammation, and make blood more likely to form clots. Trans fat consumption has been linked to heart disease, cancer, and diabetes.

Trans fats are found in foods such as margarine, French fries, potato chips, cookies, crackers, baked goods, and frozen foods. Trans fats don't occur naturally. They're manufactured by taking oils—mainly vegetable oils—and putting them through a process called hydrogenation, and were developed so that foods could last longer on the shelf without becoming rancid.

The biggest problem with the American diet is that we consume too much saturated fat and trans fat. In fact, certain countries have actually banned trans fat from their food supply! Until America does the same, the best course of action is to pay attention to nutrition labels, avoid food that contains trans fat or partially hydrogenated oil, and limit our consumption of saturated fat.

Omega-3 Deficiency: The Scurvy of Our Time

It has been suggested that up to 90% of Americans are omega-3 deficient. How can that be? Prior to the Industrial Revolution and the migration from the farm to the city, the vast majority of our food was grown locally. Our fruits and vegetables were good sources of omega-3 fat, and since cattle were free-roaming and grass-fed, they too consumed naturally occurring omega-3, which we took in when we ate beef. Today we live in a different world. Food is shipped from farms to grocery stores, and thus requires the inclusion of preservatives. Our soil has been depleted of its nutrients, and cattle are sedentary grain-fed creatures, woefully deficient in omega-3.

Why should this matter? The ratio of omega-3 to omega-6 in our body is important to health maintenance: omega-3 fat is anti-inflammatory, whereas omega-6 fat is pro-inflammatory. The omega-6/omega-3 ratio should be 1/1; however, due to the decrease in omega-3 intake and an increase in omega-6 intake (especially via corn oil and red meat), the omega-6/omega-3 ratio in the average American is somewhere between 10/1 to 20/1. This imbalance is associated with an increase in:

- Acne
- Allergies
- Arthritis
- Asthma
- Cancer
- Depression
- Diabetes
- Disorder of the heart rhythm
- Heart disease
- Hypertension
- Inflammatory bowel disease
- Sudden cardiac death

The Mediterranean diet alters this ratio by providing your body with ample amounts of omega-3 fat and limiting the amount of omega-6 fat you consume.

Carbohydrates: Simple and Complex

Carbohydrates are a source of energy and nutrition that is essential to good health. Simple carbohydrates like candy and soda are sugars, which are quickly absorbed into our bloodstream and provide an immediate source of energy. Complex carbohydrates like whole grain bread and cereal, oatmeal, and apples (also known as polysaccharides or starches) are made of long strands of sugars and are broken down and metabolized more slowly, providing the body with energy over a longer period of time. Consequently, they are more filling and help curb appetite.

A good way to think of this is in terms of foods' glycemic index. The glycemic index is a ranking of various foods based on the speed at which those foods are able to increase blood sugar or glucose compared to white bread, which was given an arbitrary glycemic index of 100. Foods that increase blood sugar faster than white bread have a glycemic index greater than 100; foods that increase blood sugar slower than white bread are assigned a glycemic index less than 100. Carbohydrates with more fiber and less sugar have glycemic indexes less than 100, meaning that they will leave you feeling full longer. Compared to simple carbohydrates, complex carbohydrates with low glycemic indexes improve blood glucose levels and decrease your likelihood of developing diabetes and heart disease. (Fortunately, you don't need to memorize the glycemic index of food; simply by following the

Mediterranean diet, you will be consuming heart-healthy non-processed food with a low glycemic index.)

Foods to Avoid: The Hidden Danger of High-Fructose Corn Syrup

Most of us know to avoid excess sugar, whether in the form of table sugar or in candy or sweet syrups. But there's another sinister sweetener present in much of the food you consume: high-fructose corn syrup. This is a favorite of the food industry since it is inexpensive and prolongs the shelf life of a product. It is found in many beverages and foods, including soft drinks, sports drinks, packaged cookies, and other baked goods.

The real danger posed by high-fructose corn syrup and table sugar is more than just the added calories—it's the metabolic havoc they cause. Both of these sweeteners contain an equal amount of glucose and fructose. Fructose is not utilized by our muscles as an energy source; it goes directly to the liver, where it spikes triglyceride production, a major risk factor for heart disease.

And that's not all. New research presented at the American Society of Nephrology's 42nd Annual Meeting and Scientific Exposition in San Diego, California, shows that people who ate or drank more than seventy-four grams per day of fructose (the equivalent of only 2.5 soft drinks) increased their risk of developing high blood pressure or hypertension. A normal blood pressure reading is below 120/80 mmHg, but consuming more than seventy-four grams of fructose per day led to a 28 percent, 36 percent, and 87 percent higher risk of blood pressure levels of 135/85, 140/90, and 160/100 mmHg, respectively, in a study population of 4,528 adults eighteen years of age or older with no prior history of hypertension.

While the controversy regarding high-fructose corn syrup continues, what isn't controversial is that excess consumption of sugar, in any form, should be avoided. What should you use instead? Many nutritionists believe that natural non-caloric sweeteners, such as those derived from the stevia plant, are preferable.

Coincidence? High-Fructose Corn Syrup and Obesity

Since its introduction in 1970, the amount of high-fructose corn syrup in our food has steadily increased. Currently the average American consumes about seventy-five pounds of this sweetener each year. During the same time period, American obesity rates jumped from 15 to 30 percent. Many nutritionists believe this is no coincidence.

Water: The Fountain of Youth

It is essential to consume an adequate amount of water each day: at least six to eight glasses, or 48 ounces. When we don't drink enough water we become dehydrated. This causes our blood to become thicker and more likely to clot, which can result in a sudden heart attack or stroke. People who live in tropical climates need to drink even more water because they lose fluid through perspiration.

Not only is drinking water throughout the day a healthful thing to do, it can also help you lose weight. Sometimes it's difficult to distinguish whether you are hungry or thirsty. If you drink a glass of water, and then wait twenty to thirty minutes before eating, you may find that your hunger has been eliminated, or at least diminished. Furthermore, water is important to your body's ability to function properly, gives your skin a healthy glow, and improves muscle tone. Refreshing water indeed is a fountain of youth.

But water is not the only drink available to us. What about our other options?

Fruit and Vegetable Juices

Although higher in calories than water, fruit juice, enjoyed in moderation, also has its place in the Mediterranean diet. Fruit juice doesn't replace the need to eat whole fruit, which has fiber and makes you feel full, but it can still be a refreshing source of nutrients and disease-fighting antioxidants.

Which fruit juice to choose? Drinking a wide variety of juices can bring a host of disease-fighting vitamins, minerals, and antioxidants to the table. Purple grape juice and cranberry juice are particularly good sources of antioxidants. Orange juice has vitamin C, potassium, and folic acid. Grapefruit juice also has vitamin C and potassium, but also contains a chemical that can interfere with the metabolism or breakdown of certain medications (check with your doctor or pharmacist if you take any medications).

Pomegranate juice is also a great choice. The pomegranate's popularity is on the rise lately, thanks mostly to the growing interest in its health benefits. Like many other fruit juices, this sweet-and-tangy drink is loaded with a combination of antioxidants for a particularly potent effect. Research studies have found that pomegranate juice helps lower blood pressure, reduce the buildup of atherosclerotic plaque, and preserve nitric oxide, key in keeping the coronary arteries healthy. Pomegranate juice is also a great source of vitamin C and potassium, and it contains less sugar than some other fruit juices. (Don't let the enthusiasm for pomegranate juice discourage you from trying the fruit itself, though; it's perfect for eating and cooking.)

Vegetable juices offer many of the same benefits as their fruity counterparts. Tomato juice and V-8, for example, are great low-calorie sources of vitamins and minerals. These juices contain a significant amount of sodium, however, which can lead to high blood pressure and fluid retention. Low-sodium tomato juice or V-8 is preferable—you can add potassium salt for taste, if desired.

Finally, when it comes to fruit and vegetable juices, just don't go overboard—moderation is the key!

Fruit Drinks—Caution!

Many people consume fruit drinks thinking that they are healthy. Beware—these drinks are often nothing more than flavored sugar water and have little to no nutritional value. Also, these beverages are often marketed to children and can contribute to childhood obesity. Remember, whole fruit paired with a glass of good old-fashioned water is still your best nutritional bet!

Enjoy Your Morning Coffee, but Don't Forget Your Afternoon Tea!

Though drinking anything containing caffeine can worsen dehydration (because it has a diuretic effect that can lead to fluid loss), one or two cups of coffee a day is fine, as long as you avoid rich, blended coffee drinks. Don't let your love affair with coffee blind you from the possibility of enjoying a cup of tea, however. Both coffee and tea can be enjoyed hot or iced, and both also contain antioxidants and chemicals that have been found to reduce the risk of diabetes, gallstones, and kidney stones. But it is tea that contains substances that help reduce the risk of heart disease and cancer.

Green tea, for instance, is rich in catechin polyphenols such as ECGC, a potent antioxidant that has been shown to be twice as powerful as resveratrol (another powerful antioxidant found in red wine). In addition, ECGC lowers bad (LDL) cholesterol, inhibits blood clot formation, and inhibits the growth of cancer cells. Finally, green tea has been shown to aid in weight loss and also help prevent dental plaque.

Does the color of the tea matter? Both black tea and green tea come from the same source: the white-flowered *Camellia sinensis* plant, which is loaded with antioxidants and gives tea its cardiovascular benefits. Green tea may have an edge because it's made from young tea leaves, providing more antioxidant power and boosting its health benefits. But if you prefer black tea, or it's the type you have handy, don't be dissuaded from enjoying it because it's a healthy brew as well. The same goes for white tea.

To release tea's strongest health benefits, brew it yourself, using either the leaves or a tea bag, and let it steep in the cup for three to five minutes (though different color teas may require different brewing times; check the packaging). Bear in mind that although you may enjoy herbal teas, pure tea provides more antioxidant punch.

Wine, Whiskey, or Beer?

It used to be said that wine was preferable to whiskey or beer for heart health. Clinical studies, however, have shown that all forms of alcohol are beneficial for cardiovascular disease prevention—providing they are consumed in moderation! Moderation is defined as one drink a day for a woman and two drinks a day for a man (one drink: 5 ounces of wine; 1.5 ounces of whiskey; 12 ounces of beer). Nevertheless, several studies have suggested that red wine (rich in the antioxidant resveratrol) does have additional health benefits beyond beer or whiskey. As the debate continues regarding the optimal form of alcohol, however, the following remains clear:

- Alcohol, in any form, is not encouraged for cardiovascular disease prevention in those who already abstain from drinking—there are better ways to prevent heart disease (such as a healthy lifestyle and medical therapy if required).
- There is a dark side to alcohol consumption, especially when consumed in excess (addiction, liver disease, increased incidence of certain cancers, cardiomyopathy and heart rhythm disorders, accidents—especially automobile accidents, etc.).
- If you choose to consume alcohol, do so in moderation!

Wine consumption has been enjoyed since antiquity in the Mediterranean regions of the world. Nevertheless, it was never consumed in isolation—it was enjoyed with delicious food and shared among family and friends.

Milk: Friend or Foe?

One of our most prevalent American myths is the health benefit of drinking three or more glasses of whole milk per day. Besides increasing cholesterol due to its saturated fat content, whole milk has been a big contributor to the obesity epidemic in America and developed nations worldwide. Note that three 8-ounce glasses of milk a day deliver 450 calories and 15 grams of saturated fat. In addition, the hormones cows are given to increase their milk production, as well as the antibiotics they're fed to prevent infection, have also been found in blood samples of milk drinkers.

Regular milk consumption may increase the risk of:

- Diabetes
- GI disturbances (due to lactose intolerance)
- Heart disease

- Multiple sclerosis
- Ovarian cancer
- Prostate cancer

If you must consume milk, enjoying fat-free milk or almond milk in moderation makes more sense. Likewise, choose low-fat or fat-free cheese, select low-fat or fat-free yogurt, and switch from butter and margarine to olive oil or a trans fat–free vegetable spread for your other dairy needs. Finally, for all you ice cream junkies out there, consider fat-free ice milk or a fresh fruit sorbet—your heart will thank you!

Don't Lose Your Whey

Dairy isn't all bad, however. Whey, once considered a waste byproduct of cheese manufacturing, is now prized as a high-quality, protein-packed snack that is low in fat and easily digested.

Known as a "fast" protein, whey provides a host of health benefits beyond the speed at which it's absorbed. Amino acids, the body's "building blocks," are necessary for the growth and repair of tissue, and whey's specific combination of these substances helps stabilize blood sugar and boosts the immune system. When it comes to heart health, whey has been found to benefit cholesterol by raising good (HDL) cholesterol and lowering triglycerides. Whey protein also promotes the growth of lean muscle and helps burn abdominal fat.

Regular dairy products contain lactose, which is milk sugar, but whey is lactose-free and a good choice for people who are lactose intolerant. Whey protein is generally safe; however, it should be consumed in moderation, as excessive protein consumption can lead to kidney impairment. For most people, a whey protein smoothie or shake as a substitute meal or snack several times a week, in addition to a healthy diet and lifestyle, is perfectly acceptable; however, be sure to discuss this with your doctor.

Free Radicals: The Result of a Toxic American Diet and Lifestyle

If you cut an apple in half and let it sit on your countertop, it turns brown in a matter of minutes. A metal pipe left outside in the rain and elements begins to rust in due time. This process is called oxidation—and it happens in our bodies, too.

Free radicals are a key part of this. Free radicals are unstable atoms continuously produced as a byproduct of oxygen, as oxygen is used for fuel in the human body. In a stable atom, the nucleus is surrounded by a cloud of paired electrons. Free radicals, in contrast, are atoms that contain an odd number of electrons, meaning that one pair is missing an electron. Because of this, free radicals are highly unstable and very reactive. As free radicals come into contact with other, normal atoms, they steal their electrons to replace the missing one, creating new free radicals and starting an ongoing chain reaction. This is the same process of oxidation that makes apples turn brown and metal rust. In the human body, it causes tissue damage at the cellular level, affecting DNA, the cell mitochondria, and the cell membrane, and eventually causing cell death. This, in turn, leads to both aging and disease. In addition, free radical production can lead to the buildup of fatty deposits in the artery wall (atherosclerosis), as well as blood clot formation and coronary artery spasm.

Today, the human body is exposed to many more external environmental toxins than in the past. These toxins act as catalysts, multiplying the free radical chain reaction in our bodies by several thousand, perhaps even several million.

Examples of toxins that lead to free radical formation:

- Pollutants in our air (such as carbon monoxide from cigarette smoke and automobile exhaust)
- Ultraviolet rays from the sun
- Pesticides
- Ionizing radiation from X-rays and procedures like CAT scans
- Radiation exposure from television and computer screens
- Excess alcohol consumption
- Processed foods
- Trans fats

It has also been shown that consuming a high-fat diet leads to elevated levels of free radicals called lipid peroxides (free radicals formed from fat); a low-fat diet, on the other hand, reduces the production of lipid peroxides.

Where Do Antioxidants Come From, and How Do They Work?

The natural internal production of free radicals is an inevitable byproduct of life, and our body has evolved a natural array of antioxidant nutrients to help rein free radicals in, keeping them from doing extensive damage. However, we are adding thousands more free radicals into our bodies through environmental toxins, and our body isn't equipped to handle them alone. That's why it's so important to take in additional antioxidants in the form of fruits and vegetables. If we don't get enough antioxidants, our bodies are in danger.

Antioxidants are the body's defense system—they combat and quench the biochemical fires that result from free radical formation. In fact, antioxidants can deactivate free radicals before extensive damage can been done. Antioxidants are capable of donating an electron to free radicals, thereby neutralizing them and ending the electron-stealing chain reaction that would otherwise take place. The antioxidants themselves do not become free radicals because they are stable even when they are missing an electron.

Foods to Avoid: My Beef with Red Meat

Americans eat too much red meat—they have bacon or sausage for breakfast, a hamburger or hot dog for lunch, steak for dinner, and then wake up and do it all over again. This is not healthy!

Excessive consumption of red meat has been linked to:

- Cancer (including colorectal cancer, breast cancer, prostate cancer, and pancreatic cancer)
- Diabetes
- Elevated cholesterol
- Heart disease
- Hypertension
- Chronic inflammation

In addition, red meat may contain:

- Bacteria
- Heterocyclic amines (which have been linked to cancer)
- Hormones
- PCBs (which are toxic)
- Protein prions (which have been linked to bovine spongiform encephalopathy, also known as mad cow disease)
- Viruses

Americans and other Western societies should follow the example set by people living in the Mediterranean: if you consume meat, do so less frequently (weekly or monthly, not daily), and when you do, utilize lean cuts of meat. Meat is often used as flavoring in a Mediterranean meal rather than the meal itself.

So enjoy your occasional meat dish—just not to excess!

The principal micronutrient (or vitamin) antioxidants are vitamin E, vitamin C, and beta-carotene. But since our bodies do not manufacture these micronutrients, they must be supplied externally through the food we eat. The best way to protect ourselves from the ravages of oxidation and free radicals is nutrition. Consumption of a wide variety of fruits and vegetables provides thousands of antioxidants and phytonutrients that work in concert with one another to fight disease.

It is recommended that you eat at least five to nine servings of fruits and vegetables per day. I recommend that you select a wide variety of colors when choosing those fruits and vegetables, since this ensures you'll be consuming lots of different phytonutrients and antioxidants. For example:

- Oranges provide vitamin C
- Tomatoes provide lycopene
- Carrots provide beta-carotene
- Blueberries provide anthocyanins
- Spinach provides lutein and zeaxanthin
- Purple grapes provide resveratrol

In addition to fruits and vegetables, whole grains, nuts, beans, fish, and other foods common to a Mediterranean diet help to reduce free radical damage in our bodies. They contain a variety of different antioxidants such as selenium, zinc, and other minerals and essential amino acids. All of these antioxidants work in different areas of cells to control and neutralize free radicals and prevent disease. It is the full spectrum of antioxidants working together with one another that promotes good health. And all the thousands of antioxidants that you need can be obtained by eating a healthy diet.

What About Vitamins?

The processing of food unfortunately removes many of the vitamins, phytochemicals, and micronutrients that we need for our long-term health. The best way to take in these vitamins and nutrients is by eating non-processed whole foods. But might vitamins be an acceptable substitute?

Despite our best efforts, we are unable to duplicate what Mother Nature provides with a healthy diet by simply taking vitamin pills. Taking a few vitamins in high doses to stay healthy just doesn't work. Clinical trials have failed to show any benefit to taking large doses of select vitamins; in fact, vitamins can actually be detrimental to our health if taken in large doses. Vitamin A and niacin, for example, can be toxic in large amounts. We need the whole package, thousands of antioxidant vitamins and minerals, to stay healthy. A daily multivitamin can be beneficial as an "insurance policy" against gaps in nutrition, but only provided it is taken *in addition* to a healthy diet—not in place of it!

Fish oil capsules, to increase omega-3 intake, may be an exception. Several large clinical trials have demonstrated the value of consuming an adequate amount of fish, but in one large Italian study, more than 10,000 men and women with pre-existing heart disease were given fish oil or a placebo, and those taking fish oil capsules had a 45% reduction in their risk of sudden cardiac death. Other clinical trials have also demonstrated cardiovascular benefits from fish oil. A Japanese study demonstrated that the addition of fish oil to statin medication in patients with elevated cholesterol resulted in a reduced risk of heart attacks and death from heart disease as compared to patients who were placed on statins without fish oil.

So should you take omega-3 laden fish oil supplements? If your intake of cold-water fish is limited, it might be worth considering. But since high doses of fish oil may thin the blood, they should not be taken without medical supervision.

Cinnamon: The Spice of Life

Too often in America, we remove cinnamon from the cupboard only on special occasions, to flavor pumpkin pies for Thanksgiving or bake cookies during the Christmas holidays. No more! It's time to steal a secret that other countries like China and India know: that cinnamon not only flavors food, but offers health benefits as well.

Ground cinnamon is made from the bark of the cinnamon tree, and it contains three types of essential oils (cinnamaldehyde, cinnamyl acetate, and cinnamyl alcohol), which provide it with health-boosting properties, as well as a wide range of other active substances. These oils have different beneficial effects: they act as an anti-coagulant, preventing blood from forming heart-attack-causing clots; they have anti-inflammatory properties; and they enhance the ability of diabetics to metabolize sugar. There's even some research indicating the smell of cinnamon can help improve brain activity.

And you don't have to down copious amounts of cinnamon to reap its benefits; research shows that less than a half-teaspoon of cinnamon a day lowers blood glucose levels and improves the cholesterol balance in people at high risk for diabetes and coronary heart disease.

Cinnamon tastes great, so it's also an inexpensive, easy way to brighten up a vast variety of recipes. Use cinnamon to spice up hot beverages, like tea or apple cider, or sprinkle it on top of sugar-free cocoa. Dust it on squash or carrots, or swirl it into yogurt and add a dash of honey for a quick dessert. Just leaf through this book and you'll find many recipes in the Mediterranean diet that utilize this versatile and healthful spice. But perhaps the best tip of all is to take that container of cinnamon down from the shelf, transfer its contents to a shaker, and leave it on the kitchen table. That way, you'll keep it on hand and use it often.

The Mediterranean "Salt Shaker"

Forget table salt—it contains sodium, which increases your risk of high blood pressure, stroke, and heart attack. Instead, take a salt shaker and fill it with equal parts potassium salt, garlic powder, onion powder, and black pepper. Your heart will thank you!

Dark Chocolate: It Tastes Too Good to Be Healthy!

Not everything that tastes good is bad for you. Take chocolate!

Chocolate can be enjoyed on the Mediterranean diet, as long as it is dark chocolate. Chocolate is made from cocoa beans, which are one of the richest sources of beneficial antioxidants, especially flavanols. Flavanols help lower blood pressure, balance cholesterol, and maintain a favorable blood glucose level. But it is flavanols that give chocolate a bitter taste, so confectioners remove them and then add refined sugar and fat. *Voilà*! The result is unhealthy milk chocolate.

Dark chocolate, however, is the darling of chocolate connoisseurs, who prefer its less sweet, more interesting taste. And thanks to its flavanols, dark chocolate also makes the grade for inclusion in the Mediterranean diet, as long as it's enjoyed in moderation. Confectionary companies are catching on and touting dark chocolate's health merits. But always read the nutrition label, and choose dark chocolates that are low in saturated fat and sugar, have no trans fats, and contain at least 70% cocoa flavanols.

Remember, no matter how it's touted, dark chocolate still has plenty of calories, so enjoy it in moderation and, when you do indulge, don't gobble it up. Instead, savor a piece or two, perhaps with a glass of red wine, as a delightful ending to a Mediterranean meal.

There Is No Need to Desert the Dessert

You don't need to be deprived; you can enjoy scrumptious desserts while on the Mediterranean diet. In this book you will find a variety of new and exciting desserts that will satisfy even the most discriminating palate.

The problem with most traditional American desserts is their use of high fructose corn syrup, saturated fats, and trans fats—all unhealthy ingredients that have a high calorie content. Not so for the desserts found in the second half of this book. These desserts are not only delicious but have no trans fats, are very low in saturated fat content, and do not contain high fructose corn syrup. There's even a 5-calorie cookie!

It's Your Choice!

You've seen the dangers of the American diet—and you've seen the benefits of the alternative. In particular, you've seen the threat that cardiovascular disease poses. Now you have to make a choice.

There are two different pathways that you can travel in the war against cardiovascular disease. The first pathway is called the dead-end road. Those who travel down the dead-end road refuse to learn about cardiovascular disease prevention. Their attitude is, "I'll wait until I have chest pain and then I'll worry about it." They frequently criticize people who take medications, saying, "The medications have adverse side effects that can cause serious problems, and I simply won't take them." They refuse to exercise or eat a heart-healthy diet. The dead-end road eventually leads to the number one cause of death in the United States and most developed countries in the world—cardiovascular disease.

The second pathway is called progress road. People who travel down progress road refuse to succumb to cardiovascular disease without a fight. They understand the basic principles of cardiovascular disease prevention. They maintain a heart-healthy diet and exercise on a regular basis. They have appropriate blood tests to screen for cardiovascular disease, and they understand the current guidelines for cholesterol and triglyceride management. If they have an elevated cholesterol or triglyceride level, they seek out appropriate medical attention so they can receive proper treatment. Those who travel down the progress road have a much lower likelihood of being hospitalized with a heart attack or undergoing expensive and risky procedures such as bypass surgery or stent placement. Progress road ultimately leads to cardiovascular health!

Let us not underestimate our enemy. Cardiovascular disease claims more lives than any other disease: every thirty seconds someone will die from a heart attack in America. Certainly if we were fighting an external enemy this formidable, we would do whatever it took to win the war.

If you're ready to fight, read on. The next section will provide you with all the information you need to begin the Mediterranean diet, and start you on a journey of lifelong health.

Robert's Story

I was a forty-eight-year-old male executive who often worked a sixty-hour week and played tennis occasionally, whenever I could fit it into my hectic schedule. I was divorced and tended to eat out, often just grabbing two double cheeseburgers with bacon and super-sized fries at the nearest fast-food restaurant. I also ate potato chips for snacks. I seldom saw a doctor, except for an occasional bad cold. Other than being fifteen pounds overweight, I considered myself to be in fairly good health. When I was a young boy, my parents always encouraged me to eat foods high in protein and fat because they thought those foods would make me strong and healthy. Except for in my ice cream or on my pizza, I seldom consumed either fruit or vegetables. Also, fish was just not part of my vocabulary.

One Sunday afternoon about six months ago, I was playing a grueling game of tennis when I suddenly developed tightness in my chest. It was severe enough to cause me to stop and take notice. Two days later I saw a doctor who led me to a heart evaluation by a cardiologist. I underwent a heart catheterization and a stent was placed in one of my coronary arteries. While I was hospitalized, I heard about Dr. Ozner from the nurses taking care of me. He had just given a lecture on heart disease prevention and they were all buzzing about his approach of preventive care. It was then that I decided to make an appointment to see him.

Dr. Ozner educated me about cardiovascular health and the role that diet, exercise, and stress management play in maintaining good health. He said that I could significantly reduce my likelihood of having a heart attack if I changed my current lifestyle and eating habits. He gave me a copy of his Mediterranean diet book. After reading the book, it became clear to me that a diet of high protein and saturated fat actually contributed to my chances of dying from a heart attack. So I tried the Mediterranean diet and realized it was not only a healthy and nutritious way to eat, but also a delicious one! Although I still take medications, I have improved my diet, and I exercise on a regular basis. I am confident that these measures will decrease my chances of having a heart attack or dying prematurely from heart disease.

PART TWO

RECIPES

A 14-Day Menu Plan

The Mediterranean diet is not a quick weight-loss diet plan but rather a healthy nutritional plan that will help you reach and maintain your optimal weight, and this sample 14-day menu plan will help get you started.

You may substitute any Mediterranean recipe for those listed in the 14-day menu plan. In addition, you are encouraged to eat a wide variety of fruits and vegetables of many different colors. All of the recipes in this book are made from fresh, healthy, non-processed foods. The fat content included in these recipes is mainly unsaturated fat (especially monounsaturated fat and omega-3 fat), with limited saturated fat and no trans fat. The sodium content of recipes that call for canned beans can be significantly reduced if you drain and cold water rinse the beans before using them. Remember to exercise daily and adjust your portion size to achieve ideal body weight.

For cooking tutorials and more information on creating these recipes at home, please visit www.drozncr.com/mediterranean-recipes.html and watch the video series, "The Mediterranean Diet Comes Alive: Cooking with Chris."

Bon appetit!

DAY 1

BREAKFAST

4 ounces vegetable or fruit juice

1 slice whole wheat toast with extra-virgin olive oil or 1 teaspoon vegetable spread (trans fat–free canola/olive oil spread)

1 teaspoon jam

½ cup plain low-fat yogurt (sweetened with non-caloric sweetener, if desired)

½ cup blueberries or strawberries

8 ounces water

Coffee or tea (soy or non-fat milk, trans fat–free coffee creamer, and non-caloric sweetener, if desired)

- APPROX. 239 CALORIES

OPTIONAL MIDMORNING SNACK

10–20 almonds or walnuts

8 ounces water or non-caloric beverage

LUNCH

Chickpea Pita Pocket (page 370)

1 medium apple, sliced and drizzled with honey

8 ounces water or non-caloric beverage

- APPROX. 319 CALORIES

OPTIONAL MIDDAY SNACK

10–20 almonds or walnuts

8 ounces water or non-caloric beverage

DINNER

1 jumbo clove Roasted Garlic (page 445)

½ (6-inch) whole wheat pita loaf, split open, sprayed with extra-virgin olive oil and herb seasonings of choice, and toasted in the microwave or oven until crispy

Goat Cheese Stuffed Tomatoes (page 68)

Linguine and Mixed Seafood (page 197)

Fresh vegetable of choice (flavor with olive oil or vegetable spread, as desired)

Drunken Apricots (page 407)

8 ounces water

1 or 2 (4-ounce) glasses of red wine or purple grape juice

Coffee or tea (soy milk or non-fat, trans fat–free coffee creamer and non-caloric sweetener, if desired)

- APPROX. 761 CALORIES

OPTIONAL EVENING SNACK

1 apple or orange
8 ounces water

DAY 2

BREAKFAST

4 ounces vegetable or fruit juice
½ cup egg whites with diced onions, tomato, and green bell peppers cooked into an omelet
1 slice whole wheat toast with extra-virgin olive oil or 1 teaspoon vegetable spread (trans fat–free canola/olive oil spread)
1 teaspoon fruit jam
½ small banana
8 ounces water
Coffee or tea (soy or non-fat milk, trans fat–free coffee creamer, and non-caloric sweetener, if desired)

- APPROX. 230 CALORIES

OPTIONAL MIDMORNING SNACK

10–20 almonds or walnuts
8 ounces water or non-caloric beverage

LUNCH

Greek Olive and Feta Cheese Pasta (page 67)
½ (6-inch) whole wheat pita loaf, toasted, if desired
⅛-inch fresh cantaloupe
8 ounces water or non-caloric beverage

- APPROX. 354 CALORIES

OPTIONAL MIDDAY SNACK

1 apple
8 ounces water or non-caloric beverage

DINNER

1 jumbo clove Roasted Garlic (page 445)

½ (6-inch) whole wheat pita loaf, split open, sprayed with extra-virgin olive oil and herb seasonings of choice, and toasted until crispy in the oven or microwave

6–8 marinated assorted olives

Grilled Citrus Salmon with Garlic Greens (page 176)

Grilled Eggplant (page 356)

Strawberries and Balsamic Syrup (page 405)

8 ounces water

1 or 2 (4-ounce) glasses of red wine or purple grape juice

Coffee or tea (soy or non-fat milk, trans fat–free coffee creamer, and non-caloric sweetener, if desired)

- APPROX. 653 CALORIES

OPTIONAL EVENING SNACK

1 apple or orange

8 ounces water

DAY 3

BREAKFAST

4 ounces vegetable or fruit juice

½ cup egg whites with diced onions, tomato, and green bell peppers

1 slice whole wheat toast with extra-virgin olive oil or 1 teaspoon vegetable spread (trans fat–free canola/olive oil spread)

1 teaspoon fruit jam

1 medium fresh peach or 1 large plum

8 ounces water

Coffee or tea (soy or non-fat milk, trans fat–free coffee creamer, and non-caloric sweetener, if desired)

- APPROX. 230 CALORIES

OPTIONAL MIDMORNING SNACK

10–20 almonds or walnuts

8 ounces water or non-caloric beverage

LUNCH

Italian Minestrone Soup with Pesto (page 126)

1 slice whole grain crusty bread with extra-virgin olive oil

½ cup fresh raspberries

½ cup plain low-fat yogurt, sweetened with non-caloric sweetener, if desired

8 ounces water or non-caloric beverage

- APPROX. 390 CALORIES

OPTIONAL MIDDAY SNACK

1 apple

8 ounces water or non-caloric beverage

DINNER

Simple Spanish Salad (page 82)

1 jumbo clove Roasted Garlic (page 445)

½ (6-inch) whole wheat pita loaf, split open, sprayed with extra-virgin olive oil and herb
    seasonings of choice, and toasted until crispy in the oven or microwave

1 slice soft goat cheese

6–8 marinated mixed olives

Fresh vegetable of choice (flavor with olive oil or vegetable spread, as desired)

Chicken Piccata (page 207)

Honeydew Sorbet (page 405)

8 ounces water

1 or 2 (4-ounce) glasses of red wine or purple grape juice

Coffee or tea (soy or non-fat milk, trans fat–free coffee creamer, and non-caloric sweetener,
    if desired)

- APPROX. 725 CALORIES

OPTIONAL EVENING SNACK

2 Meringue Cookies (page 427)

Green tea or 8 ounces water

DAY 4

BREAKFAST

4 ounces vegetable or fruit juice

2 slices whole wheat toast

2 tablespoons fresh chunky peanut butter

2 teaspoons honey

½ ruby red grapefruit, sweetened with non-caloric sweetener, if desired

8 ounces water

Coffee or tea (soy or non-fat milk, trans fat–free coffee creamer, and non-caloric sweetener, if desired)

- APPROX. 385 CALORIES

OPTIONAL MIDMORNING SNACK

10–20 almonds or walnuts

8 ounces water or non-caloric beverage

LUNCH

Light Caesar Salad (page 78)

1 slice Pizza Margherita (page 142)

10–20 seedless grapes

8 ounces water or non-caloric beverage

- APPROX. 302 CALORIES

OPTIONAL MIDDAY SNACK

1 apple

8 ounces water or non-caloric beverage

DINNER

1 clove jumbo Roasted Garlic (page 445)

½ (6-inch) whole wheat pita loaf, split open, sprayed with extra-virgin olive oil and herb seasonings of choice, and toasted until crispy in the oven or microwave

Chilly Tomato Soup (page 125)

Fennel Salad (page 75)

Fresh vegetable of choice (flavor with olive oil or vegetable spread, as desired)

Spicy Whole Wheat Capellini with Garlic (page 180)

8 ounces water

Sweet Plum Compote (page 430)

1 or 2 (4-ounce) glasses of red wine or purple grape juice

Coffee or tea (soy or non-fat milk, trans fat–free coffee creamer, and non-caloric sweetener, if desired)

- APPROX. 786 CALORIES

OPTIONAL EVENING SNACK

1 apple or orange

8 ounces water

DAY 5

BREAKFAST

4 ounces vegetable or fruit juice

1 slice whole wheat toast with extra-virgin olive oil or 1 teaspoon vegetable spread (trans fat–free canola/olive oil spread)

1 teaspoon fruit jam

½ cup plain low-fat yogurt, sweetened with non-caloric sweetener, if desired

½ cup blueberries or strawberries

8 ounces water

Coffee or tea (soy or non-fat milk, trans fat–free coffee creamer, and non-caloric sweetener, if desired)

• APPROX. 289 CALORIES

OPTIONAL MIDMORNING SNACK

10–20 almonds or walnuts

8 ounces water or non-caloric beverage

LUNCH

Hearty Bean Soup (page 129)

1 slice whole grain bread with extra-virgin olive oil or 1 teaspoon vegetable spread (trans fat–free canola/olive oil spread)

3 fresh apricots

8 ounces water or non-caloric beverage

• APPROX. 414 CALORIES

OPTIONAL MIDDAY SNACK

1 apple

8 ounces water or non-caloric beverage

DINNER

4 tablespoons hummus

½ (6-inch) whole wheat pita loaf, split open, sprayed with extra-virgin olive oil and herb seasonings of choice, and toasted until crispy in the oven or microwave

4 tomato wedges topped with slivers of red onion, freshly grated mozzarella cheese, and chopped fresh cilantro, and drizzled with aged balsamic vinegar and 1 teaspoon extra-virgin olive oil.

Fettuccine with Smoked Salmon and Basil Pesto (page 230)

Peach Marsala Compote (page 399)

1 or 2 (4-ounce) glasses of red wine or purple grape juice

8 ounces water

Coffee or tea (soy or non-fat milk, trans fat–free coffee creamer, and non-caloric sweetener, if desired)

- APPROX. 774 CALORIES

OPTIONAL EVENING SNACK

2 Meringue Cookies (page 427)

Green tea or 8 ounces water

DAY 6

BREAKFAST

4 ounces vegetable or fruit juice

½ cup dry oatmeal, cooked and sweetened with non-caloric sweetener, if desired

1 tablespoon seedless black raisins

1 medium orange, sliced

8 ounces water

Coffee or tea (soy or non-fat milk, trans fat–free coffee creamer, and non-caloric sweetener, if desired)

- APPROX. 292 CALORIES

OPTIONAL MIDMORNING SNACK

10–20 almonds or walnuts

8 ounces water or non-caloric beverage

LUNCH

Veggie Wrap (page 365)
Roasted Peppers (page 311)
6–8 marinated mixed olives
1 medium fresh pear, peach, or apple
8 ounces water or non-caloric beverage

• Approx. 601 calories

OPTIONAL MIDDAY SNACK

1 apple
8 ounces water or non-caloric beverage

DINNER

1 jumbo clove Roasted Garlic (page 445)
½ (6-inch) whole wheat pita loaf, split open, sprayed with extra-virgin olive oil and herb seasonings, and toasted until crispy in the oven or microwave
Mediterranean Mixed Greens (page 72)
Baked Tilapia (page 195)
Classic Spinach and Pine Nuts (page 312)
Strawberries Amaretto (page 419)
8 ounces water
1 or 2 (4-ounce) glasses of red wine or purple grape juice coffee or tea (soy or non-fat milk, trans fat–free coffee creamer, and non-caloric sweetener, if desired)

• approx. 597 calories

OPTIONAL EVENING SNACK

2 Meringue Cookies (page 427)
Green tea or 8 ounces water

DAY 7

BREAKFAST

4 ounces vegetable or fruit juice
½ cup egg whites with diced red onion, tomato, and green bell peppers cooked into an omelet
1 slice whole wheat toast with extra-virgin olive oil or 1 teaspoon vegetable spread (trans fat–free canola/olive oil spread)

1 teaspoon fruit jam

1 purple plum

8 ounces water

Coffee or tea (soy or non-fat milk, trans fat–free coffee creamer, and non-caloric sweetener, if desired)

- APPROX. 230 CALORIES

OPTIONAL MIDMORNING SNACK

10–20 almonds or walnuts

8 ounces water or non-caloric beverage

LUNCH

Eggplant Soup with Dry Sherry and Feta Cheese (page 134)

1 slice whole grain crusty bread, drizzled with extra-virgin olive oil and herb seasonings of choice

1 large kiwi fruit, sliced

½ cup fresh strawberries, sliced

8 ounces water or non-caloric beverage

- APPROX. 420 CALORIES

OPTIONAL MIDDAY SNACK

1 apple

8 ounces water or non-caloric beverage

DINNER

1 slice whole grain bread with extra-virgin olive oil and herb seasonings of choice

6–8 marinated assorted olives

Broccoli with Fresh Garlic (page 317)

Fettuccine with Sundried Tomatoes and Goat Cheese (page 204)

Fresh Fruit Kabobs and Cinnamon Honey Dip (page 401)

8 ounces water

1 or 2 (4-ounce) glasses of red wine or purple grape juice

Coffee or tea (soy or non-fat milk, trans fat–free coffee creamer, and non-caloric sweetener, if desired)

- APPROX. 1050 CALORIES

OPTIONAL EVENING SNACK

1 apple or orange

8 ounces water

DAY 8

BREAKFAST

4 ounces vegetable or fruit juice

½ cup dry oatmeal, cooked and sweetened with non-caloric sweetener, if desired

1 tablespoon seedless dark raisins

1 small banana, sliced

8 ounces water

Coffee or tea (soy or non-fat milk, trans fat–free coffee creamer, and non-caloric sweetener, if desired)

• APPROX. 323 CALORIES

OPTIONAL MIDMORNING SNACK

10–20 almonds or walnuts

8 ounces water or non-caloric beverage

LUNCH

Easy Couscous Parsley Salad (page 83)

½ (6-inch) whole wheat pita loaf, split open, sprayed with extra-virgin olive oil and herb seasonings, and toasted until crispy in the oven or microwave

Fresh fruit in plain low-fat yogurt

8 ounces water or non-caloric beverage

• APPROX. 331 CALORIES

OPTIONAL MIDDAY SNACK

1 apple

8 ounces water or non-caloric beverage

DINNER

4 large pre-cooked shrimp with tails

2 tablespoons cocktail sauce

Avocado Salad (page 75)

½ (6-inch) whole wheat pita loaf, split open, sprayed with extra-virgin olive oil and herb seasonings of choice, and toasted until crispy in the oven or microwave

1 tablespoon mustard, if desired

1 tablespoon catsup, if desired

1 slice raw onion

1 slice tomato

Mom's Turkey Burgers (page 229)

½-inch slice honeydew or cantaloupe

8 ounces water

1 or 2 (4-ounce) glasses of red wine or purple grape juice

*Coffee or tea (soy or non-fat milk, trans fat–free coffee creamer, and non-caloric sweetener,
if desired)*

- APPROX. 714 CALORIES

OPTIONAL EVENING SNACK

1 apple or orange

8 ounces water

DAY 9

BREAKFAST

4 ounces vegetable or fruit juice

2 slices whole wheat toast

2 tablespoons fresh chunky peanut butter

2 teaspoons honey

½ ruby red grapefruit, sweetened with non-caloric sweetener

8 ounces water

*Coffee or tea (soy or non-fat milk, trans fat–free coffee creamer, and non-caloric sweetener,
if desired)*

- APPROX. 385 CALORIES

OPTIONAL MIDMORNING SNACK

10–20 almonds or walnuts

8 ounces water or non-caloric beverage

LUNCH

Chicken Escarole Soup (page 132)

1 slice whole grain crusty bread

⅛ wedge honeydew

8 ounces water or non-caloric beverage

- APPROX. 259 CALORIES

OPTIONAL MIDDAY SNACK

1 apple

8 ounces water or a non-caloric beverage

DINNER

2 Stuffed Grape Leaves (Dolmas) with lemon slices (page 446)

½ (6-inch) whole wheat pita loaf, split open, sprayed with extra-virgin olive oil and herb seasonings of choice, and toasted until crispy in the oven or microwave

6–8 marinated assorted olives

Baked Eggplant with Garlic and Basil (page 353)

Steamed Sea Bass (page 188)

Cantaloupe Sorbet (page 404)

8 ounces water

1 or 2 (4-ounce) glasses of red wine or purple grape juice

Coffee or tea (soy or non-fat milk, trans fat–free coffee creamer, and non-caloric sweetener, if desired)

- APPROX. 662 CALORIES

OPTIONAL EVENING SNACK

2 Meringue Cookies (page 427)

Green tea or 8 ounces water

DAY 10

BREAKFAST

4 ounces vegetable or fruit juice

1 slice whole wheat toast with extra-virgin olive oil or 1 teaspoon vegetable spread (trans fat–free canola/olive oil spread)

1 teaspoon fruit jam

½ cup plain low-fat yogurt, sweetened with non-caloric sweetener

½ cup fresh blueberries or strawberries

8 ounces water

Coffee or tea (soy or non-fat milk, trans fat–free coffee creamer, and non-caloric sweetener, if desired)

- APPROX. 289 CALORIES

OPTIONAL MIDMORNING SNACK

10–20 almonds or walnuts

8 ounces water or non-caloric beverage

LUNCH

Chilled Stuffed Pasta Shells (page 313)

10–20 seedless grapes

1 large fresh tangerine

8 ounces water or non-caloric beverage

- APPROX. 292 CALORIES

OPTIONAL MIDDAY SNACK

1 apple

8 ounces water or non-caloric beverage

DINNER

1 jumbo clove Roasted Garlic (page 445)

½ (6-inch) whole wheat pita loaf, split open, sprayed with extra-virgin olive oil and herb seasonings of choice, and toasted until crispy in the oven or microwave

Roasted Peppers (page 311)

Spicy Shrimp with Angel Hair Pasta (page 183)

Crème de Banana Baked Apples (page 403)

8 ounces water

1 or 2 (4-ounce) glasses of red wine or purple grape juice

Coffee or tea (soy or non-fat milk, trans fat–free coffee creamer, and non-caloric sweetener, if desired)

- APPROX. 735 CALORIES

OPTIONAL EVENING SNACK

1 apple or orange

8 ounces water

DAY 11

BREAKFAST

4 ounces vegetable or fruit juice

½ cup dry oatmeal, cooked and sweetened with non-caloric sweetener, if desired

1 tablespoon seedless dark raisins

1 medium orange, sliced

8 ounces water

Coffee or tea (soy or non-fat milk, trans fat–free coffee creamer, and non-caloric sweetener, if desired)

- APPROX. 292 CALORIES

OPTIONAL MIDMORNING SNACK

10–20 almonds or walnuts

8 ounces water or non-caloric beverage

LUNCH

Garlicky Cannellini Beans (page 355)

½ (6-inch) whole wheat pita loaf, split open, sprayed with extra-virgin olive oil and herb seasonings of choice, and toasted in the oven or microwave

1 medium apple sliced and drizzled with 1 teaspoon honey

8 ounces water or non-caloric beverage

- APPROX. 389 CALORIES

OPTIONAL MIDDAY SNACK

10–20 almonds or walnuts

8 ounces water or non-caloric beverage

DINNER

Light Caesar Salad (page 78)

1 slice whole grain bread or whole grain dinner roll

1 tablespoon extra-virgin olive oil and a splash of aged balsamic vinegar for dipping, seasoned with freshly ground pepper, if desired

Lemon Garlic Asparagus (page 343)

Meatless Lasagna (page 227)

Strawberry and Poached Pears (page 395)

8 ounces water

1 or 2 (4-ounce) glasses of red wine or purple grape juice

Coffee or tea (soy or non-fat milk, trans fat–free coffee creamer, and non-caloric sweetener, if desired)

- APPROX. 790 CALORIES

OPTIONAL EVENING SNACK

2 Meringue Cookies (page 427)

Green tea or 8 ounces water

DAY 12

BREAKFAST

4 ounces vegetable or fruit juice

½ cup egg whites with diced onions, tomato, and green bell peppers cooked into an omelet

1 slice whole wheat toast with extra-virgin olive oil or 1 teaspoon vegetable spread (trans fat–free canola/olive oil spread)

1 teaspoon fruit jam

½ small banana

8 ounces water

Coffee or tea (soy or non-fat milk, trans fat–free coffee creamer, and non-caloric sweetener, if desired)

- APPROX. 230 CALORIES

OPTIONAL MIDMORNING SNACK

10–20 almonds or walnuts

8 ounces water or non-caloric beverage

LUNCH

Smoked Fish and Roasted Pepper Sandwich (page 373)

½ cup fresh raspberries

½ cup plain low-fat yogurt, non-caloric sweetener, if desired

8 ounces water or non-caloric beverage

- APPROX. 322 CALORIES

OPTIONAL MIDDAY SNACK

1 apple

8 ounces water or non-caloric beverage

DINNER

Mediterranean Mixed Greens (page 72)

Tomato and Fresh Parmesan Cheese Bruschetta (page 448)

1 slice crusty toasted French bread with extra-virgin olive oil

Fresh vegetable of choice (flavor with olive oil or trans fat–free canola/olive oil, as desired)

Bow Tie Pasta with Eggplant and Black Olives (page 200)

Sweet Italian Rice Pudding (page 402)

8 ounces water

1 or 2 (4-ounce) glasses of red wine or purple grape juice

Coffee or tea (soy or non-fat milk, trans fat–free coffee creamer, and non-caloric sweetener, if desired)

- APPROX. 984 CALORIES

OPTIONAL EVENING SNACK

1 apple or orange

8 ounces water

DAY 13

BREAKFAST

4 ounces vegetable or fruit juice

2 slices whole wheat toast

2 tablespoons fresh chunky peanut butter

2 teaspoons honey

½ ruby red grapefruit, sweetened with non-caloric sweetener, if desired

8 ounces water

Coffee or tea (soy or non-fat milk, trans fat–free coffee creamer, and non-caloric sweetener, if desired)

- APPROX. 385 CALORIES

OPTIONAL MIDMORNING SNACK

10–20 almonds or walnuts

8 ounces water or non-caloric beverage

LUNCH

Chickpeas and Garden Vegetables (page 91)

½ (6-inch) whole wheat pita loaf, split open, sprayed with extra-virgin olive oil and herb seasonings of choice, and toasted in the oven or microwave

1 medium orange, sliced

8 ounces water or non-caloric beverage

- APPROX. 325 CALORIES

OPTIONAL MIDDAY SNACK

1 apple

8 ounces water or non-caloric beverage

DINNER

1 jumbo clove Roasted Garlic (page 445)

*½ (6-inch) whole wheat pita loaf, split open, sprayed with extra-virgin olive oil and herb
seasonings of choice, and toasted until crispy in the oven or microwave*

6–8 marinated assorted olives

Steamed Artichokes (page 358)

Trout Almandine (page 233)

Strawberries and Balsamic Syrup (page 405)

8 ounces water

1 or 2 (4-ounce) glasses of red wine or purple grape juice

*Coffee or tea (soy or non-fat milk, trans fat–free coffee creamer, and non-caloric sweetener,
if desired)*

- APPROX. 578 CALORIES

OPTIONAL EVENING SNACK

2 Meringue Cookies (page 427)

Green tea or 8 ounces water

DAY 14

BREAKFAST

4 ounces vegetable or fruit juice

½ cup dry oatmeal, cooked and sweetened with non-caloric sweetener, if desired

1 tablespoon seedless dark raisins

1 medium orange, sliced

8 ounces water

*Coffee or tea (soy or non-fat milk, trans fat–free coffee creamer, and non-caloric sweetener,
if desired)*

- APPROX. 292 CALORIES

OPTIONAL MIDMORNING SNACK

10–20 almonds or walnuts

8 ounces water or non-caloric beverage

LUNCH

Spicy Mushroom Wrap (page 371)
1 medium fresh peach
8 ounces water or non-caloric beverage

- APPROX. 544 CALORIES

OPTIONAL MIDDAY SNACK

1 apple
8 ounces water or non-caloric beverage

DINNER

1 jumbo clove Roasted Garlic (page 445)
½ (6-inch) whole wheat pita loaf, split open, sprayed with extra-virgin olive oil and herb
  seasonings of choice, and toasted until crispy in the oven or microwave
Goat Cheese Stuffed Tomatoes (page 68)
Fresh vegetable of choice (flavor with olive oil or vegetable spread, as desired)
Pasta with Red Clam Sauce (page 201)
Drunken Peaches (page 406)
8 ounces water
1 or 2 (4-ounce) glasses of red wine or purple grape juice
Coffee or tea (soy or non-fat milk, trans fat–free coffee creamer, and non-caloric sweetener,
  if desired)

- APPROX. 830 CALORIES

OPTIONAL EVENING SNACK

2 Meringue Cookies (page 427)
Green tea or 8 ounces water

A Guide to
Cooking Method Terminology

Boiling......................cooking in water or other liquid at 212 degrees

Simmering ....cooking in water or other liquid at a temperature less than boiling point (around 180–210 degrees)

Steaming....................cooking by steam that is generated by a small amount of water or other liquid

Stewing.....................simmering in just enough liquid to cover food (usually used to cook tender cuts of beef)

Broiling.....................cooking in an oven, either over or under direct heat, with the oven door slightly ajar

Pan broiling ....cooking in a ridged heavy skillet oiled only enough to keep the food from sticking

Baking or *Roasting* .....these are the same thing, cooking in a closed-door oven

Sautéing....................rapid cooking in a pan on a stovetop using very little oil

Frying......................cooking in a pan on a stovetop where the food is bathed in oil

Fricasseeing ....a combination of sautéing and stewing or steaming

Salads

GREEK OLIVE AND FETA CHEESE PASTA
MAKES 4 SERVINGS

4½ ounces ziti pasta

3 ounces crumbled feta cheese

10 small Greek olives, pitted and coarsely chopped

¼ cup fresh, coarsely chopped basil leaves

2 cloves fresh garlic, finely minced

1 tablespoon extra-virgin olive oil + more to drizzle

¼ teaspoon finely chopped hot pepper

½ red bell pepper, diced

½ yellow bell pepper, diced

2 plum tomatoes, seeded and diced

Bring water to a boil, add pasta, and cook pasta until *al dente*. Remove from heat, drain pasta, and return to pot, drizzling with scant amount of olive oil to keep pasta from sticking together. Set aside. In a large serving bowl combine feta cheese, olives, basil, garlic, olive oil, and hot pepper, then set aside for 30 minutes. Add cooked pasta, red and yellow bell peppers, and tomatoes; toss ingredients well. Cover and refrigerate for at least 1 hour, until well chilled. Toss again before serving.

This salad goes well as a side dish to grilled lamb or fish.

Approx. 235 calories per serving
7g protein, 10g total fat, 1g saturated fat, 0 trans fat,
27g carbohydrates, 18mg cholesterol, 98mg sodium, 2g fiber

GOAT CHEESE STUFFED TOMATOES

MAKES 2 SERVINGS

6–8 leaves arugula
2 medium ripe tomatoes
3 ounces crumbled feta cheese
Salt and freshly ground pepper to taste
Balsamic vinegar to drizzle
Extra-virgin olive oil to drizzle
1 red onion, very thinly sliced for garnish
Fresh chopped parsley for garnish

Place 3–4 leaves arugula in the center of each salad plate. Cut tops (about ¼ inch) off the tomatoes. With a paring knife, core out the center of the tomatoes, about ½ inch deep. Fill tomatoes with crumbled feta cheese, add salt and pepper to taste, and drizzle with balsamic vinegar and olive oil. Garnish with red onion slices and chopped parsley. Serve at room temperature.

Approx. 142 calories per serving
7g protein, 13g total fat, 3g saturated fat, 0 trans fat,
7g carbohydrates, 37mg cholesterol, 485mg sodium, 1g fiber

SYRIAN CUCUMBER AND YOGURT SALAD

MAKES 4 SERVINGS

1½ teaspoons crushed fresh garlic
⅛ teaspoon minced fresh dill
Salt to taste
1 quart plain low-fat yogurt
2 English cucumbers, peeled and diced
2 tablespoons dried mint

In a bowl combine garlic, dill, and salt. Add yogurt and mix well. Stir in cucumbers and mint. Cover and refrigerate until well chilled before serving.

Approx. 167 calories per serving
13g protein, 4g total fat, <0.5g saturated fat, 0 trans fat,
21g carbohydrates, 10mg cholesterol, 183mg sodium, 1g fiber

CLASSIC TABBOULEH

MAKES 4–6 SERVINGS AS DINNER SALAD OR 8–10 AS APPETIZER

¾ cup bulgur

1½ cups water

2 cups freshly chopped parsley

¾ cup chopped scallions, white and green parts

½ red bell pepper, diced

½ green bell pepper, diced

½ cup finely chopped fresh mint

½ cup fresh lemon juice

½ cup extra-virgin olive oil

Sea salt and freshly ground pepper to taste

3 ripe plum tomatoes, peeled, seeded, and diced

1 large cucumber, peeled, seeded, and diced

Handful of greens for serving

Seasoned pita wedges

In a small saucepan soak bulgur in water for 30 minutes. Drain bulgur through a sieve and allow it to dry thoroughly. Clean parsley under cold running water and press gently between paper towels to dry. Place bulgur, parsley, scallions, peppers, and mint in a large bowl. Stir to mix well. In a separate bowl whisk together lemon juice and olive oil. Season bulgur mixture with salt and pepper to taste. Add lemon mixture to bulgur—only enough to make salad moist (not runny)—and toss. Fold in tomatoes and cucumber, then cover and chill. Serve on a bed of greens, with seasoned pita wedges for dipping.

This salad goes well with toasted, herb-seasoned whole wheat pita triangles.

Approx. 177 calories per serving
3g protein, 21g total fat, 2g saturated fat, 0 trans fat,
19g carbohydrates, 0 cholesterol, 23mg sodium, 4g fiber

SAVORY GREEK WHITE FAVA BEAN SALAD

MAKES 4 SERVINGS

1¼ cups dried white fava beans

2–3 fresh sage leaves

Salt to taste

2 cloves fresh garlic, finely minced

1 small onion, finely chopped

1 celery stalk, finely chopped

3 tablespoons fresh lemon juice

½ teaspoon dried oregano

3 tablespoons extra-virgin olive oil

4½ tablespoons red wine vinegar

Freshly ground pepper to taste

Soak the beans overnight in fresh water (water must cover the beans by twice their volume). In the morning, drain beans, rinse with fresh water, and drain a second time. Combine drained beans and 1 quart of fresh water in a large pot; bring to a boil. Add sage, cover pot, and cook for about 45 minutes. Gently stir and add salt to taste. Continue cooking for about another 15 minutes, until beans are soft but not mushy. Remove from heat and drain. Let beans cool slightly, then toss with garlic, onion, celery, lemon juice, oregano, olive oil, and vinegar. Add pepper to taste, and chill for 1 hour or more before serving.

Approx. 253 calories per serving
12g protein, 11g total fat, 1g saturated fat, 0 trans fat,
28g carbohydrates, 0 cholesterol, 15mg sodium, 12g fiber

TANGY ORANGE ROASTED ASPARAGUS SALAD

MAKES 6 SERVINGS

1 pound fresh asparagus, trimmed and cut into ½-inch diagonal pieces

4 tablespoons extra-virgin olive oil

Salt to taste

4 tablespoons fresh, sweet, no-pulp orange juice

1 tablespoon freshly squeezed lime juice

2 cloves finely minced garlic

Salt and freshly ground pepper to taste

6 cups chopped fresh romaine lettuce

3 tablespoons toasted pine nuts

1 tablespoon minced fresh basil leaf

Freshly grated Romano cheese (optional)

Toss asparagus with 2 tablespoons of olive oil and salt to taste. Arrange asparagus in a baking dish in a single layer and place in oven. Roast until tender crispy, about 10 minutes. Set aside. In a bowl, briskly whisk orange juice, lime juice, garlic, and remaining 2 tablespoons of olive oil; add salt and pepper to taste. When ready to serve, divide lettuce into 6 servings, arrange on salad plates, and top with asparagus. Briefly whisk the dressing and pour over lettuce and asparagus salad. Top with pine nuts and basil. Garnish with a small amount of Romano cheese, if desired.

To toast pine nuts in the oven:

Place the nuts in one layer on a non-stick baking sheet. Bake at 375 degrees, stirring occasionally, until lightly browned. Remove from oven and allow to cool.

Approx. 124 calories per serving

4g protein, 10g total fat, 2g saturated fat, 0 trans fat,

6g carbohydrates, 0 cholesterol, 16mg sodium, 3g fiber

MEDITERRANEAN MIXED GREENS
MAKES 4–6 SERVINGS

6 cups assorted fresh mixed greens (such as arugula, radicchio, baby spinach, watercress, and romaine)
1 small red onion, thinly sliced and separated into rings
20 firm cherry tomatoes, halved
¼ cup chopped walnuts
¼ cup dried cranberries
Crumbled feta cheese (optional)
Freshly ground pepper to taste

For Dressing:

2 tablespoons balsamic vinegar
4 tablespoons extra-virgin olive oil
1 tablespoon water
½ teaspoon crushed dried oregano
2 cloves fresh garlic, finely minced

In a large salad bowl, combine greens, onion, tomatoes, walnuts, and cranberries. Gently toss.

Dressing:

Combine vinegar, olive oil, water, oregano, and garlic; shake well. Pour dressing over salad and toss lightly to coat.

Garnish with feta cheese, if desired, and pepper to taste.

Approx. 140 calories per serving
2g protein, 12g total fat, 1g saturated fat, 0 trans fat,
6g carbohydrates, 0 cholesterol, 47mg sodium, 1g fiber

NORTH AFRICAN ZUCCHINI SALAD

MAKES 4 SERVINGS

1 pound firm green zucchini, thinly sliced
Juice from 1 large lemon
2 cloves fresh garlic, finely minced
½ teaspoon ground cumin
1 tablespoon extra-virgin olive oil
1½ tablespoons plain low-fat yogurt
Salt and freshly ground pepper to taste
Finely chopped parsley for garnish
Crumbled feta cheese (optional)

Steam zucchini until crispy tender, roughly 2–5 minutes. Rinse under cold water and drain well. In a large salad bowl, mix the lemon juice, garlic, cumin, olive oil, yogurt, and salt and pepper to taste. Add zucchini and gently toss. Chill in the refrigerator for 45 minutes to 1 hour before serving. Garnish with parsley and feta cheese, if desired.

Approx. 66 calories per serving
4g protein, 4g total fat, <0.5g saturated fat, 0 trans fat,
6g carbohydrates, 0 cholesterol, 22mg sodium, 1g fiber

GREENS WITH CHEESE MEDALLIONS

MAKES 6 SERVINGS

6 ounces soft goat cheese, log style

½ cup extra-virgin olive oil, divided in half

¼ cup plain bread crumbs

2 tablespoons freshly crushed garlic

Olive oil cooking spray

6 cups (roughly 16–18 ounces) mixed greens such as escarole, red and green leaf lettuce, radicchio, and endive, washed and well dried

1 cup halved cherry tomatoes

2 tablespoons red wine vinegar

2 teaspoons Dijon mustard

Salt and freshly ground pepper to taste

Finely chopped pecans (optional)

Preheat broiler. Cut goat cheese log into 6 equal pieces and place cheese medallions in a bowl containing ¼ cup olive oil; lightly swish mixture. Transfer the oil-laden cheese medallions to a bowl containing a mixture of bread crumbs and crushed garlic. Coat medallions on both sides with bread crumbs and garlic mixture. Lightly spray a baking sheet with cooking oil and place medallions on sheet; broil until golden brown and crisp, 1–2 minutes per side. Toss greens with tomatoes, divide into 6 portions, and top each portion with a cheese medallion. Combine the remaining ¼ cup olive oil, red wine vinegar, and Dijon mustard in a bottle and shake to mix well. Drizzle mixture over salads. Add salt and pepper to taste. Garnish with pecans, if desired, before serving.

Approx. 204 calories per serving
6g protein, 25g total fat, 6.9g saturated fat, 0 trans fat,
6g carbohydrates, 0 cholesterol, 159mg sodium, 1g fiber

FENNEL SALAD
MAKES 4–6 SERVINGS

1 large clove fresh garlic, halved
1 large fennel bulb, thinly sliced
½ English cucumber, thinly sliced
1 tablespoon minced fresh chives
8 large radishes, thinly sliced
3 tablespoons extra-virgin olive oil
2½ tablespoons freshly squeezed lemon juice
Salt and freshly ground pepper to taste
Marinated mixed olives (optional)

Rub the inside of a large bowl with garlic. Add fennel, cucumber, chives, and radishes. In a separate bowl whisk together olive oil, fresh lemon juice, and salt and pepper to taste. Pour olive oil mixture over salad and toss to mix. Garnish with marinated olives, if desired.

Approx. 76 calories per serving
0 protein, 10g total fat, 1g saturated fat, 0 trans fat,
3g carbohydrates, 2mg cholesterol, 20mg sodium, 1g fiber

AVOCADO SALAD
MAKES 3 SERVINGS

1 large ripe avocado, pitted and peeled
1 cup halved cherry tomatoes
2 tablespoons chopped fresh parsley
1 small onion, finely chopped
½ small hot pepper, finely chopped (optional)
2 teaspoons fresh lime juice
Salt and freshly ground pepper to taste

Cut avocado into bite-sized chunks. Combine tomatoes, parsley, onion, hot pepper, and lime juice. Toss well; add salt and pepper to taste. Add avocado and toss gently. Divide into 3 equal portions and serve.

Approx. 130 calories per serving
2g protein, 10g total fat, 2g saturated fat, 0 trans fat,
10g carbohydrates, 0 cholesterol, 110mg sodium, 4g fiber

TUNISIAN CARROT SALAD
MAKES 6 SERVINGS

10 medium carrots, peeled and sliced into ½-inch-thick slices
5 teaspoons freshly minced garlic
Salt to taste
2 teaspoons caraway seed
1 tablespoon Harissa (page 476)
6 tablespoons cider vinegar
¼ cup extra-virgin olive oil
1 cup crumbled feta cheese, divided
20 pitted Kalamata olives, reserving some for garnish

In a medium saucepan filled with water, cook carrots until tender. Drain and cool under cold running water, then drain again and place in a bowl. Combine garlic, salt, and caraway seed in a mortar and grind until it forms a rough paste, then pulse the paste in a food processor. Add Harissa and vinegar to the bowl with the carrots and mix well. Mash the carrots. Add the garlic-caraway mixture to Harissa-carrot mixture, blend well, and mix in olive oil. Add ¾ cup feta cheese and olives and toss again. Place salad in a shallow bowl and garnish with remaining feta cheese and olives.

Approx. 138 calories per serving
7g protein, 15g total fat, 5g saturated fat, 0 trans fat,
13g carbohydrates, 0 cholesterol, 643mg sodium, 17g fiber

CLASSIC GREEK SALAD

MAKES 6 SERVINGS

¼ cup extra-virgin olive oil

3 tablespoons red wine vinegar

2 cloves fresh garlic, finely minced

1 tablespoon dried oregano

Pinch of low-calorie baking sweetener

Salt and freshly ground pepper to taste

½ head of escarole, shredded

6 large firm tomatoes, quartered

½ English cucumber, peeled, seeded, and thinly sliced

1 medium red bell pepper, seeded and sliced

½ red onion, sliced

½ pound Greek feta cheese, cut into small cubes

20 Greek black olives

¼ cup freshly chopped Italian parsley

Whisk together olive oil, vinegar, garlic, oregano, sweetener, and salt and pepper to taste, and set aside. Combine escarole, tomatoes, cucumber, bell pepper, onion, and cheese in a large salad bowl and toss. Drizzle oil mixture over salad and toss again. Scatter olives and parsley over salad and serve.

Approx. 268 calories per serving
23g protein, 17g total fat, 7g saturated fat, 0 trans fat,
44g carbohydrates, 0 cholesterol, 595mg sodium, 3g fiber

LIGHT CAESAR SALAD

MAKES 6 SERVINGS

1–2 bunches packaged pre-cleaned romaine lettuce, torn in pieces
½ cup non-fat plain yogurt
2 teaspoons lemon juice
2½ teaspoons balsamic vinegar
1 teaspoon Worcestershire sauce
2 cloves freshly minced garlic
½ teaspoon anchovy paste
½ cup grated Parmesan cheese
10 small pitted black olives, chopped

Clean and pat dry romaine lettuce and place in a large salad bowl. In a blender mix yogurt, lemon juice, vinegar, Worcestershire sauce, garlic, anchovy paste, and ¼ cup Parmesan cheese until smooth. Pour mixture over lettuce and toss. Garnish with remaining cheese and olives.

Approx. 49 calories per serving
4g protein, 1g total fat, <0.1g saturated fat, 0 trans fat,
4g carbohydrates, 4mg cholesterol, 112mg sodium, 1g fiber

MOROCCAN EGGPLANT SALAD

MAKES 4–6 SERVINGS

1 large unpeeled eggplant (about 1 pound), cubed

3 cloves fresh garlic, finely chopped

5 cups water

1 teaspoon salt

3 tablespoons extra-virgin olive oil

2 large tomatoes, chopped

1 teaspoon cumin

1 teaspoon paprika

¼ cup lemon juice

In a pot, place eggplant cubes, roughly ⅓ of the garlic, water, and salt. Cover and boil for about 5–10 minutes or until the eggplant is cooked but still firm. Drain cubes in a strainer and allow to cool. In a large skillet, heat 2 tablespoons olive oil. Add tomatoes, remaining garlic, cumin, and paprika. Stir while mashing with a fork until mixture is somewhat smooth. Remove from heat. Combine eggplant cubes with tomato mixture in a bowl; allow to slightly cool before covering. Refrigerate and chill for about 2 hours. Before serving, add lemon juice and remainder of olive oil, and toss gently.

Approx. 128 calories per serving
1g protein, 7g total fat, 1g saturated fat, 0 trans fat,
13g carbohydrates, 0 cholesterol, 561mg sodium, 4g fiber

TUNISIAN TUNA SALAD

MAKES 4 SERVINGS

3 large ripe tomatoes, peeled

2 medium green bell peppers, seeded and sliced into thin rings

1 large cucumber, sliced

1 sweet onion, thinly sliced and separated into rings

2 hard-boiled eggs, shelled and divided into quarters

2 tablespoons fresh lemon juice

2 cloves fresh garlic, minced

2 tablespoons red wine vinegar

1 tablespoon water

1 teaspoon Dijon mustard

2 tablespoons chopped fresh basil

¼ cup extra-virgin olive oil

1 (12-ounce) can water-packed white albacore tuna, drained and divided into 4 equal parts

Salt and freshly ground pepper to taste

Capers, rinsed and drained, for garnish

Kalamata olives, chopped, for garnish

Divide tomatoes, bell peppers, cucumber, onion, and eggs into 4 portions. On 4 individual salad platters first layer tomatoes, then cover with layers of pepper rings, cucumber slices, and onion rings. Arrange eggs around edges of platters. In a small bowl, whisk the lemon juice, garlic, vinegar, water, mustard, and basil together until smooth. Gradually whisk in olive oil. Pour dressing over each salad platter. Place a scoop of tuna on the center of each salad, and add salt and pepper to taste. Garnish with capers and olives.

Approx. 306 calories per serving
27g protein, 17g total fat, 3g saturated fat, 0 trans fat,
13g carbohydrates, 132mg cholesterol, 332mg sodium, 3g fiber

FRESHLY CHOPPED SALAD WITH WALNUT DRESSING

MAKES 6 SERVINGS

3 medium ripe tomatoes, seeded and chopped

1 medium cucumber, peeled, seeded, and diced

1 large green bell pepper, seeded and diced

5 scallions, finely chopped

1 head iceberg lettuce

¼ cup fresh spearmint leaves, finely chopped

20 pitted Kalamata black olives

For Walnut Dressing:

2 slices Italian bread, soaked in water, squeezed dry, and crumbled

¼ cup finely minced shelled walnuts

½ teaspoon finely crushed garlic

¼ cup extra-virgin olive oil

Lemon juice, freshly squeezed, to taste

Salt to taste (optional)

Red hot pepper sauce to taste (optional)

In a large mixing bowl combine tomatoes, cucumber, green bell pepper, and scallions. Add Walnut Dressing and toss thoroughly. Add salt to taste. Line a serving platter with lettuce leaves. Spoon salad mixture over cleaned and separated lettuce leaves, sprinkle with spearmint, and garnish with olives. Serve immediately.

Walnut Dressing:

In a blender or food processor add bread, walnuts, and garlic and blend while slowly adding olive oil. Gradually add lemon juice and beat until mixture is smooth. Add salt and hot pepper sauce to taste.

Approx. 195 calories per serving of salad plus dressing
4g protein, 16g total fat, 1g saturated fat, 0 trans fat,
13g carbohydrates, 0 cholesterol, 227mg sodium, 3g fiber

SIMPLE SPANISH SALAD

MAKES 6 SERVINGS

1 bag (2 bunches) cleaned and trimmed romaine lettuce, torn into bite-sized pieces

3 medium ripe tomatoes, cut into ¼-inch wedges

1 large sweet onion, thinly sliced

1 green bell pepper, seeded and thinly sliced

1 red bell pepper, seeded and thinly sliced

¼ cup chopped and pitted marinated green olives

¼ cup chopped and pitted black olives

¼ cup extra-virgin olive oil

3 tablespoons balsamic vinegar

Salt and freshly ground pepper to taste (optional)

Place a bed of romaine lettuce on 6 chilled salad plates. Arrange tomatoes, onion, peppers, and olives on top of the lettuce on each plate. Mix olive oil and vinegar together; drizzle over salad. Add salt and pepper, if desired, and serve.

Approx. 107 calories per serving
2g protein, 9g total fat, 1g saturated fat, 0 trans fat,
7g carbohydrates, 0 cholesterol, 145mg sodium, 3g fiber

EASY COUSCOUS PARSLEY SALAD

MAKES 4 SERVINGS

¼ cup couscous

¼ cup water

2 tablespoons fresh lemon juice

2 teaspoons extra-virgin olive oil

¼ cup finely chopped fresh flat parsley leaves

2 tablespoons finely chopped fresh mint leaves

2 teaspoons lemon zest

2 tablespoons pine nuts

Salt and freshly ground pepper to taste

1 medium ripe tomato, peeled, seeded, and diced

2 heads Belgian endive, leaves for scooping

Whole wheat pita rounds, cut into wedges and toasted until crispy (optional)

Combine couscous with water and lemon juice in a medium bowl, and let stand for 1 hour. After 1 hour, add olive oil, parsley, mint, lemon zest, pine nuts, and salt and pepper to taste. Mix well. Mold couscous mixture into a mound in the center of a serving platter and garnish with tomato. Surround with endive leaves or toasted pita wedges, if desired. Serve at room temperature.

Approx. 120 calories per serving
5g protein, 2g total fat, <0.5g saturated fat, 0 trans fat,
18g carbohydrates, 0 cholesterol, 65mg sodium, 9g fiber

SARDINE SALAD

MAKES 4–6 SERVINGS

8 ounces spiral-shaped pasta

¼ cup extra-virgin olive oil + more to drizzle

1 medium onion, thinly sliced

2 cloves fresh garlic, minced

½ small hot pepper, seeded and finely chopped

⅓ cup freshly squeezed orange juice

¼ cup golden raisins

¼ cup toasted sliced almonds

16 jumbo pitted green olives, chopped

7½ ounces (2 cans) sardines in olive oil

Salt and freshly ground pepper to taste

Splash of lemon juice

4 tablespoons finely chopped fresh parsley for garnish

Finely shredded Parmesan cheese (optional)

Bring water to a boil, add pasta, and cook pasta until tender. Remove from heat, drain pasta, and return to pot, drizzling with scant amount of olive oil to keep pasta from sticking together. Heat olive oil in a large skillet; add onion, garlic, and hot pepper, and sauté until golden brown. Add orange juice and raisins, and bring to a boil. Remove from heat but keep warm. Combine toasted almonds and olives with onion mixture; stir together. Add sardines but try not to break them into pieces. Pour sardine mixture over pasta. Add salt and pepper and a splash of lemon juice to taste. Garnish with parsley and a small amount of Parmesan cheese, if desired. Serve at room temperature.

Approx. 467 calories per serving
31g protein, 26g total fat, 2g saturated fat, 0 trans fat,
38g carbohydrates, 60mg cholesterol, 288mg sodium, 1g fiber

PASTA AND SHRIMP SALAD
MAKES 6 SERVINGS

½ pound whole wheat fettuccine
16 large (about 1 pound) pre-cooked shrimp
12 pitted black olives, halved
6 cherry tomatoes, halved
½ cup diced roasted red peppers
¼ cup chopped fresh parsley
¼ cup chopped fresh basil
4 scallions, trimmed and sliced
¼ pound feta cheese, crumbled
Salt and freshly ground pepper to taste
Extra-virgin olive oil to drizzle

Fill a large pot with water and heat to boiling, add pasta, and cook until *al dente*. When ready, drain pasta well and transfer to a large serving bowl. Add cooked shrimp, olives, tomatoes, peppers, parsley, basil, scallions, and feta cheese to pasta. Toss to mix. Add salt and pepper and drizzle with olive oil to lightly moisten pasta; serve.

Approx. 411 calories per serving
32g protein, 6g total fat, 2g saturated fat, 0 trans fat,
57g carbohydrates, 150mg cholesterol, 206mg sodium, 3g fiber

TANGY TANGERINE CRESS SALAD

MAKES 4 SERVINGS

4 large sweet tangerines
Juice from 1 fresh lemon
¼ cup extra-virgin olive oil
Sea salt and freshly ground pepper to taste
2 large bunches watercress (washed, with tough stems removed)
10 cherry tomatoes, halved
16 pitted Kalamata olives

Peel tangerines and separate sections. Remove any pits and squeeze sections to get ¼ cup of juice. Set sections aside. In a large bowl, whisk together tangerine juice, lemon juice, olive oil, and salt and pepper to taste. Pat watercress dry with paper towels to remove any excess water. Add watercress, tomatoes, and olives to tangerine sections in a large bowl and toss with oil mixture. Serve immediately on chilled salad plates.

Approx. 195 calories per serving
3g protein, 16g total fat, 2g saturated fat, 0 trans fat,
14g carbohydrates, 0 cholesterol, 125mg sodium, 3g fiber

TOASTED CAPRI SALAD

MAKES 4 SERVINGS

1 large firm ripe tomato, cut into 8 thin slices
8 thin slices of red onion
1 (roughly 8-ounce) ball of fresh mozzarella cheese, cut into 8 slices
12 pitted Kalamata olives, halved
8 whole fresh basil leaves, garnish for plates
Aged balsamic vinegar to drizzle
Extra-virgin olive oil to drizzle
Sea salt and freshly ground pepper to taste
Freshly chopped basil for garnish

Preheat oven to broil. Divide first 4 ingredients into 4 equal portions. Alternate ingredients starting with tomato, onion, and cheese, and top with a few olives to make 4 separate stacks. Place stacks in an oven-safe dish about 4 inches under broiler, and broil for about 2–3 minutes or until cheese partially melts. Remove from oven. Place 2 whole basil leaves on each plate and top with toasted salad stack. Drizzle small amount of vinegar and olive oil over each salad, add salt and pepper, if desired, garnish with chopped basil, and serve.

Approx. 111 calories per serving
6g protein, 8g total fat, 4g saturated fat, 0 trans fat,
3g carbohydrates, 20mg cholesterol, 117mg sodium, <1g fiber

ENDIVE SPINACH SALAD

MAKES 6 SERVINGS

Olive oil cooking spray
½ cup chopped walnuts
¼ cup extra-virgin olive oil
4 tablespoons freshly chopped shallots
2 tablespoons white wine vinegar
1 tablespoon pure maple syrup
Salt to taste
¼ teaspoon freshly ground pepper
1 (10-ounce) bag cleaned fresh spinach
2 heads Belgian endive
1½ tablespoons chopped dried cranberries
¼ cup crumbled Danish blue cheese

Spray a small heavy-bottomed skillet with cooking oil and lightly toast walnuts over medium heat. Stir constantly to keep from burning. Remove from heat and set aside. In a small bowl, whisk together olive oil, shallots, vinegar, syrup, salt, and pepper. Set aside to marry flavors. Place cleaned spinach in a large salad bowl. Cut endive on the diagonal into thin slices with a sharp knife and add to spinach. Add cranberries and walnuts to spinach, and toss all ingredients with dressing. Sprinkle salad with blue cheese and serve.

Approx. 244 calories per serving
6g protein, 18g total fat, 3g saturated fat, 0 trans fat,
29g carbohydrates, 4mg cholesterol, 108mg sodium, 3g fiber

ARUGULA AND ASIAN PEAR SALAD

MAKES 4 SERVINGS

⅓ cup fresh grapefruit juice

⅓ cup fresh orange juice

3 tablespoons extra-virgin olive oil + enough to drizzle

1 small shallot, finely chopped

16 raw almonds, chopped

Dash of garlic powder

1 (6-ounce) bag arugula

1 ripe but firm Asian pear, halved and cored

¼ cup crumbled blue cheese

Salt and freshly ground pepper to taste

Whisk together both juices, olive oil, and shallot, and set aside to marry flavors. In a small skillet over medium heat, add chopped almonds, garlic powder, and a drizzle of olive oil. Toast almonds but do not burn; set aside. Divide arugula into 4 portions on salad plates. Slice pear into 16 slices, and top each plate of arugula with 4 pear slices. Drizzle each salad with dressing, including bits of shallot. Scatter on blue cheese, toasted almonds, and salt and pepper to taste, and serve.

Approx. 208 calories per serving
5g protein, 16g total fat, 3g saturated fat, 0 trans fat,
10g carbohydrates, 6mg cholesterol, 101mg sodium, 3g fiber

FIG AND PROSCIUTTO SALAD

MAKES 4 SERVINGS

1 (10–12-ounce) package fresh baby spinach
1 carton figs, stems removed and quartered
4 slices prosciutto, cut into strips
½ cup walnuts, coarsely chopped
Shaved Parmesan cheese for garnish

For Dressing:

1 tablespoon fresh orange juice
1 tablespoon honey
1 small hot red chili pepper, finely diced

Divide spinach into 4 equal portions. Place on individual salad plates. Top each with quartered figs, prosciutto, and walnuts.

Dressing:

In a separate small bowl combine orange juice, honey, and diced pepper. Whisk to blend. Drizzle dressing over salad.

Toss each salad to coat, garnish with Parmesan cheese, and serve immediately.

Approx. 190 calories per serving
26g protein, 9g total fat, 0 saturated fat, 0 trans fat,
17g carbohydrates, 9mg cholesterol, 316mg sodium, 5g fiber

BROILED ARTICHOKE SALAD

MAKES 4 SERVINGS

Olive oil cooking spray
1 cup marinated artichoke hearts, quartered and drained, reserve 1 tablespoon and 2
*   teaspoons of liquid*
6 flat anchovy fillets, minced
8 cups torn Boston lettuce
Finely grated Parmesan cheese (optional)

Preheat broiler. Lightly spray a small rimmed baking sheet with cooking oil. Toss artichokes with anchovy pieces and spread mixture in a single layer on baking sheet. Broil artichoke mixture about 3–5 minutes or until they start to brown. Remove from heat and allow to cool slightly, then toss mixture with lettuce and reserved marinade to coat and serve. Sprinkle with Parmesan cheese, if desired.

Approx. 96 calories per serving
4g protein, 5g total fat, 0 saturated fat, 0 trans fat,
5g carbohydrates, 5mg cholesterol, 435mg sodium, 5g fiber

CHICKPEAS AND GARDEN VEGETABLES

MAKES 4 SERVINGS

2 tablespoons freshly squeezed lemon juice
2 cloves fresh garlic, finely minced
1 tablespoon fresh basil leaf, snipped
⅛ teaspoon freshly ground pepper
1 (15-ounce) can chickpeas, rinsed and well drained
2 cups coarsely chopped fresh broccoli
½ cup sliced fresh carrots
1 (7½-ounce) can diced tomatoes, undrained
1 cup cubed part-skim mozzarella cheese

In a large serving bowl combine lemon juice, garlic, basil, and ground pepper. Stir in chickpeas, broccoli, carrots, tomatoes with juice, and mozzarella cheese. Toss ingredients, mixing well. Cover and refrigerate for at least 4 hours.

Approx. 195 calories per serving
16g protein, 7g total fat, 2g saturated fat, 0 trans fat,
24g carbohydrates, 17mg cholesterol, 411mg sodium, 2g fiber

PEPPERY WATERCRESS SALAD
MAKES 4–6 SERVINGS

2 bunches (about 8 cups) watercress, rinsed and rough stems removed
2 teaspoons champagne vinegar
Salt and freshly ground pepper to taste
2 tablespoons extra-virgin olive oil

Allow watercress to drain. In a small bowl, whisk together vinegar, salt and pepper, and olive oil. Place watercress in a salad bowl and toss well with olive oil mixture to coat evenly. Serve immediately.

Approx. 67 calories per serving
4g protein, 7g total fat, 1g saturated fat, 0 trans fat,
1g carbohydrates, 0 cholesterol, 28mg sodium, 1g fiber

HERBED POTATO SALAD
MAKES 4 SERVINGS

2 pounds red skin potatoes, cubed
14 ounces low-sodium, fat-free chicken broth
2 cloves fresh garlic, minced
½ cup plain low-fat yogurt
1 tablespoon chopped fresh dill
1 tablespoon chopped fresh oregano
2 tablespoons light mayonnaise
2 tablespoons extra-virgin olive oil
2 tablespoons white wine vinegar
Salt and freshly ground pepper to taste

In a large saucepan, add 2 cups water, potatoes, chicken broth, and garlic. Cook over medium-high heat for about 20 minutes or until potatoes are tender. Drain and allow to cool. Whisk together yogurt, dill, oregano, mayonnaise, olive oil, vinegar, and salt and pepper. Gently fold potatoes into yogurt mixture and chill for at least 2 hours before serving.

Approx. 274 calories per serving
8g protein, 10g total fat, 2g saturated fat, 0 trans fat,
41g carbohydrates, 3mg cholesterol, 702mg sodium, 4g fiber

WATERMELON SALAD

MAKES 4 SERVINGS

2 cups cubed seedless watermelon
Salt and freshly ground pepper to taste
2 cups arugula
1 cup sliced cucumber, with skin on
4 ounces fresh feta cheese, cut into bite-sized pieces
3 tablespoons extra-virgin olive oil
2 teaspoons white balsamic vinegar

Add watermelon to a large salad bowl and sprinkle with salt and pepper to taste. Add arugula, cucumber, and feta; toss to mix. Combine olive oil and vinegar, and drizzle over salad. Toss to coat salad and serve.

Approx. 94 calories per serving
5g protein, 16g total fat, 5g saturated fat, 0 trans fat,
7g carbohydrates, 25mg cholesterol, 320mg sodium, 0 fiber

SUMMER PASTA SALAD

MAKES 4 SERVINGS

5 ounces whole wheat Fusilli pasta
4 cups loosely packed baby arugula
⅓ cup sundried tomatoes, chopped
2 tablespoons capers, rinsed and drained
2 tablespoons shaved Parmesan cheese
Low-calorie dressing of choice

Cook pasta as per package instructions and drain. Combine pasta with arugula, tomatoes, and capers. Gently toss to mix. Add Parmesan cheese and dressing of choice.

Approx. 250 calories per serving
10g protein, 2g total fat, 0 saturated fat, 0 trans fat,
47g carbohydrates, 0mg cholesterol, 121mg sodium, 7g fiber

ESCAROLE WITH ANCHOVY DRESSING

MAKES 4 SERVINGS

4 cups bite-sized escarole

3 scallions, chopped

½ (6.5-ounce) can sliced black olives, well drained

Shaved Parmesan cheese for garnish

For Anchovy Dressing:

2 tablespoons red wine vinegar

1 teaspoon Dijon mustard

Juice from 1 lemon

1 clove fresh garlic, minced

3 flat anchovies, mashed

6 tablespoons extra-virgin olive oil

Salt and freshly ground pepper to taste

Tear and clean escarole, drain, and set aside.

Dressing:

In a small bowl, whisk together vinegar, mustard, and lemon juice. Stir in garlic and anchovies and slowly whisk in olive oil. Add salt and pepper to taste. Refrigerate to chill.

In a large salad bowl, combine escarole, scallions, and olives, toss with chilled dressing, top with Parmesan shavings, and serve.

Approx. 153 calories per serving
1g protein, 18g total fat, 1g saturated fat, 0 trans fat,
9g carbohydrates, 0 cholesterol, 403mg sodium, 5g fiber

PEAR AND WALNUT SALAD

MAKES 6 SERVINGS

2 cups low-sodium, fat-free chicken broth
1 cup white grain quinoa
2 tablespoons canola oil
1 tablespoon raspberry vinaigrette
¼ cup snipped fresh chives
Salt and freshly ground pepper to taste
2 ripe-but-firm pears, cored and diced
½ cup toasted walnuts for garnish

In a large saucepan, heat broth to a boil. Stir in quinoa, cover and reduce to a simmer, and cook until liquid is absorbed, about 15–20 minutes. While quinoa simmers, in a bowl whisk together canola oil, vinaigrette, chives, and salt and pepper. Add pears and toss to coat. Drain any excess remaining liquid from quinoa and add quinoa to pears. Toss to mix well. Place pear-quinoa mixture in refrigerator and chill for about 15 minutes. Serve cold with a sprinkling of walnuts.

Approx. 244 calories per serving
6g protein, 13g total fat, 2g saturated fat, 0 trans fat,
27g carbohydrates, 0 cholesterol, 24mg sodium, 5g fiber

CRUNCHY CHICKEN AND FRUIT SALAD

MAKES 4 SERVINGS

¼ cup pecans, chopped

3 cups chopped roasted chicken, breast meat only

1 large head Bibb lettuce

2 ripe tangerines, peeled and sectioned

2 small Granny Smith apples, cored and coarsely chopped

For Dressing:

⅓ cup light mayonnaise

1 orange, halved

Salt and freshly ground pepper to taste

In a small skillet over low heat, toast pecans, stirring frequently until golden brown, and set aside. Divide chicken, lettuce, tangerine slices, and apples into 4 portions. Arrange on individual plates. Add a sprinkling of toasted pecans and drizzle each serving with dressing.

Dressing:

In a small bowl add mayonnaise. Squeeze juice from orange. Stir enough juice into mayonnaise until it has a dressing consistency. Add salt and pepper to taste.

Approx. 286 calories per serving

34g protein, 11g total fat, 3g saturated fat, 0 trans fat,

12g carbohydrates, 89mg cholesterol, 143mg sodium, 3g fiber

PEAR AND WATERCRESS SALAD

MAKES 4 SERVINGS

4 ripe-but-firm smooth-skin pears
2 cups watercress
2 tablespoons toasted pecan halves
2 ounces crumbled blue cheese
¼ cup vinaigrette dressing
Juice from 1 lemon
Honey to drizzle

Core each pear from the bottom up leaving stem intact. In a bowl add watercress, pecans, blue cheese, and vinaigrette. Toss well to coat and set aside. Slice each pear in 4 horizontal slices. Brush cut sides with lemon juice. Reassemble pears into original shape, adding salad mixture between each slice. Drizzle pears with honey and serve.

Approx. 143 calories per serving
4g protein, 4g total fat, 1g saturated fat, 0 trans fat,
25g carbohydrates, 3mg cholesterol, 110mg sodium, 6g fiber

MUSHROOM AND BARLEY SALAD

MAKES 6 SERVINGS

½ cup extra-virgin olive oil, divided
1½ pounds assorted mushrooms, halved and divided
Salt and freshly ground pepper to taste
2 heads Bibb lettuce, leaves separated
1½ cups cooked barley
½ cup toasted chopped hazelnuts
½ cup fresh flat leaf parsley

For Dressing:

1 shallot, minced
3 tablespoons sherry vinegar, divided
½ cup low-fat sour cream
3 tablespoons chopped fresh chives
3 teaspoons fresh thyme
Salt and freshly ground pepper to taste

Heat 1 tablespoon olive oil in a large skillet over medium heat. Add half of the mushrooms and sauté until golden brown, stirring often. Transfer to a large salad bowl. Repeat for remainder of mushrooms. Add salt and pepper to taste to mushrooms in bowl. In the same bowl, add lettuce, barley, hazelnuts, and parsley. Add dressing, tossing to coat, and while serving toss occasionally to continue to coat.

Dressing:

Add 1 tablespoon olive oil and shallots to a skillet (you can use the same skillet) and cook shallots on low heat until softened. Add 2 tablespoons vinegar and let simmer until reduced by half. Remove from heat and whisk in sour cream and the rest of the vinegar. Add the balance of the olive oil and whisk to combine. Add chives, thyme, and salt and pepper to taste and allow mixture to cool.

Approx. 238 calories per serving
6g protein, 16g total fat, 3g saturated fat, 0 trans fat,
17g carbohydrates, 7mg cholesterol, 75mg sodium, 3g fiber

FRESH CHOPPED GARDEN SALAD

MAKES 4 SERVINGS

½ head iceberg lettuce, shredded
1 large carrot, cleaned and finely chopped
3 stalks celery, cleaned and finely chopped
½ small red onion, finely diced
4 large red radishes, chopped
½ (6.5-ounce) can sliced black ripe olives, well drained
½ (6.5-ounce) can chickpeas, well drained
4 teaspoons julienne-cut sundried tomatoes in olive oil
4 tablespoons oil from the sundried tomato jar
½ medium ripe-but-firm tomato, diced
½ large avocado, cut into ½-inch cubes
Salt and freshly ground pepper to taste
Seasoned croutons for garnish (optional)

In a large salad bowl, combine lettuce, carrot, celery, onion, radishes, black olives, chickpeas, and sundried tomatoes. Drizzle salad with the oil from sundried tomato. Gently toss salad until well mixed. Scatter diced tomato and avocado pieces over top of salad, and season with salt and pepper. Garnish with croutons, if desired, and serve.

Approx. 119 calories per serving
2g protein, 4g total fat, 0 saturated fat, 0 trans fat,
16g carbohydrates, 0 cholesterol, 195mg sodium, 6g fiber

CUCUMBER SALAD

MAKES 2 SERVINGS

1 large cucumber, thinly sliced
1 small red onion, thinly sliced
Aged red wine vinegar
Salt and freshly ground black pepper to taste

Place cucumber and onion slices in a bowl and cover them with vinegar. Cover and chill for at least 1–2 hours. Before serving, sprinkle with salt and pepper to taste.

Approx. 38 calories per serving
1g protein, <0.5g total fat, <0.05g saturated fat, 0 trans fat,
4g carbohydrates, 0 cholesterol, 1mg sodium, 0.05g fiber

CORN AND BEAN SALAD

MAKES 4 SERVINGS

1 (10-ounce) bag frozen corn, steamed and well drained
1 (15-ounce) can red small kidney beans, drained
½ cup chopped green bell pepper
1 (28-ounce) can diced tomatoes with chipotle, drained
2 tablespoons chopped fresh cilantro
1 clove fresh garlic, minced
Salt and freshly ground pepper to taste
8 large iceberg lettuce leaves
Extra-virgin olive oil to drizzle

In a bowl, combine all ingredients except lettuce leaves and olive oil. Cover and refrigerate for roughly 2 hours. To serve, place 2 lettuce leaves each onto 4 salad plates. Divide salad mixture into 4 portions. Mound salad mixture on top of lettuce. Drizzle salad with scant amount of olive oil and serve.

Approx. 203 calories per serving
8g protein, 0 total fat, 0 saturated fat, 0 trans fat,
30g carbohydrates, 0 cholesterol, 388mg sodium, 12g fiber

EXOTIC PEAR SALAD

MAKES 6 SERVINGS

2 heads Belgian endive, sliced diagonally in ½-inch wide strips

1 large bunch watercress, cleaned and trimmed

1 medium head of radicchio, torn into small pieces

¼ cup fresh Italian parsley leaves

2 ripe Anjou pears, cored and thinly sliced

½ cup toasted walnut pieces

½ cup chopped dried cherries

½ cup crumbled Danish blue cheese for garnish

For Dressing:

3 tablespoons sherry wine vinegar

1 tablespoon chopped shallots

2 teaspoons Dijon mustard

6 tablespoons walnut oil

Salt and freshly ground pepper to taste

In a large salad bowl, combine endive, watercress, radicchio, and parsley. Add pear slices, walnuts, and cherries, set aside.

Dressing:

Whisk vinegar, shallots, and mustard together in a small bowl. Gradually add in walnut oil. Add salt and pepper to taste. Add dressing to salad bowl and gently toss to coat. Divide onto 6 individual plates, garnish each serving with crumbled blue cheese, and serve.

Approx. 349 calories per serving
6g protein, 24g total fat, 4g saturated fat, 0 trans fat.
24g carbohydrates, 5mg cholesterol, 228mg sodium, 7g fiber

TOMATO PASTA SALAD

MAKES 4 SERVINGS

8 ounces penne pasta, cooked
1 pint grape tomatoes, halved
4–6 ounces fresh mozzarella cheese
1 medium red bell pepper, coarsely chopped
1 small sweet onion, diced
2 cloves fresh garlic, minced
½ cup fresh basil leaves, torn into pieces

For Dressing:

2 tablespoons balsamic vinegar
2 tablespoons extra-virgin olive oil
1 teaspoon Dijon mustard
Salt and freshly ground pepper to taste

In a large salad bowl, combine cooked pasta, tomatoes, mozzarella cheese, red bell pepper, onion, garlic, and basil.

Dressing:

In a salad dressing carafe, combine vinegar, olive oil, mustard, and salt and pepper, and shake well. Pour dressing over salad to coat and gently toss. Cover and chill overnight before serving.

Approx. 292 calories per serving
14g protein, 7g total fat, 4g saturated fat, 0 trans fat,
45g carbohydrates, 22mg cholesterol, 504mg sodium, 4g fiber

SPINACH SALAD

MAKES 4 SERVINGS

4 cups fresh spinach leaves, rinsed and well drained
1 (8-ounce) package sliced fresh cremini mushrooms
⅓ cup thinly sliced red onion
¼ cup sweet balsamic vinegar
2–3 tablespoons shredded fresh Parmesan cheese for garnish

In a large salad bowl, toss spinach, mushrooms, onion, and vinegar. Sprinkle with Parmesan cheese and serve.

Approx. 35 calories per serving
4g protein, 1g total fat, 1g saturated fat, 0 trans fat,
3g carbohydrates, 3mg cholesterol, 94mg sodium, 1g fiber

SWEET RED CABBAGE SALAD

MAKES 6 SERVINGS

1 small head red cabbage
1 tablespoon balsamic vinegar
2 tablespoons olive oil
½ cup raisins
⅓ cup water
¾ teaspoon freshly squeezed lemon juice
Salt and freshly ground pepper to taste

Cut cabbage head in half and remove stem. Slice cabbage halves into thin slices and place in a large bowl. Add vinegar, olive oil, and raisins and toss to coat cabbage. In a large saucepan add cabbage mixture and water and cook over medium high heat until tender, about 15 minutes. Stir occasionally. Add lemon juice and salt and pepper to taste, and serve.

Approx. 85 calories per serving
1g protein, 2g total fat, 1g saturated fat, 0 trans fat,
16g carbohydrates, 0 cholesterol, 25mg sodium, 2g fiber

BEET AND TOMATO SALAD

MAKES 4 SERVINGS

2 pounds tomatoes (preferably heirloom), sliced
1 pint cherry tomatoes, halved
2 (15-ounce) cans sliced red beets, well drained
¼ cup crumbled reduced-fat feta cheese
¼ cup torn fresh cilantro leaves, no stems
¼ cup extra-virgin olive oil
Salt and freshly ground pepper to taste

Arrange tomatoes and beets on a platter. Scatter feta cheese and cilantro over top and drizzle on olive oil. Season with salt and pepper to taste.

Approx. 225 calories per serving
7g protein, 11g total fat, 2g saturated fat, 0 trans fat,
25 g carbohydrates, 3mg cholesterol, 565mg sodium, 4g fiber

SNOW PEA SALAD

MAKES 4 SERVINGS

2 tablespoons aged white wine vinegar
2 teaspoons Dijon mustard
¼ cup extra-virgin olive oil
Salt and freshly ground pepper to taste
2 tablespoons minced shallots
1 pound fresh snow peas, thinly sliced
2 tablespoons chopped fresh tarragon

In a large serving bowl, whisk together vinegar, mustard, and olive oil. Add salt and pepper to taste. Add shallots, snow peas, and tarragon. Toss and refrigerate for 4–6 hours before serving.

Approx. 138 calories per serving
3g protein, 10g total fat, 1g saturated fat, 0 trans fat,
8g carbohydrates, 0 cholesterol, 4mg sodium, 2g fiber

TOMATO SALAD WITH BASIL, CAPERS, AND VINAIGRETTE
MAKES 6 SERVINGS

5 large ripe beefsteak tomatoes, cut into ½-inch slices
2 tablespoons capers, rinsed and drained
Salt and freshly ground black pepper to taste
10 medium fresh basil leaves, chopped

For Vinaigrette:

3 tablespoons minced shallots
3 tablespoons aged white wine vinegar
½ teaspoon garlic salt
1 tablespoon pure maple syrup
½ cup extra-virgin olive oil

Arrange tomatoes on a large platter. Sprinkle on capers and season with salt and pepper to taste. Scatter basil over tomatoes. Whisk vinaigrette again and drizzle over salad.

Vinaigrette:

Combine shallots, vinegar, garlic salt, syrup, and olive oil in a small bowl. Whisk to blend ingredients and set aside.

Approx. 148 calories per serving
2g protein, 14g total fat, 2g saturated fat, 0 trans fat,
6g carbohydrates, 0 cholesterol, 92mg sodium, 2g fiber

SPICY COLE SLAW

MAKES 4 SERVINGS

1 teaspoon canola oil

2 jalapeño peppers, seeded and finely chopped

2 large tomatoes, seeded and diced into small pieces

3 Napa cabbage leaves, shredded

1 small red onion, finely chopped

Sea salt to taste

1 tablespoon grated lime zest

1 teaspoon smoked paprika

⅛ teaspoon cayenne pepper

1 avocado, peeled, pitted, and sliced into 8 wedges

2 limes, 1 to juice and 1 cut into 4 wedges

In a small heavy skillet over medium heat, add canola oil and jalapeños. Stir-fry until peppers are browned and softened. Remove from heat and set aside. In a medium bowl, combine tomatoes, cabbage, onion, and stir-fried jalapeños. In a separate small pinch bowl, combine sea salt, lime zest, paprika, and cayenne. Stir to mix. Add small pinches of seasoning mixture to the tomato-slaw mixture to taste. Divide slaw onto 4 plates, add avocado, and drizzle with lime juice. Garnish with lime wedges and serve.

Approx. 112 calories per serving
1g protein, 8g total fat, 1g saturated fat, 0 trans fat,
6g carbohydrates, 0 cholesterol, 6mg sodium, 4g fiber

Soups

EGG-LEMON PASTA SOUP

MAKES 4 SERVINGS

4 cups low-sodium, fat-free chicken broth
4 ounces ditalini pasta
½ cup egg substitute or 2 large whole eggs, if desired
½ cup fresh lemon juice
Salt and freshly ground pepper to taste
4 tablespoons chopped fresh parsley for garnish
1 lemon, thinly sliced for garnish

In a medium saucepan, bring chicken broth to a boil. Add pasta; return to a boil, stirring once. Reduce to low, and simmer for 3–5 minutes. Remove from heat. Beat the eggs in a bowl, then beat in the lemon juice. Add a ladle of soup to this mixture and stir; transfer to soup pot. Heat soup on low heat, being careful not to curdle the eggs. Add salt and pepper to taste. Divide soup into 4 portions, garnish with parsley and lemon slices, and serve.

Approx. 161 calories per serving
10g protein, 2g total fat, <0.5g saturated fat, 0 trans fat,
65g carbohydrates, 5mg cholesterol, 197mg sodium, 1g fiber

FRESH CHICKEN BROTH
MAKES 6–6½ SERVINGS

2 pounds skinless, bone-in chicken

2 stalks celery with leaves, cut into chunks

1 large white onion, quartered

2 medium carrots, cut into chunks

2 cloves fresh garlic, diced

1 teaspoon dry Italian seasoning mix

9 cups cold water

Put all the ingredients into a large pot and bring to a boil. Using a slotted spoon, skim foam from the surface. Reduce heat to a gentle simmer, cover, and cook for 2 hours. Remove chicken and set aside to cool. Strain liquid through a strainer, discarding vegetables and seasonings. Refrigerate remaining strained broth for several hours to chill. Before using broth, skim fat from surface. Refrigerated, broth can be stored up to 3–4 days or it can be frozen and stored up to 3 months. Cooled chicken can be deboned and used for other recipes.

Approx. 201 calories per serving
32g protein, 5g total fat, 1g saturated fat, 0 trans fat,
4g carbohydrates, 106mg cholesterol, 147mg sodium, <0.5g fiber

CREAMY GREEN GARDEN SOUP

MAKES 6 SERVINGS

4 tablespoons trans fat–free canola/olive oil spread

1 white onion, chopped

4 cloves fresh garlic, minced

1 large leek, thinly sliced white parts and sliced green parts, keep separate

8 ounces fresh brussels sprouts, sliced

5 ounces fresh green beans, thinly sliced

5 cups low-sodium, fat-free vegetable broth

1½ cups frozen peas, defrosted

1 tablespoon freshly squeezed lemon juice

1 teaspoon ground coriander

1 cup low-fat milk

4 teaspoons all-purpose flour

Salt and freshly ground pepper to taste

Herb-flavored croutons for garnish (optional)

In a large skillet, melt canola/olive oil spread over low heat. Add onion and garlic and cook until soft and fragrant, but do not brown. Add the green parts of the leek, brussels sprouts, and green beans to the skillet. Add broth and bring to a boil. Reduce heat and let simmer for 10 minutes. Add peas, lemon juice, and coriander and continue to let simmer for 10–15 minutes more or until vegetables are tender. Remove vegetable mixture from heat and allow to cool slightly, then transfer to a blender or food processor and process until smooth. Return to a saucepan and add white parts of leek. Bring to a boil over medium-high heat, then reduce to a simmer for about 5 minutes, and reduce again to keep warm. In a separate small bowl, whisk together milk and flour until smooth. Add flour mix to soup, stirring to incorporate, and add salt and pepper to taste. Serve with a scattering of croutons on top, if desired.

Approx. 163 calories per serving
4g protein, 8g total fat, 2g saturated fat, 0 trans fat,
15g carbohydrates, 3mg cholesterol, 240mg sodium, 3g fiber

LEMONY CHICKEN AND ORZO SOUP

MAKES 4 SERVINGS

1 tablespoon olive oil
½ cup chopped white onion
½ cup chopped celery
6 cups low-sodium, fat-free chicken broth
½ cup sliced carrot
12 ounces skinless, boneless chicken breasts
Salt and freshly ground pepper to taste
½ cup orzo
¼ cup chopped fresh dill
Lemon halves to squeeze

In a large pot, heat olive oil over medium heat. Add onion and celery and cook until vegetables are soft. Add chicken broth, carrot, chicken, and salt and pepper to taste. Bring to a boil, then reduce heat to a simmer, and cook for roughly 20 minutes until chicken is cooked. Remove chicken from broth, allow to cool, then shred chicken into bite-sized pieces and set aside. Keep broth pot covered and on very low heat to keep warm while shredding chicken. Add orzo to broth, return broth to a boil, and cook for about 8 minutes. Remove pot from heat, add chicken and dill to broth, and serve with a healthy squeeze of fresh lemon juice.

Approx. 248 calories per serving
25g protein, 4g total fat, 1g saturated fat, 0 trans fat,
23g carbohydrates, 49mg cholesterol, 237mg sodium, 1g fiber

CHILLED AVOCADO SOUP

MAKES 4–6 SERVINGS

3 medium ripe avocados, halved, seeded, peeled, and cut to chunks
½ cucumber, peeled and chopped
½ cup chopped white onion
¼ cup finely diced carrot
2 cloves fresh garlic, minced
2 cups low-sodium, fat-free chicken broth, divided
Hot red pepper sauce to taste
Salt and freshly ground pepper to taste
Paprika to sprinkle
Thin avocado slices for garnish
Low-fat sour cream (optional)

Chill 4–6 soup bowls. In a food processor or blender, combine avocados, cucumber, onion, carrot, garlic, and 1 cup broth, process until almost smooth. Add remaining broth, hot sauce, and salt and pepper to taste, and process again until almost smooth. Pour into chilled bowls, cover tops, and chill for at least 1 or more hours. To serve, remove chilled bowls and sprinkle each serving with paprika. Add slices of avocado and a dollop of sour cream, if desired. Serve chilled.

Approx. 255 calories per serving
4g protein, 22g total fat, 3g saturated fat, 0 trans fat,
15g carbohydrates, 0 cholesterol, 70mg sodium, 10g fiber

POTATO-BROCCOLI SOUP WITH GREENS

MAKES 4 SERVINGS

3 medium red-gold potatoes, chopped

2 cloves fresh garlic, minced

2 cups low-sodium, fat-free chicken broth

3 cups fresh broccoli florets

3 scallions, sliced

2 cups 2% milk

3 tablespoons all-purpose flour

2 cups smoked Gouda cheese, shredded + more for garnish

Salt and freshly ground pepper to taste

2 cups coarsely torn escarole leaves, rinsed and drained

1 cup peppered seasoned croutons for garnish

In a large pot, combine potatoes, garlic, and broth. Bring to a boil, then reduce heat, and let simmer uncovered until potatoes start to soften. With a heavy fork, slightly mash potatoes. Add broccoli, scallions, and milk, and heat to a simmer until florets are crispy tender. Reduce heat to very low, then add flour and Gouda cheese, gently stirring until cheese melts and sauce is thickened. Season with salt and pepper to taste. Divide soup into 4 portions. Top each serving with escarole, additional cheese, and a scattering of croutons, and serve.

Approx. 350 calories per serving

17g protein, 14g total fat, 8g saturated fat, 0 trans fat,

42g carbohydrates, 30mg cholesterol, 349mg sodium, 7g fiber

VEGETABLE AND TORTELLINI SOUP

MAKES 8–10 SERVINGS

1 large white onion, chopped

4 cloves fresh garlic, chopped

3 celery stalks, chopped

2 tablespoons olive oil

32 ounces low-sodium, fat-free chicken broth

1 cup frozen corn

1 cup chopped carrot

1 cup frozen cut green beans

1 cup diced raw potato

1 teaspoon dried sweet basil

1 teaspoon dried thyme

1 teaspoon minced chives

2 (14.5-ounce) cans diced tomatoes, undrained

3 cups fresh chicken-filled tortellini

Shredded fat-free or low-fat cheddar cheese (optional)

Crusty croutons for garnish (optional)

In a large pot, sauté onion, garlic, celery, and olive oil until soft and fragrant. Add broth, corn, carrot, beans, potato, basil, thyme, and chives. Bring to a boil. Reduce heat, cover, and let simmer for about 15 minutes or until vegetables are tender. Add tomatoes and tortellini and let simmer uncovered for another 5 minutes or until heated through. Serve hot with a sprinkling cheddar cheese and a few crusty croutons, if desired.

Approx. 213 calories per serving
7g protein, 7g total fat, 1g saturated fat, 0 trans fat,
26g carbohydrates, 12mg cholesterol, 331mg sodium, 2g fiber

OLD-FASHIONED OYSTER STEW

MAKES 6 SERVINGS

2 pints fresh shucked oysters (about 32 ounces), undrained
4 tablespoons trans fat–free canola/olive oil spread
1 cup finely chopped celery
6 tablespoons minced shallots
3 (12-ounce) cans low-fat 2% evaporated milk
Salt and freshly ground pepper to taste
2 pinches of cayenne pepper
Bread squares, toasted

Drain liquid from the oysters, reserving the liquid. Strain the liquid through a wire strainer to remove any grit or sand. In a large heavy pot, melt canola/olive oil spread over medium heat. Reduce heat to a simmer and add oysters, celery, and shallots. Let simmer gently for about 4 minutes until edges of oysters begin to curl. While oysters are simmering, heat milk and oyster liquid in a separate pan over low heat until warm. When warmed, add milk mixture to oysters, gently stirring. Add salt and pepper to taste and cayenne pepper. Serve soup warm in warmed soup bowls with toasted bread squares.

Approx. 311 calories per serving
23g protein, 11g total fat, 2g saturated fat, 0 trans fat,
22g carbohydrates, 63mg cholesterol, 516mg sodium, 3g fiber

EGGPLANT SOUP

MAKES 2 SERVINGS

3 tablespoons olive oil
1 small eggplant, halved and sliced thinly (about 2 cups)
½ cup chopped white onion
2 cloves fresh garlic, minced
1 (14-ounce) can low-sodium tomato and basil pasta sauce
2 cups low-sodium, fat-free chicken broth
½ cup shredded reduced-fat mozzarella cheese
2 tablespoons Italian bread crumbs
2 tablespoons freshly grated Parmesan cheese for garnish
Crusty bread

In a large non-stick pan, heat olive oil over medium-high heat and cook eggplant for about 5 minutes, stirring occasionally. Add onion and garlic and continue cooking until eggplant is golden brown. Add sauce and broth, bring to a boil, then reduce heat to a simmer, and continue to cook until soup thickens.

Heat oven to broil. Line a cookie sheet with tin foil and place 2 oven-safe crock bowls on sheet. Divide soup into both bowls, top with mozzarella cheese, bread crumbs, and a sprinkling of Parmesan cheese. Broil for about 2–3 minutes or until cheese is melted and golden. Serve hot with chunks of crusty bread, if desired.

Approx. 274 calories per serving
7g protein, 17g total fat, 3g saturated fat, 0 trans fat,
23g carbohydrates, 7mg cholesterol, 476mg sodium, 5g fiber

SPINACH TORTELLINI SOUP

MAKES 4 SERVINGS

4 cups low-sodium, fat-free chicken broth
2 cloves fresh garlic, minced
4 scallions, chopped
¼ teaspoon ground pepper
5 ounces fresh cheese-filled tortellini
2 cups coarsely chopped fresh spinach leaves
Fresh grated Parmesan cheese (optional)

Heat broth in a pot and add garlic, scallions, and pepper. Bring to a boil, then reduce to medium heat. Add tortellini and cook for 10 minutes. Add spinach and cook for an additional 5 minutes or until pasta is tender. Transfer to 4 bowls and serve with a sprinkle of Parmesan cheese, if desired.

Approx. 97 calories per serving
6g protein, 4g total fat, 1g saturated fat, 0 trans fat,
14g carbohydrates, 11mg cholesterol, 129mg sodium, <0.5g fiber

RED CLAM CHOWDER
MAKES 8–10 SERVINGS

3 large stalks celery, chopped

1 large white onion, chopped

4 (8-ounce) jars clam juice

4 cloves fresh garlic, chopped

Creole seasoning of choice to taste

Tabasco sauce to taste

¼ cup Worcestershire sauce

¼ cup freshly squeezed lemon juice

3–4 cups water

1½ (14.5-ounce) cans crushed tomatoes

6 cups raw diced potatoes

4 (10-ounce) cans whole baby clams

Hot sauce (optional)

Crusty country bread

Combine all ingredients, except for clams, hot sauce, and bread, in a large pot. Bring to a low simmer, cover, and cook for 25–30 minutes. Add clams and continue to cook on a low simmer for another 15–20 minutes. Serve hot with hot sauce, if desired, and crusty country bread.

Approx. 181 calories per serving
13g protein, 3g total fat, 0 saturated fat, 0 trans fat,
18g carbohydrates, 54mg cholesterol, 311mg sodium, 3g fiber

SPICY VEGETABLE STEW

MAKES 4 SERVINGS

4 cups fresh cauliflower florets

2 teaspoons curry powder

½ teaspoon cumin

1 (14.5-ounce) can fiery roasted diced tomatoes, undrained

2 cloves fresh garlic, finely minced

1 tablespoon finely chopped Serrano chili pepper

1 (15-ounce) can chickpeas, drained

¾ cup solid packed canned pumpkin mash

¾ cup water

Salt and freshly ground pepper to taste

1 cup frozen baby peas

1 cup frozen corn

Couscous or *brown rice, cooked*

Place cauliflower florets in a pot and cover partially with water. Bring to a boil, cover, and steam until florets are almost tender. Remove from heat, drain well, and cut large florets into smaller sizes. Set aside. In a large, non-stick skillet over medium heat, add curry powder and cumin and heat until fragrant. Add tomatoes with juices, garlic, chili pepper, chickpeas, pumpkin, and water. Bring to a boil, then reduce heat to a simmer. Add florets and salt and pepper to taste and let simmer for about 15 minutes. Add peas and corn and let simmer for 5 minutes longer. Remove from heat and serve over cooked couscous or brown rice.

Approx. 228 calories per serving
12g protein, 2g total fat, 0 saturated fat, 0 trans fat,
43g carbohydrates, 0 cholesterol, 555mg sodium, 13g fiber

CAULIFLOWER SOUP

MAKES 6 SERVINGS

2 tablespoons olive oil
1 large yellow onion, coarsely chopped
2 teaspoons finely chopped fresh garlic
6 cups fresh cauliflower florets (about 1 large head)
½ cup chopped carrot
½ cup chopped celery
1 small jalapeño pepper, seeds removed and diced
3½ cups low-sodium, fat-free chicken broth
1 (14.5-ounce) can diced tomatoes
1 bay leaf
½ teaspoon ground cumin
Salt and freshly ground pepper to taste
Large croutons (optional)
Crumbled feta cheese for garnish

Heat olive oil in a large pot over medium heat, add onion and garlic, and sauté until soft. Add cauliflower florets, carrot, celery, and jalapeño. Cook until florets begin to brown. Add broth, tomatoes, bay leaf, cumin, and salt and pepper, and bring to a boil. Reduce heat to low and cook for 20–25 minutes, stirring occasionally, until cauliflower is tender. Remove from heat, discard bay leaf, and serve with croutons, if desired, and feta cheese.

Approx. 68 calories per serving
2g protein, 5g total fat, 1g saturated fat, 0 trans fat,
4g carbohydrates, 0 cholesterol, 57mg sodium, 1g fiber

TOMATO TORTELLINI SOUP

MAKES 8 SERVINGS

1 tablespoon olive oil
1 white onion, chopped
½ teaspoon crushed red hot pepper flakes
2 teaspoons chopped fresh garlic
2 cups low-sodium, fat-free chicken broth
1 cup water
2 teaspoons beef bouillon base
1 (14.5-ounce) can diced low-sodium tomatoes with basil and garlic
1 (15-ounce) can low-sodium tomato sauce
1 tablespoon dry Italian seasoning mix
Salt and freshly ground pepper to taste
1 (16-ounce) bag cheese tortellini
Crusty bread

In a large skillet over medium heat, add olive oil, onion, hot pepper flakes, and garlic. Sauté until onion and garlic are soft. Transfer to a large soup pot. Add broth, water, and beef base to the pot, and bring to a boil, then reduce heat to a simmer. Add tomatoes, tomato sauce, Italian seasoning, and salt and pepper to taste. Let simmer for 15 minutes, then add tortellini, and let simmer for another 5 minutes or until tortellini is soft. Serve while hot with crusty bread.

Approx. 148 calories per serving
4 g protein, 5g total fat, 0 saturated fat, 0 trans fat,
20g carbohydrates, 7mg cholesterol, 456mg sodium, 2g fiber

STRACCIATELLA (ITALIAN EGG DROP SOUP)

MAKES 4 (2-CUP) SERVINGS

6 cups low-sodium, fat-free chicken broth
2 tablespoons minced fresh garlic
8 cups chopped escarole, cut into bite-sized pieces
¾ cup liquid eggs
⅓ cup freshly grated Parmesan cheese
Pinch of freshly grated nutmeg
2 tablespoons freshly squeezed lemon juice
Salt and freshly ground pepper to taste
Extra-virgin olive oil to drizzle
Scant amount freshly grated Parmesan cheese for garnish

Heat chicken broth and garlic in a large pot over medium heat. Cover and bring to a simmer, then add escarole and cook until tender, about 5 minutes. Slowly add in liquid eggs. As they solidify, break into pieces. Add in Parmesan cheese and nutmeg, stirring soup gently. Reduce heat to medium-low and cook for roughly 2–3 minutes, then add lemon juice and salt and pepper to taste. Serve in bowls with a drizzle of olive oil and a sprinkle of Parmesan cheese.

Approx. 88 calories per serving
9g protein, 2g total fat, 1g saturated fat, 0 trans fat,
3g carbohydrates, 7mg cholesterol, 191mg sodium, 2g fiber

BASIC LENTIL SOUP

MAKES 6–8 SERVINGS

4 cups low-sodium, fat-free chicken broth

4 cups water

1 cup split brown lentils, rinsed and drained

Salt and freshly ground pepper to taste

2 teaspoons ground cumin

¼ cup extra-virgin olive oil

2 medium yellow onions, finely chopped

4 large cloves fresh garlic, finely chopped

2 ounces ditalini pasta

1 large firm ripe tomato, seeded and cut into chunks

10 ounces fresh escarole, washed and chopped

1 cup finely chopped fresh parsley

½ cup fresh lemon juice

Shredded Parmesan cheese for garnish (optional)

In a large pot add chicken broth and water, and bring to a boil. Add lentils, salt and pepper, and cumin, reduce heat to medium, and cook until lentils are tender. Do not overcook; beans should be tender but firm. While lentils are cooking, add olive oil to a skillet and sauté onions and garlic until golden brown. Stir mixture often to prevent burning; when browned, set aside. When lentils are almost tender, add pasta and cook until both are tender but not mushy. Reduce heat to a low simmer, and add garlic mixture, tomato, escarole, parsley, and lemon juice. Simmer until escarole is cooked. Serve garnished with a small amount of Parmesan cheese, if desired.

Approx. 195 calories per serving
8g protein, 11g total fat, 1g saturated fat, 0 trans fat,
26g carbohydrates, 3mg cholesterol, 152mg sodium, 6g fiber

SAVORY MEDITERRANEAN CHICKPEA SOUP

MAKES 6 SERVINGS

2 cups water

4 cups low-sodium, fat-free chicken broth

4 cups canned chickpeas, rinsed with fresh water and drained

1 tablespoon extra-virgin olive oil

1 large onion, chopped

4–5 cloves fresh garlic, minced

1 medium green bell pepper, chopped

1 teaspoon cayenne

2 teaspoons dried sage

2 teaspoons dried rosemary

1 teaspoon ground cinnamon

Salt and freshly ground pepper to taste

¼ cup crumbled low-fat feta cheese (optional)

2 tablespoons finely chopped fresh parsley for garnish

In a large pot combine water, broth, chickpeas, olive oil, onion, garlic, green bell pepper, cayenne, sage, rosemary, and cinnamon. Bring mixture to boil over medium heat, lower temperature, and simmer for 20 minutes, uncovered. Add salt and pepper to taste. Garnish with feta cheese, if desired, and parsley.

Approx. 163 calories per serving
9g protein, 3g total fat, <0.5g saturated fat, 0 trans fat,
32g carbohydrates, 3mg cholesterol, 560mg sodium, 8g fiber

FRESH GARDEN GAZPACHO

MAKES 4 SERVINGS

4 cups chopped ripe peeled tomatoes

4 cloves fresh garlic, chopped

½ red onion, chopped

1 green bell pepper, seeded and diced

¼ cup extra-virgin olive oil

2 tablespoons red wine vinegar

2 slices stale French sourdough bread

½ cup canned tomato juice

½ teaspoon cumin

½ small hot pepper, finely chopped

1 tablespoon chopped fresh basil

Salt and freshly ground pepper to taste

¼ cup green bell peppers and cucumbers for garnish, finely diced

Croutons (optional)

Plain low-fat sour cream or yogurt (optional)

In a food processor or blender, add tomatoes, garlic, onion, and green pepper. Blend until pureed. Add olive oil and vinegar, blend about 1 minute to mix. Soak bread in tomato juice, then add soaked bread mixture to blender. Add cumin, hot peppers, and basil. Blend for 2–3 minutes to mix well. Adjust with salt and pepper to taste. Chill for several hours. Serve very chilled, garnished with diced green peppers and cucumber. If desired, add croutons and a dollop of sour cream or yogurt.

Approx. 210 calories per serving
4g protein, 14g total fat, 2g saturated fat, 0 trans fat,
20g carbohydrates, 0 cholesterol, 201mg sodium, 3g fiber

CHILLY TOMATO SOUP

MAKES 4 SERVINGS

10 medium ripe tomatoes
½ tablespoon extra-virgin olive oil
4–5 cloves fresh garlic, minced
2 tablespoons chopped onion
2 cups low-sodium, fat-free chicken broth
2 teaspoons low-calorie baking sweetener
½ teaspoon chopped fresh basil
Salt and freshly ground pepper to taste
8 scallions, chopped (optional)
2 cucumbers, diced (optional)
1 large green zucchini, diced (optional)

In a large pot of boiling water, dip tomatoes for 30 seconds, then immediately place tomatoes in cold water. Allow to sit until they can be handled. Skin tomatoes with a paring knife, cut in half crosswise, and remove seeds. Core and then cut into quarter pieces. In a blender or food processor, process tomatoes until pureed. In a skillet, heat olive oil and sauté garlic and onion until tender. Remove from heat. In a large bowl, combine pureed tomatoes, sautéed onion mixture, chicken broth, sweetener, basil, and salt and pepper, stirring to mix ingredients together. Refrigerate soup for 4–6 hours until well chilled. Garnish with scallion, cucumbers, and zucchini, if desired.

Approx. 161 calories per serving
10g protein, <0.5g total fat, 0 saturated fat, 0 trans fat,
65g carbohydrates, 5mg cholesterol, 197mg sodium, 1g fiber

ITALIAN MINESTRONE SOUP WITH PESTO
MAKES 6–8 SERVINGS

1 cup dried cannellini beans
4 cups low-sodium, fat-free chicken broth
4 cups water
2 medium white potatoes, peeled and diced
2 ounces ditalini pasta
2 large carrots, chopped
3 stalks celery, chopped
½ cup chopped white onion
2 cloves fresh garlic, minced
1 cup tomato juice
3 plum tomatoes, chopped
1 large zucchini, chopped
Freshly shredded Parmesan cheese for garnish (optional)

For pesto:

1 cup fresh basil leaves
1 teaspoon crumbled dried basil leaves
4 cloves fresh garlic, finely minced
3 tablespoons extra-virgin olive oil
½ cup grated Parmesan cheese
Salt and freshly ground pepper to taste

Rinse dried cannellini beans and place in a large covered pot. Add chicken broth and water and bring to a boil. Uncover pot, reduce heat, and simmer until beans are tender; roughly 1 hour. Add potatoes, pasta, carrots, celery, onion, garlic, and tomato juice. Return mixture to a boil, then reduce heat and simmer uncovered for 10 minutes. Add tomato and zucchini and simmer until all are tender. Process pesto ingredients in a food processor or blender until finely chopped. Remove soup from heat and stir in pesto mixture, and serve garnished with Parmesan cheese, if desired.

Approx. 182 calories per serving without pesto
10g protein, 1g total fat, 0 saturated fat, 0 trans fat,
20g carbohydrates, 3mg cholesterol, 204mg sodium, 4g fiber

Approx. 254 calories per serving with pesto added
12g protein, 8g total fat, 2g saturated fat, 0 trans fat,
20g carbohydrates, 10mg cholesterol, 291mg sodium, 4g fiber

CHUNKY CHICKEN AND CABBAGE SOUP

MAKES 4–6 SERVINGS

4 cups low-sodium, fat-free chicken broth

2 cups water

8 ounces skinless, boneless chicken, cubed

2 medium potatoes, peeled and cubed

1 cup chopped carrots

2 bay leaves

4–6 whole peppercorns

½ teaspoon cumin

1 cup chopped celery

1 medium onion, chunked

3 cloves fresh garlic, chopped

1 small head of cabbage, torn

2 medium tomatoes, peeled and quartered

¼ cup fresh parsley, finely chopped

Salt and freshly ground pepper to taste

1 tablespoon plain non-fat yogurt (optional)

In a large pot, bring chicken broth, water, chicken, potatoes, carrots, bay leaves, peppercorns, and cumin to boil. Reduce heat, simmer for 30–40 minutes or until chicken is cooked. Add celery, onion, garlic, cabbage, tomatoes, and parsley; cook for additional 15 minutes or until vegetables are tender. Add salt and pepper to taste. Garnish each serving with yogurt, if desired.

Approx. 143 calories per serving
15g protein, 2g total fat, <0.3g saturated fat, 0 trans fat,
21g carbohydrates, 21mg cholesterol, 50mg sodium, 3g fiber

FRENCH PISTOU SOUP

MAKES 6 SERVINGS

1 tablespoon extra-virgin olive oil
1 medium onion, finely chopped
½ cup dry kidney beans
2 medium potatoes, diced
1 stalk celery, chopped
2 cups chopped carrots
8 cups water
8 ounces fresh green beans cut into 1-inch pieces
1 leek, green part only, thinly sliced
2 medium tomatoes, peeled and chopped
2 small zucchini cut into 1-inch cubes
1 cup whole wheat elbow macaroni
Salt and freshly ground pepper to taste

For Pistou Mix:

3 cloves fresh garlic
2 cups fresh basil leaves
1 tablespoon hot liquid from soup
Salt and freshly ground pepper to taste
3 tablespoons extra-virgin olive oil
Freshly grated Gruyere cheese for garnish

In large saucepan heat olive oil, add onion, and cook to soften. Add kidney beans, potatoes, celery, carrots, and water. Bring to a boil, reduce heat, and simmer covered for about 15 minutes. Add green beans, leek, tomatoes, zucchini, and pasta; cook another 10 minutes or until the vegetables are tender. Season mixture with salt and pepper to taste. Reduce heat to very low, cover to keep warm.

Pistou:

In a food processor, finely chop garlic and basil. Add soup liquid, salt and pepper to taste, and olive oil. Ladle soup into individual soup bowls, then spoon in some pistou and garnish with cheese.

Approx. 248 calories per serving
10g protein, 9g total fat, 1g saturated fat, 0 trans fat,
35g carbohydrates, 0 cholesterol, 28mg sodium, 8g fiber

HEARTY BEAN SOUP

MAKES 6–8 SERVINGS

2 cups water

2 medium potatoes, peeled and coarsely chopped

2 large carrots, coarsely chopped

2 stalks celery, coarsely chopped

1 bay leaf

1 tablespoon fresh thyme

Salt and freshly ground pepper to taste

3 tablespoons extra virgin olive oil

5 cloves fresh garlic, minced

1 medium onion, finely chopped

½ small hot pepper, finely chopped

5 cups low-sodium, fat-free chicken broth

4 (15-ounce) cans Great Northern beans

Grated Parmesan cheese (optional)

Chopped fresh flat leaf parsley (optional)

In a heavy pot, combine water, potatoes, carrots, celery, bay leaf, thyme, and salt and pepper. Bring to a boil, reduce heat, cover, and simmer until vegetables are tender. While vegetables are cooking, combine olive oil, garlic, onion, and hot pepper in a large skillet, and sauté until tender and lightly browned. Add 1 cup of chicken broth and beans to garlic mixture, mix together well, cover, and simmer for about 10 minutes to allow flavors to blend. Add salt and pepper to taste. Combine bean mixture and 4 cups of chicken broth, and add to vegetable pot. Stir to mix, then keep at a low simmer for about 10–15 minutes, allowing flavors to blend. Garnish with Parmesan cheese and parsley, if desired.

Approx. 220 calories per serving
11g protein, 6g total fat, 0.7g saturated fat, 0 trans fat,
36g carbohydrates, 3mg cholesterol, 663mg sodium, 9g fiber

SPINACH FETA CHEESE SOUP

MAKES 6–8 SERVINGS

10 ounces spinach, washed under running water, divided

6 cups low-sodium, fat-free chicken broth, divided

¼ cup fresh cilantro, chopped

2 tablespoons extra-virgin olive oil

1 large white onion, coarsely chopped

2 medium potatoes, peeled and diced

4 cloves fresh garlic, minced

1 teaspoon ground cumin

1 (10-ounce) package frozen baby lima beans, thawed

⅓ cup couscous

6 ounces feta cheese, cut into chunks

½ teaspoon freshly ground pepper to taste

Finely chopped fresh parsley for garnish

Lemon wedges for garnish

Cut half of the spinach leaves into thin ribbons, reserving stems, and set aside. Using a food processor or blender, combine the reserved stems and the remaining spinach with 1 cup of broth and cilantro. Process until smooth and set aside. In a large pot, heat olive oil over medium heat, add onion, sauté until golden brown, and then add potatoes, garlic, and cumin; stir to make sure potatoes are well coated. Add remaining 5 cups of broth. Reduce heat to medium and cook until potatoes are tender, roughly 15 minutes. Add ribbon spinach, spinach-cilantro puree, lima beans, couscous, and feta cheese. Cook until lima beans are crispy tender and cheese has melted through soup. Season soup with freshly ground pepper. Divide soup into 6–8 servings. For garnish, sprinkle parsley over soup and add a lemon wedge on the side.

Approx. 226 calories per serving
10g protein, 10g total fat, 4g saturated fat, 0 trans fat,
24g carbohydrates, 15mg cholesterol, 157mg sodium, 4g fiber

CHUNKY FISH CHOWDER WITH SAFFRON

MAKES 6 SERVINGS

1 pound fresh grouper fillets

1 pound fresh tuna or cod fillets

2 tablespoons extra-virgin olive oil

8–10 diced scallions

1 cup chopped celery

3 large cloves fresh garlic, crushed

1 small yellow bell pepper, diced

1 small red bell pepper, diced

1 teaspoon turmeric

¼ teaspoon ground saffron

1¼ cup dry white wine

8 ounces bottled clam juice

4 cups water

2 bay leaves

½ teaspoon fresh thyme

¼ teaspoon crushed red hot pepper flakes

Salt to taste

¾ cup small elbow macaroni

2 tablespoons lemon juice

4 tablespoons chopped fresh parsley for garnish

Rinse and cut fish fillets into 1-inch cubes; refrigerate. In a large heavy-bottomed skillet, heat olive oil and sauté scallions, celery, garlic, and yellow and red bell peppers. Add turmeric and saffron and cook a few more minutes. Stir in wine, clam juice, and water. Add in bay leaves, thyme, hot pepper flakes, and salt, then bring to boil. Reduce heat and simmer for 10 minutes. Add pasta and cook until pasta is tender. Add fish and simmer for 10–15 minutes longer, until fish is cooked. Remove bay leaves. Add lemon juice and stir to mix. Serve garnished with parsley.

Approx. 296 calories per serving
35g protein, 8g total fat, 2g saturated fat, 0 trans fat,
11g carbohydrates, 27mg cholesterol, 187mg sodium, 3g fiber

CHICKEN ESCAROLE SOUP

MAKES 4–6 SERVINGS

3 cups water (enough to cover chicken)
5 skinless, boneless chicken breasts, cut into chunks
1 small white onion, cut in half
⅛ cup black peppercorns
1 bay leaf
4 cloves fresh garlic, finely minced
3 cups canned low-sodium, fat-free chicken broth
2 medium carrots, sliced
1 celery stalk, sliced
½ head escarole, cut into 1-inch strips, stems removed
Salt and freshly ground pepper to taste
Freshly grated Parmesan cheese for garnish

In a large saucepan, combine water, chicken, onion, peppercorns, bay leaf, and garlic. Bring to a boil, reduce heat to low, cover, and simmer 1 hour or until chicken is tender. Remove chicken from broth and strain out bay leaf and peppercorns; set aside. In a separate saucepan, combine canned chicken broth with strained broth, add carrots and celery, bring to a rapid boil, reduce to low, and simmer for 10 minutes or until vegetables are crispy tender. Stir in escarole and chicken, heat through, add salt and pepper to taste, and serve. Garnish each serving with a sprinkling of Parmesan cheese.

Approx. 153 calories per serving
28g protein, 2g total fat, <0.4g saturated fat, 0 trans fat,
4g carbohydrates, 62mg cholesterol, 129mg sodium, 5g fiber

CHILLED CUCUMBER SOUP

MAKES 4–6 SERVINGS

2 large English cucumbers, peeled and coarsely chopped
1 medium yellow onion, coarsely chopped
5 cups canned low-sodium, fat-free chicken broth
2 cups plain low-fat yogurt
2 scallions, white and green parts, finely minced
Salt to taste
Freshly ground pepper to taste
Fresh dill, finely chopped

Combine cucumbers and onion in a large saucepan; add chicken broth. Heat on high heat to rapid boil, immediately reduce to low, cover, and simmer until vegetables are just tender. Remove from heat, allow to cool slightly, then refrigerate to chill for several hours. To serve, blend in yogurt, scallions, and salt to taste. Sprinkle with pepper and dill.

Approx. 91 calories per serving
7g protein, 3g total fat, <0.4g saturated fat, 0 trans fat,
10g carbohydrates, 4mg cholesterol, 164mg sodium, 1g fiber

EGGPLANT SOUP WITH DRY SHERRY AND FETA CHEESE
MAKES 4–6 SERVINGS

2 tablespoons extra-virgin olive oil

2 cloves fresh garlic, minced

½ medium onion, thinly sliced and separated into rings

1 medium eggplant, peeled and cut into ½-inch cubes

½ teaspoon oregano

¼ teaspoon fresh thyme

4 cups canned low-sodium, fat-free chicken broth

½ cup dry sherry

Salt and freshly ground pepper to taste

1 large tomato, sliced

10 ounces crumbled non-fat feta cheese

Freshly grated Parmesan cheese (optional)

Heat olive oil in large skillet over medium heat; add garlic and onion, and sauté until lightly golden. Add eggplant, oregano, and thyme; continue cooking until eggplant browns slightly, stirring constantly. Reduce heat to low, add broth, cover, and simmer for roughly 5 minutes. Add sherry, cover, and continue to simmer for another 2–3 minutes. Stir in salt and pepper to taste, if needed, and remove from heat. Allow to cool slightly. Preheat broiler, and pour slightly cooled soup into an oven-safe bowl. Top soup with tomato slices and feta cheese, place soup under broiler, and heat until feta melts into soup. Garnish with Parmesan cheese, if desired, and broil until cheese is browned.

Approx. 146 calories per serving
9g protein, 5g total fat, <1g saturated fat, 0 trans fat,
10g carbohydrates, 3mg cholesterol, 538mg sodium, 2g fiber

PASTA e FAGIOLI SOUP

MAKES 14 1-CUP SERVINGS

2 tablespoons extra-virgin olive oil

6 cloves fresh garlic, minced

1½ cups chopped carrots

1½ cups chopped celery

1½ cups chopped white onion

3 cups water

3 (14.5-ounce) cans low-sodium, fat-free chicken broth

3 teaspoons dried parsley

1½ teaspoons dried mixed Italian seasoning

¼ teaspoon crushed hot red pepper flakes

1 (14.5-ounce) can diced tomatoes with liquid

½ cup ditalini pasta

½ cup dried kidney beans

½ cup dried cannellini beans

Salt and freshly ground pepper to taste

Freshly grated Parmesan cheese for garnish

In a large skillet, add olive oil and sauté garlic, carrots, celery, and onion. Transfer to a large heavy-bottomed pot; add water, broth, parsley, Italian seasoning, hot pepper flakes, tomatoes, pasta, beans, and salt and pepper to taste. Bring soup to a boil, cover, and reduce to a simmer for about 2–3 hours or until beans are soft. Serve with a sprinkling of Parmesan cheese.

Approx. 150 calories per 1 cup serving
6g protein, 0.5g total fat, 0 saturated fat, <0.1g trans fat,
18g carbohydrates, 0 cholesterol, 5mg sodium, 4g fiber

MOM'S CHICKEN SOUP

MAKES 8–10 SERVINGS

3 (5–6-ounce) skinless, boneless chicken breasts cut into 1-inch cubes

2 cups water

4 cloves fresh garlic, chopped

3 large carrots, cut into small chunks

4–6 celery stalks, cut into small chunks

1 medium yellow onion, cut into chunks

8 cups canned fat-free, low-sodium chicken broth

½ cup orzo

1 tablespoon extra-virgin olive oil

Freshly ground pepper to taste

Tabasco sauce (optional)

In a large pot, add chicken cubes, water, and garlic. Bring to a boil, cover, and reduce heat to a simmer. Simmer for about 10 minutes. Add carrots, celery, and onion, and cook for an additional 5–10 minutes. Add chicken broth, orzo, olive oil, and pepper to taste. Continue to simmer on low heat, covered, until orzo is soft. Serve with a drizzle of Tabasco sauce, if desired.

Approx. 131 calories per serving
16g protein, 3g total fat, 0.4g saturated fat, 0 trans fat,
12g carbohydrates, 29mg cholesterol, 513mg sodium, 1g fiber

POTATO LEEK SOUP WITH SMOKED SALMON
MAKES 8 SERVINGS

1 tablespoon extra-virgin olive oil

2 tablespoons trans fat–free canola/olive oil spread

2 large leeks, white and light green parts only, cut in half lengthwise and thinly sliced

2 medium fennel bulbs, trimmed and chopped

1 teaspoon fennel seeds

6 cups canned low-sodium, low-fat chicken broth

2 pounds red potatoes, peeled and cubed (2-inch cubes)

2 ounces thinly sliced nova lox, cut into pieces

Salt and freshly ground pepper to taste

Freshly chopped chives for garnish

In a heavy-bottomed pan, heat olive oil over medium-high heat; add spread and allow to melt. Add leeks, fennel, and fennel seeds, and sauté until translucent (about 7 minutes). Add broth and potatoes to skillet and bring to a boil. Reduce to medium-low heat and simmer until potatoes are tender (about 20–25 minutes). Transfer soup in batches to a blender and puree. Return to pot to warm on low heat. When soup is warm, add nova lox pieces, salt and pepper to taste, and serve, garnished with fresh-chopped chives.

Approx. 144 calories per serving
10g protein, 10g total fat, 0.89g saturated fat, 0 trans fat,
23g carbohydrates, 0 cholesterol, 92mg sodium, 4g fiber

Pizza, Pizza Sauces, and Pizza Crusts

In the Mediterranean regions, a pizza made at home is a well-balanced modern meal, made from complex carbohydrate pizza dough, fresh vegetables, small amounts of animal protein, and monounsaturated fat in the form of extra-virgin olive oil. In contrast, the fast-food pizza made in the United States is loaded with saturated fat, trans fats, refined sugar, and sodium.

For healthy, quick, and easy pizzas, just top Toufayan's round whole grain wraps or Flat Out's oval, light whole grain wraps (both are trans fat free and make great quick pizza crusts) with your favorite pizza ingredients and bake in the oven at 350 degrees for about 5 minutes or until cheese melts and edges of wrap become crispy.

SMOKED SALMON AND MOZZARELLA CHEESE PIZZA
MAKES AN 8-INCH PERSONAL PIZZA

1 flat wrap
1 tablespoon fresh Basil Pesto Sauce (page 488) or a market-fresh basil pesto
4 slices of smoked nova (about 2 ounces)
2 tablespoons coarsely chopped red onion
¼ cup shredded part-skim mozzarella cheese
Dried oregano flakes to sprinkle

Preheat oven to 350 degrees. Place wrap on a baking sheet and spread pesto sauce lightly over surface of wrap. Arrange salmon over pesto and scatter on onion and mozzarella cheese. Sprinkle with oregano and bake at 350 degrees until cheese melts and begins to bubble. Remove from oven and serve.

Approx. 325 calories per pizza
28g protein, 16g total fat, 3g saturated fat, 0 trans fat,
17g carbohydrates, 30mg cholesterol, 145mg sodium, 8g fiber

BROCCOLI AND PECORINO FLATBREAD PIZZAS
MAKES 4 SERVINGS

4 oval, trans fat–free whole grain flatbreads
30 fresh broccoli florets, thinly sliced
2 tablespoons olive oil
3 cloves fresh garlic, thinly sliced
½ teaspoon crushed red hot pepper flakes or to taste
Salt and freshly ground pepper to taste
1 cup shaved fresh Pecorino Romano (about 4 ounces)

Preheat oven to 400 degrees. Place flatbreads on 2 rimmed baking sheets. In a bowl, toss together broccoli, olive oil, garlic, hot pepper flakes, and salt and pepper to taste. Scatter broccoli mixture evenly on flatbreads and sprinkle with Pecorino shavings. Bake at 400 degrees until flatbreads are crispy and broccoli is browning, about 15 minutes. Serve warm.

Approx. 405 calories per serving
16g protein, 17g total fat, 9g saturated fat, 0 trans fat,
46g carbohydrates, 30mg cholesterol, 622mg sodium, 3g fiber

ASSORTED MUSHROOM AND SWISS CHEESE PIZZA

MAKES AN 8-INCH PERSONAL PIZZA

1 flat wrap
1 tablespoon extra-virgin olive oil
½ cup sliced assorted mushrooms
2 tablespoons chopped scallions, white and green parts
2 teaspoons fresh garlic paste
Freshly ground pepper to taste
1 ounce shredded light Swiss cheese
1 tablespoon dried thyme, finely crushed

Preheat oven to 350 degrees. Place wrap on a baking sheet and set aside. Heat a small amount of olive oil in a heavy-bottomed skillet. Add mushrooms, scallions, garlic paste, and pepper. Sauté for 2–3 minutes, stirring often, until mushrooms and scallions soften. Remove from heat and spread mixture out evenly over wrap. Distribute Swiss cheese over mushroom mixture and sprinkle on thyme. Place in oven and bake at 350 degrees until cheese melts. Remove from oven and serve.

Approx. 262 calories per pizza
24g protein, 8g total fat, 4g saturated fat, 0 trans fat,
18g carbohydrates, 20mg cholesterol, 607mg sodium, 8g fiber

FRESH BASIL AND MOZZARELLA CHEESE PIZZA

MAKES AN 8-INCH PERSONAL PIZZA

1 flat wrap
1 teaspoon finely minced fresh garlic
¼ cup fresh Traditional Pizza Sauce (page 147) or a market sauce like Del Fratelli
¼ cup shredded part-skim mozzarella cheese
4 slices fresh tomato
4–6 fresh whole basil leaves

Preheat oven to 350 degrees. Place wrap on a baking sheet. Stir garlic into pizza sauce and spread evenly over wrap. Top sauce first with mozzarella cheese, then tomato slices and basil leaves. Bake at 350 degrees until cheese melts. Remove from oven and serve.

Approx. 270 calories per pizza
23g protein, 9g total fat, 4g saturated fat, 0 trans fat,
25g carbohydrates, 15mg cholesterol, 888mg sodium, 10g fiber

BABY SHRIMP AND MOZZARELLA CHEESE PIZZA

MAKES AN 8-INCH PERSONAL PIZZA

1 flat wrap
1 tablespoon fresh Basil Pesto Sauce (page 488) or a market-fresh basil pesto
½ cup cooked baby salad shrimp, defrosted (if frozen) and well drained
4 small pitted black olives, drained and sliced
¼ cup shredded part-skim mozzarella cheese
Dried chives to sprinkle

Preheat oven to 350 degrees. Place wrap on a baking sheet and spread pesto evenly over surface of wrap. Scatter shrimp over pesto, add olives, and top with mozzarella cheese. Sprinkle chives over cheese and bake at 350 degrees until cheese melts and begins to bubble. Remove from oven and serve.

Approx. 371 calories per pizza
37g protein, 18g total fat, 5g saturated fat, 0 trans fat,
18g carbohydrates, 70mg cholesterol, 121mg sodium, 9g fiber

PIZZA MARGHERITA

MAKES AN 8-SLICE, 15-INCH PIZZA

Thin Crust Pizza Dough (page 152)
4 Roma tomatoes, thinly sliced
Salt and freshly ground pepper to taste
½ cup yellow sweet pepper, thinly sliced
¾ cup shredded part-skim mozzarella cheese, about 3 ounces
4–5 snipped fresh basil leaves
¼ cup freshly grated Parmesan cheese
1 tablespoon extra-virgin olive oil

Preheat oven to 450 degrees. Follow directions for pizza dough and roll out to a 12–15-inch round. Place dough on a scantly oiled pizza pan. Spread tomatoes on rolled-out dough almost to the edge of the crust. Sprinkle with salt and pepper to taste. Top tomatoes with yellow peppers, mozzarella cheese, basil, and Parmesan cheese, and drizzle olive oil over the top. Bake at 450 degrees for 8–10 minutes or until crust is crisp and cheeses are melted.

Approx. 202 calories per slice
11g protein, 7g total fat, 3g saturated fat, 0 trans fat,
28g carbohydrates, 7mg cholesterol, 375mg sodium, 1g fiber

TOMATO, EGGPLANT, AND BASIL PIZZA

MAKES AN 8-SLICE, 15-INCH PIZZA

Crispy Thin Whole Wheat Pizza Dough (page 150)
1 large eggplant
6 cloves fresh garlic, minced
2 tablespoons extra-virgin olive oil
5 medium tomatoes, seeded and chopped
3 tablespoons chopped fresh basil
Pinch of crushed red hot pepper flakes
3 cups crumbled non-fat feta cheese
Salt and freshly ground pepper to taste
⅓ cup freshly grated Parmesan cheese for garnish
Fresh rosemary, finely chopped (optional)

Preheat oven to 425 degrees. Follow directions for pizza dough and roll out to a 12–15-inch round. Place pizza round on scantly oiled pizza pan. Cut eggplant in half the long way, slashing down the middle but not through the skin. Place on separate pan and bake for 20–30 minutes. Skin should be shriveled and eggplant tender. Remove to a plate and reserve; when cooled, slice crosswise into thin slices. In a skillet, sauté garlic in 1 tablespoon of olive oil over low heat until softened. Add tomatoes, basil, and hot pepper flakes. Brush pizza dough lightly with ½ teaspoon olive oil, top with tomato mixture, then feta cheese, and arrange eggplant slices in a pinwheel pattern, slightly overlapping the slices. Season pizza with salt and pepper and drizzle remaining olive oil over eggplant. Bake at 425 degrees for 10–15 minutes until pizza crust is crisp. Garnish top of pizza with Parmesan cheese and rosemary, if desired.

Approx. 166 calories per slice
20g protein, 4g total fat, <0.5g saturated fat, 0 trans fat,
21g carbohydrates, 0 cholesterol, 185mg sodium, 1g fiber

SPICY SWEET PEPPER PIZZA

MAKES AN 8-SLICE, 15-INCH PIZZA

Whole Wheat Pizza Dough (page 151)
1 tablespoon extra-virgin olive oil
3 large red bell peppers, seeded and thinly sliced
3 large yellow bell peppers, seeded and thinly sliced
2 cloves fresh garlic, minced
1 tablespoon chopped fresh thyme
Salt and freshly ground pepper to taste
Crushed red hot pepper flakes to taste
1 cup shredded part-skim mozzarella cheese

Preheat oven to 500 degrees. Follow directions for pizza dough and roll out to 12–15-inch round. Place dough on scantly oiled pizza pan. Heat olive oil in heavy-bottomed pan and sauté the red and yellow bell peppers and garlic, about 10 minutes until soft. Stir in thyme, salt and pepper to taste, and hot pepper flakes. Spread pepper mixture over pizza dough, sprinkle mozzarella cheese over pepper mixture, and bake at 500 degrees for 20–25 minutes until crust is crisp and cheese has melted.

Approx. 209 calories per slice
9g protein, 7g total fat, 3g saturated fat, 0 trans fat,
25g carbohydrates, 7mg cholesterol, 78mg sodium, 4g fiber

WILD MUSHROOM PIZZA

MAKES AN 8-SLICE, 15-INCH PIZZA

Thin Crust Pizza Dough (page 152)
3 ounces dried porcine mushrooms
1 quart warm water
2 tablespoons extra-virgin olive oil
4 cloves fresh garlic, finely minced
1 cup fresh button mushrooms, cleaned and thinly sliced
1 cup fresh shiitake or other wild mushrooms
4 tablespoons white wine
1 tablespoon low-sodium soy sauce
½ teaspoon dried thyme
½ teaspoon dried rosemary
Salt and freshly ground pepper to taste
3 tablespoons chopped fresh parsley
8 ounces shredded smoked provolone cheese

Preheat oven to 425 degrees. Follow directions for pizza dough; when ready, roll it out to a 15-inch round. Place on scantly oiled pizza pan. Soak the dried mushrooms in warm water for 30 minutes. After soaking, squeeze excess liquid from mushrooms and chop coarsely. Strain soaking water through a cheesecloth and set aside. Heat 1 tablespoon of olive oil over medium heat in a heavy-bottomed skillet and add half of the garlic. Sauté garlic, stirring often until it becomes golden. Add both dried and fresh mushrooms, sauté for about 5 minutes until they begin to release their liquid, and then add wine and soy sauce. Continue to sauté until wine evaporates. Add soaking liquid to mushrooms, thyme, rosemary, remaining garlic, and salt and pepper to taste. Increase heat; continue cooking and stirring until most of the liquid has evaporated and mushrooms have become glazed. Add parsley and remove from heat. Brush pizza dough with remaining olive oil. Evenly spread provolone cheese over crust. Spread mushroom mixture over cheese and bake at 425 degrees for roughly 8–10 minutes, until crust is crisp and cheese is melted.

Approx. 208 calories per slice
9g protein, 10g total fat, 0.5g saturated fat, 0 trans fat,
22g carbohydrates, 0 cholesterol, 351mg sodium, 2g fiber

SUNDRIED TOMATO AND ANCHOVY PIZZA
MAKES AN 8-SLICE, 15-INCH PIZZA

Crispy Thin Whole Wheat Pizza Dough (page 150)
1 red onion, thinly sliced
8 sundried tomatoes in oil, chopped
1 tablespoon fresh basil leaves, broken in pieces
1 can (2 ounces) anchovy fillets, chopped, oil reserved
1 clove fresh garlic, minced
1 cup fresh part-skim mozzarella cheese, shredded
Salt and freshly ground pepper to taste
Finely chopped fresh parsley for garnish (optional)

Preheat oven to 425 degrees. Follow directions for pizza dough; when ready, roll out to 15-inch round. Place on scantly oiled pizza pan. Top pizza crust dough with onion, sundried tomatoes, basil, anchovies, garlic, and mozzarella cheese. Salt and pepper to taste and bake at 425 degrees until crust is crisp and cheese is melted. Garnish with parsley, if desired.

Approx. 137 calories per slice
6g protein, 5g total fat, 3g saturated fat, 0 trans fat,
18g carbohydrates, 10mg cholesterol, 119mg sodium, 1g fiber

Pizza Sauces

TRADITIONAL PIZZA SAUCE

MAKES ENOUGH FOR A 15-INCH CRUST

2 tablespoons extra-virgin olive oil

3 cloves fresh garlic, peeled and sliced

5 medium tomatoes, seeded and chopped

2 sprigs fresh rosemary

Salt and freshly ground pepper to taste

Pinch of sugar

In a heavy skillet over medium-high heat, add olive oil and garlic and cook until soft. Add tomatoes, rosemary, salt and pepper, and sugar; raise heat slightly and cook rapidly, stirring often until juices thicken (about 15–20 minutes). Put sauce through a food mill, letting pulp pass through. If sauce is too thin, return to low heat and cook until desired consistency.

Approx. 63 calories per serving, based on a 2-inch slice
1g protein, 4g total fat, <0.5g saturated fat, 0 trans fat,
4g carbohydrates, 0 cholesterol, 390mg sodium, 1g fiber

FIERY TOMATO AND BASIL PIZZA SAUCE

MAKES ENOUGH FOR A 15-INCH CRUST

1 tablespoon extra-virgin olive oil
4 cloves fresh garlic, chopped
5 medium tomatoes, seeded and chopped
3 tablespoons fresh chopped basil
Salt and freshly ground pepper to taste
Pinch of sugar
¼ teaspoon crushed red hot pepper flakes

In skillet, heat olive oil over medium-high heat and sauté garlic. Add tomatoes, cook, and stir for about 5 minutes. In a separate bowl, combine basil, salt and pepper, sugar, and hot pepper flakes, and add to tomato mixture.

Approx. 38 calories per serving, based on a 2-inch slice
1g protein, 2g total fat, <0.5g saturated fat, 0 trans fat,
3g carbohydrates, 0 cholesterol, 7mg sodium, 1g fiber

SPICY GARLIC, OLIVE OIL,
AND SUNDRIED TOMATO PIZZA SAUCE

MAKES ENOUGH FOR A 12-INCH CRUST

¼ cup extra-virgin olive oil
4 cloves fresh garlic, minced
¼ teaspoon crushed red hot pepper flakes
6 jumbo pitted black olives, diced
8 sundried tomatoes in oil, drained and diced
Salt and freshly ground pepper to taste

In a medium-sized skillet, heat olive oil over medium-high heat, add garlic, and sauté until translucent. Add hot pepper flakes, olives, and sundried tomatoes, and salt and pepper to taste; simmer over very low heat for 3–5 minutes.

Approx. 79 calories per slice, based on a 2-inch slice
0 protein, 9g total fat, 1g saturated fat, 0 trans fat,
1g carbohydrates, 0 cholesterol, 42mg sodium, 0 fiber

EASY PIZZA SAUCE

MAKES I QUART OF SAUCE

1 teaspoon crumbled dried basil
½ teaspoon crumbled dried oregano
¼ teaspoon crumbled dried marjoram
¼ cup dry white wine
2 cloves fresh garlic, finely chopped
1 tablespoon extra-virgin olive oil
1½ cups chopped crushed plum tomato
2 tablespoons tomato paste
Salt and freshly ground pepper to taste

Add herbs to wine and marinate for 15 minutes. Meanwhile, over medium heat, sauté garlic in olive oil until soft but not brown. Add tomato, tomato paste, and herb/wine mixture. Cover and simmer for about 20 minutes. Remove from stove, put into a blender, and puree until smooth. Return to skillet uncovered and continue to simmer until sauce thickens slightly. Add salt and pepper to taste.

Approx. 19 calories per ¼ cup
0.4g protein, 1g total fat, 0 saturated fat, 0 trans fat,
2g carbohydrates, 0 cholesterol, 102mg sodium, 0.23g fiber

Pizza Crusts

CRISPY THIN WHOLE WHEAT PIZZA DOUGH
MAKES AN 8-SLICE, 15-INCH CRUST

⅔ cup + 1–2 tablespoons all-purpose unbleached flour, divided
1 package active dry yeast
⅛ teaspoon salt
½ cup warm water
1 teaspoon extra-virgin olive oil
½ cup whole wheat flour
Non-stick olive oil cooking spray

In a mixing bowl, combine ⅔ cup all-purpose flour, yeast, and salt. Add water and olive oil and beat on high speed for about 2–3 minutes. Use a wooden spoon to stir in whole wheat flour. Transfer mixture to a lightly floured surface and knead in 1–2 additional tablespoons of all-purpose flour as you form mixture into a ball that is slightly stiff, yet still smooth and elastic. Put dough into a clean bowl, cover, and place in a warm area for about 10 minutes. Spray a pizza pan lightly with cooking oil. Roll out dough on a lightly floured surface into a 15-inch round, place on pizza pan, and top with sauce and ingredients of choice. Bake at 425 degrees for about 10 minutes, or until crust is crispy.

Approx. 76 calories per slice, crust only
2g protein, 0.5g total fat, 0.5g saturated fat, 0 trans fat,
16g carbohydrates, 0 cholesterol, 35mg sodium, 1g fiber

WHOLE WHEAT PIZZA DOUGH

MAKES AN 8-SLICE, 15-INCH CRUST

2½ teaspoons active dry yeast

1½ teaspoons low-calorie baking sweetener

1 teaspoon salt

2 tablespoons extra-virgin olive oil

½ cup lukewarm water

2 cups whole wheat flour

3–4 tablespoons extra flour for kneading

In a bowl, mix together yeast, sweetener, salt, olive oil, and water. Set aside for 10 minutes; the mixture will become cloudy and thick. When this happens, make a well in the center of the whole wheat flour. Add yeast mixture and gradually fold it into the flour, adding more lukewarm water if needed. Knead dough until it becomes smooth, then place dough in a lightly oiled bowl and cover with a clean cloth. Place dough in a warm area for about 45 minutes or until it doubles its size. Roll out dough on a lightly floured surface into a 15-inch round, place on pizza pan, and top with sauce and ingredients of choice. Bake at 500 degrees until crust is crispy.

Approx. 142 calories per slice, crust only
5g protein, 3g total fat, <0.5g saturated fat, 0 trans fat,
22g carbohydrates, 0 cholesterol, 3mg sodium, 4g fiber

THIN CRUST PIZZA DOUGH

MAKES AN 8-SLICE, 15-INCH CRUST

1⅔ cups unbleached all-purpose flour
½ teaspoon salt
1 package dry active yeast
2 tablespoons extra-virgin olive oil
½ cup warm water
Olive oil to lightly coat pan

Put flour, salt, and yeast in a large bowl and mix with a wooden spoon. Make a well in the center and add olive oil and water. Gradually work in flour from the sides of the bowl as the mixture becomes smooth, pliable, soft dough. If too sticky, sprinkle a little more flour into the mixture, but don't make the dough dry. Transfer dough to a lightly floured surface and knead for about 10 minutes; add very small amounts of flour if needed until dough becomes smooth and elastic. Rub a small amount of olive oil over the surface of the dough, then return it to a clean bowl, cover it with a cloth, and place it in a warm area for about 1 hour or until dough doubles in size. Remove dough to a lightly floured surface, knead for an additional 2 minutes, then roll out into a 15-inch round. Place on pizza pan and top with sauce and ingredients of choice. Bake at 425 degrees until crust is crispy.

Approx. 115 calories per slice, crust only
2g protein, 3g total fat, <0.5g saturated fat, 0 trans fat,
18g carbohydrates, 0 cholesterol, 144mg sodium, 0 fiber

BREAD MACHINE WHOLE GRAIN THIN CRUST PIZZA DOUGH

MAKES 2 4-SLICE, 12-INCH CRUSTS

1 cup water (room temperature)
2 tablespoons canola oil
1 tablespoon low-calorie baking sweetener
½ teaspoon salt or ½ teaspoon sodium-free salt substitute
1 cup whole grain flour
1½ cups bread flour
2¼ teaspoons active dry yeast

Add water, canola oil, sweetener, salt or salt substitute, both flours, and yeast to bread machine canister, in that order. Set bread machine program to dough setting. When the machine turns off, remove dough ball from canister and place on a lightly floured flat surface. Divide ball in half and press or roll out each half to fit a 12-inch pizza pan or stone. Curl up edges of dough and prick the surface of the dough with a fork. Place pan or stone on the middle rack of an oven preheated to 400 degrees for about 10–12 minutes or until the crust turns a light golden brown. Remove baked crust from oven, top with sauce and ingredients of choice, and return to bake for additional 10–15 minutes or until cheese has melted.

Approx. 54 calories per 3-inch-wide slice, crust only
2g protein, 1g total fat, 0.75g saturated fat, 0 trans fat,
9g carbohydrates, 0 cholesterol, 49mg sodium, 1g fiber

Omelets, Eggs, Frittatas, and Cereals

CHEESY APPLE RAISIN CINNAMON OMELET
MAKES 4 SERVINGS

1 medium sweet apple (Fiji, Fuji, or Golden Delicious), peeled, cored, and sliced

1 tablespoon extra-virgin olive oil

2 tablespoons seedless black raisins

1 cup egg substitute or 1 cup egg whites or 4 whole eggs

2 tablespoons crumbled blue cheese

2 tablespoons freshly shredded Parmesan cheese

Salt and freshly ground pepper to taste

⅛ teaspoon cinnamon

Sauté apple slices in ½ tablespoon of olive oil until crispy tender; add raisins, then immediately remove apple mixture from pan and transfer to a bowl. Combine eggs, cheeses, and salt and pepper, and mix well. Heat remaining olive oil in an omelet pan; cook ¼ of egg mixture at a time, on low heat, lifting edges to allow uncooked portion to flow under and cook. Repeat process 4 times for each serving. Arrange ¼ apple mixture onto one half of cooked egg. Fold in half and sprinkle top with cinnamon. Serve as a breakfast omelet or a dessert.

Approx. 116 calories per omelet, using egg substitute
7g protein, 8g total fat, 1g saturated fat, 0 trans fat,
9g carbohydrates, 4mg cholesterol, 206mg sodium, 0 fiber

Approx. 111 calories per omelet, using egg whites
6g protein, 8g total fat, 1g saturated fat, 0 trans fat,
8g carbohydrates, 4mg cholesterol, 166mg sodium, 0 fiber

Approx. 166 calories, using fresh whole eggs
6g protein, 13g total fat, 3g saturated fat, 0 trans fat,
8g carbohydrates, 244mg cholesterol, 161mg sodium, 0 fiber

POACHED EGGS IN A GARDEN

MAKES 4 SERVINGS

2 tablespoons olive oil
2 large russet potatoes, diced
2 cups fresh broccoli florets
1 medium red bell pepper, chopped
1 medium white onion, chopped
2 cups button mushrooms, sliced
Salt and freshly ground pepper to taste
8 large eggs, poached

In a large skillet, heat olive oil over medium-high heat. Add potatoes, broccoli, red bell pepper, onion, mushrooms, and salt and pepper to taste. Cook, stirring occasionally, until vegetables are tender and potatoes start to brown. Divide into 4 portions and top each serving with 2 poached eggs and serve.

Approx. 312 calories per serving
18g protein, 17g total fat, 3g saturated fat, 0 trans fat,
20g carbohydrates, 424mg cholesterol, 57mg sodium, 2g fiber

MIXED VEGETABLE FRITTATA

MAKES 4 SERVINGS

10 large fresh asparagus spears

1½ cups egg substitute or 1½ cups egg whites or 6 whole eggs

¾ cup low-fat cottage cheese

2 teaspoons spicy brown mustard

¼ teaspoon crushed dried tarragon

¼ teaspoon marjoram

Salt and freshly ground pepper to taste

½ teaspoon extra-virgin olive oil

1 cup sliced fresh mushrooms

½ cup diced onion

¼ cup chopped seeded tomato for garnish

Boil asparagus for 8–10 minutes until crispy tender. Drain. Cut all but 3 spears into 1-inch pieces. Set aside. In a bowl mix together eggs, cottage cheese, mustard, tarragon, marjoram, and salt and pepper. Set aside. Heat olive oil in a large oven-safe skillet, and sauté mushrooms and onion until tender. Stir in asparagus pieces, pour egg mixture over top, and cook an additional 5 minutes over low heat until it bubbles and begins to set. Arrange remaining 3 uncut asparagus spears on top of mixture. Place skillet in oven and bake uncovered at 400 degrees for 10 minutes or until frittata sets. Remove from heat. Sprinkle with tomato and serve.

Approx. 169 calories per serving, using egg substitute
17g protein, 1g total fat, <0.5g saturated fat, 0 trans fat,
7g carbohydrates, 321mg cholesterol, 369mg sodium, 2g fiber

Approx. 164 calories per serving, using egg whites
16g protein, 1g total fat, <0.5g saturated fat, 0 trans fat,
6g carbohydrates, 321mg cholesterol, 329mg sodium, 2g fiber

Approx. 216 calories per serving, using fresh whole eggs
18g protein, 11g total fat, 3.5g saturated fat, 0 trans fat,
7g carbohydrates, 561mg cholesterol, 324mg sodium, 2g fiber

SPANISH OMELET

MAKES 6 MAIN-COURSE SERVINGS

2 tablespoons extra-virgin olive oil

6 whole scallions, coarsely chopped

4 cloves fresh garlic, thinly sliced

1 green bell pepper, seeded and thinly sliced

1 red bell pepper, seeded and thinly sliced

1 medium zucchini, diced

3 ripe tomatoes, peeled and cut into wedges

Salt and freshly ground pepper to taste

¼ teaspoon cayenne pepper

¾ teaspoon ground cumin

½ teaspoon ground coriander

½ teaspoon ground cinnamon

4 tablespoons chopped fresh parsley

3 cups egg substitute or 3 cups egg whites or 12 large eggs

¼ pound crumbled fresh low-fat goat cheese

Heat 2 tablespoons olive oil in an oven-safe skillet and gently sauté scallions and garlic for about 5 minutes, until they begin to soften. Add the green and red bell peppers, zucchini, and tomatoes, raise heat slightly, and continue sautéing another 5–10 minutes until the vegetables have softened and most of the juice is absorbed. Add salt and pepper to taste. Set aside at room temperature. In a large bowl combine the herbs with the eggs and mix with a fork just enough to break up the yolks. Lift the vegetables out of the skillet with a slotted spoon and combine with eggs. Return the skillet to medium heat, adding more olive oil if necessary. When the olive oil is hot, add the eggs and vegetable mixture and cook for 2–3 minutes, lifting the edges with a spatula to allow uncooked eggs to run under cooked ones. Crumble goat cheese over the top of the omelet and transfer skillet to a 400-degree oven to finish cooking for about 15–20 minutes or until omelet is set and the cheese is melted. Can also be served as a light supper.

Approx. 125 calories per serving, using egg substitute
10g protein, 9g total fat, 1g saturated fat, 0 trans fat,
6g carbohydrates, 8mg cholesterol, 190mg sodium, 1g fiber

Approx. 121 calories per serving, using egg whites
9g protein, 9g total fat, 1g saturated fat, 0 trans fat,
5g carbohydrates, 8mg cholesterol, 150mg sodium, 1g fiber

Approx. 176 calories per serving, using fresh whole eggs
11g protein, 19g total fat, 3g saturated fat, 0 trans fat,
6g carbohydrates, 248mg cholesterol, 145mg sodium, 1g fiber

BROCCOLI AND CHEESE FRITTATA
MAKES 6 MAIN COURSE SERVINGS

3 cups broccoli florets
1 tablespoon extra-virgin olive oil
½ cup finely chopped onion
½ cup chopped red bell pepper
2 cloves fresh garlic, minced
1 cup shredded mozzarella cheese
Dash of crushed red hot pepper flakes
1½ cups egg substitute or 1½ cups egg whites or 6 large eggs
Olive oil spray

Steam broccoli until crispy tender and remove from heat. In a large skillet over medium-high heat, heat olive oil and sauté onion, bell pepper, and garlic until vegetables are soft (about 5 minutes). Add broccoli and cook about 2 minutes longer. Transfer vegetable mixture to a bowl, then add mozzarella cheese and hot pepper flakes. If using whole eggs, beat in a separate bowl until blended. Stir eggs into vegetable mixture and pour into a round cake pan lightly sprayed with olive oil spray. Bake in 325-degree oven until eggs are set, about 30 minutes. Serve hot or at room temperature.

Approx. 121 calories per serving, using egg substitute
12g protein, 8g total fat, 4g saturated fat, 0 trans fat,
5g carbohydrates, 10mg cholesterol, 209mg sodium, 0 fiber

Approx. 116 calories per serving, using egg whites
11g protein, 8g total fat, 4g saturated fat, 0 trans fat,
4g carbohydrates, 10mg cholesterol, 169mg sodium, 0 fiber

Approx. 166 calories per serving, using fresh whole eggs
12g protein, 18g total fat, 8g saturated fat, 0 trans fat,
5g carbohydrates, 197mg cholesterol, 172mg sodium, 1g fiber

HAM AND ZUCCHINI FRITTATA

MAKES 6 SERVINGS

1 tablespoon olive oil

1 medium white onion, chopped

1 clove fresh garlic, minced

1 medium zucchini, halved lengthwise, cut to ¼ inch thick slices

1 cup diced low-sodium ham

1½ cups liquid eggs

¼ cup low-fat milk

1 teaspoon dry Italian seasoning mix + more to sprinkle

Salt and freshly ground pepper to taste

2 Italian plum tomatoes, sliced

1 cup shredded, part-skim milk mozzarella cheese

Preheat oven to broil. In an oven-safe skillet, heat olive oil over medium heat. Add onion, garlic, and zucchini, sauté till soft. Reduce heat to medium-low, add ham, and cook for about 2 minutes. In a bowl, combine liquid eggs, milk, Italian seasoning mix, and salt and pepper to taste. Pour mixture into skillet with ham and cook unstirred for about 5 minutes or until eggs begin to set. Arrange tomato slices on top of egg mixture and sprinkle with mozzarella cheese. Place skillet about 6 inches under broiler and broil for about 4–5 minutes until eggs set and cheese is lightly browned. Sprinkle top of frittata with a dash of Italian seasoning mix and serve.

Approx. 140 calories per serving
14g protein, 8g total fat, 2g saturated fat, 0 trans fat,
0 carbohydrates, 23mg cholesterol, 192mg sodium, 0 fiber

QUINOA AND RAISINS PORRIDGE
MAKES 2 LARGE SERVINGS

2 cups almond milk

1 cup quinoa, rinsed through a fine mesh sieve under cold water

½ teaspoon ground cinnamon

⅛ teaspoon ground nutmeg

⅛ teaspoon ground ginger

Dash of salt (optional)

2 tablespoons pure maple syrup

½ teaspoon pure vanilla extract

2 tablespoons raisins

¼ cup chopped nuts (such as pecans, walnuts, or almonds)

In a saucepan over medium heat, gently heat almond milk, stirring occasionally until it begins to bubble. Reduce heat to a simmer and add in quinoa, cinnamon, nutmeg, ginger, and salt. Cook uncovered, stirring occasionally, until quinoa is tender and begins to thicken (about 20–25 minutes). Remove from heat, add in maple syrup, vanilla extract, and raisins. Top with a sprinkling of nuts and serve.

Approx. 557 calories per serving
13g protein, 14g total fat, 1g saturated fat, 0 trans fat,
91g carbohydrates, 0 cholesterol, 172mg sodium, 9g fiber

ZUCCHINI FRITTATA
MAKES 6 SERVINGS

1½ tablespoons extra-virgin olive oil

1 medium yellow onion, chopped

2 cloves fresh garlic, minced

3 small zucchini, sliced ¼-inch thick

Salt and freshly ground pepper to taste

2 tablespoons minced fresh basil leaves

2 cups egg substitute or *2 cups egg whites* or *8 large eggs*

½ cup (2 ounces) freshly grated Parmesan cheese

In a skillet over medium-low heat, heat olive oil and sauté onion and garlic until soft and lightly browned. Add zucchini and salt and pepper to onion-garlic mixture and cook another 5–8 minutes. Remove from heat and set aside. In a bowl, add basil and eggs (beat eggs if using whole eggs) to zucchini mixture. Stir mixture to blend and pour egg mixture into a lightly greased round cake pan. Bake in oven at 325 degrees until eggs set. Remove from oven, sprinkle Parmesan cheese over top of frittata, and place under broiler for 2–3 minutes until cheese is golden brown. Remove from oven and serve immediately. Can be served as a light supper.

Approx. 126 calories per serving, using egg substitute
12g protein, 6g total fat, 2g saturated fat, 0 trans fat,
11g carbohydrates, 7mg cholesterol, 312mg sodium, 1g fiber

Approx. 121 calories per serving, using egg whites
11g protein, 6g total fat, 2g saturated fat, 0 trans fat,
4g carbohydrates, 7mg cholesterol, 244mg sodium, 1g fiber

Approx. 161 calories per serving, using whole eggs
10g protein, 10g total fat, 4g saturated fat, 0 trans fat,
4g carbohydrates, 195mg cholesterol, 242mg sodium, 1g fiber

VEGETABLE OMELET WITH PESTO
MAKES 6 SERVINGS

½ teaspoon extra-virgin olive oil

1 cup sliced white mushrooms

⅔ medium red onion, diced

½ cup fresh peas, cooked and drained

2 whole carrots, cleaned, cut julienne style, cooked, and drained
   (Option: substitute other vegetables, if desired)

2 tablespoons Basil Pesto Sauce (page 488) or a market-fresh pesto sauce

Olive oil cooking spray

3 cups egg substitute or 3 cups egg whites or 12 whole fresh eggs

¼ cup water

¼ teaspoon salt

¼ teaspoon freshly ground pepper

6 sprigs fresh basil for garnish

In a medium skillet heat olive oil and sauté mushrooms and onion, then remove from heat. Mix all other vegetables with mushrooms and onion and mix in prepared pesto. Spray a non-stick 15x10x1-inch baking pan with olive oil spray and set aside. In a mixing bowl combine eggs with water and salt and pepper. Beat until frothy. Pour egg mixture into pan, and bake uncovered at 400 degrees for about 8 minutes or until mixture is set. Cut baked eggs into 6 (5-inch) squares and remove squares from pan. Spoon ¼ cup of vegetable mixture on half of each omelet square, fold over, and garnish with basil sprigs.

Approx. 103 calories per serving, using egg substitute
7g protein, 5g total fat, 0.7g saturated fat, 0 trans fat,
6g carbohydrates, 0 cholesterol, 137mg sodium, 2g fiber

Approx. 83 calories per serving, using egg white
7g protein, 5g total fat, 0.7g saturated fat, 0 trans fat,
6g carbohydrates, 0 cholesterol, 97mg sodium, 2g fiber

Approx. 161 calories per serving, using whole eggs
7g protein, 15g total fat, 4g saturated fat, 0 trans fat,
6g carbohydrates, 34mg cholesterol, 92mg sodium, 2g fiber

Pancakes

STRAWBERRY BUTTERMILK PANCAKES

MAKES 12 PANCAKES

2 cups whole grain pastry flour
1 teaspoon baking powder
¼ teaspoon baking soda
¼ teaspoon salt (optional)
2 cups low-fat buttermilk
½ cup egg substitute
1 cup sliced fresh strawberries
Canola oil cooking spray
Sliced strawberries or other fruit or *low-sugar fruit jams as garnish (optional)*
Sugar-free syrup (optional)

In a mixing bowl whisk together flour, baking powder, baking soda, and salt, then make a well in the center of the mixture. In a separate bowl combine the buttermilk and egg and whisk to blend. Pour buttermilk mixture into the well and fold in flour with a spatula until mixture is smooth. Gently fold in strawberries and allow batter to stand for 5 minutes. In the meantime, spray a griddle with cooking oil and heat over medium heat. Drop a few droplets of water onto heated griddle. When water droplets bead, griddle is hot enough. Pour 2 tablespoons of batter onto griddle for each pancake. Cook pancakes until the surface of pancake begins to bubble and the edges turn golden brown (about 3 minutes). Flip pancake over and cook until other side is golden brown. Repeat this process until all the batter is gone. Keep cooked pancakes on a warm platter or in a low-heat oven (175 degrees) while preparing the other pancakes. Serve warm, garnished with sliced strawberries, low-sugar fruit jam, or sugar-free syrup, if desired.

Approx. 53 calories per pancake
4g protein, <0.5g total fat, 0 saturated fat, 0 trans fat,
15g carbohydrates, 1mg cholesterol, 124mg sodium, 2g fiber

BANANA BUTTERMILK PANCAKES
MAKES 12 PANCAKES

2 cups whole grain pastry flour
1 teaspoon baking powder
¼ teaspoon baking soda
¼ teaspoon salt (optional)
2 cups low-fat buttermilk
½ cup egg substitute
1 cup mashed ripe banana
Canola oil cooking spray
Sliced banana or *sugar-free or low-sugar fruit jams as garnish (optional)*
Sugar-free syrup

In a mixing bowl whisk together flour, baking powder, baking soda, and salt, then make a well in the center of the mixture. In a separate bowl combine the buttermilk and egg and whisk to blend. Pour buttermilk mixture into well and fold in flour with a spatula until mixture is smooth. Gently fold in banana and allow batter to stand for 5 minutes. In the meantime, spray a griddle with cooking oil and heat over medium heat. Drop a few droplets of water onto heated griddle. When water droplets bead, griddle is hot enough. Pour 2 tablespoons of batter onto griddle for each pancake. Cook pancakes until the surface of pancake begins to bubble and the edges turn golden brown (about 3 minutes). Flip pancake over and cook until other side is golden brown. Repeat this process until all the batter is gone. Keep cooked pancakes on a warm platter or in a low-heat oven (175 degrees) while preparing the other pancakes. Serve warm, garnished with sliced banana, low-sugar fruit jam, or sugar-free syrup, if desired.

Approx. 66 calories per pancake
4g protein, <0.5g total fat, 0 saturated fat, 0 trans fat,
18g carbohydrates, 1mg cholesterol, 124mg sodium, 2g fiber

MULTIGRAIN NUTTY BLUEBERRY PANCAKES

MAKES 6 PANCAKES

¾ cup multigrain pancake flour
½ cup + 2 tablespoons skim milk
1 tablespoon canola oil
¼ cup blueberries (either fresh or frozen)
⅛ cup chopped walnuts
Canola oil cooking spray
Fat-free sour cream or *sugar-free or low-sugar fruit jams as garnish (optional)*
Sugar-free syrup

In a mixing bowl combine pancake flour, milk, and canola oil. Using a wire whisk, mix ingredients until smooth. Add blueberries and walnuts and stir to combine all ingredients. Spray griddle with cooking spray and heat over medium heat. Drop a few droplets of water onto the heated griddle. If droplets bead, then griddle is hot enough. Pour about 1 tablespoon of batter per pancake onto griddle. Cook pancake until it begins to bubble up and edges turn brown, then flip over and continue cooking until the other side is golden brown. Remove cooked pancakes to a warmed platter or hold in a low-heat oven (175 degrees) while preparing other pancakes. Repeat this process until all the batter is gone. Serve with a dollop of fat-free sour cream, low-sugar fruit jam, or your favorite sugar-free syrup, if desired.

Approx. 85 calories per pancake
3g protein, 2g total fat, 0.5g saturated fat, 0 trans fat,
15g carbohydrates, 3mg cholesterol, 130mg sodium, 2g fiber

MULTIGRAIN APPLE AND NUT PANCAKES
MAKES 6 PANCAKES

¾ cup multigrain pancake flour

½ cup + 2 tablespoons skim milk

1 tablespoon canola oil

½ medium sweet apple, cored, peeled, and diced

⅛ cup chopped walnuts

Canola oil cooking spray

Fat-free sour cream or sugar-free or low-sugar fruit jams as garnish (optional)

Sugar-free syrup

In a mixing bowl combine pancake flour, milk, and canola oil. Using a wire whisk, mix ingredients until smooth. Add apple and walnuts and stir to combine all ingredients. Spray griddle with cooking spray and heat over medium heat. Drop a few droplets of water onto the heated griddle. If droplets bead, then griddle is hot enough. Pour about 1 tablespoon of batter per pancake onto griddle. Cook pancake until it begins to bubble up and edges turn brown, then flip over and continue cooking until the other side is golden brown. Remove cooked pancakes to a warmed platter or hold in a low-heat oven (175 degrees) while preparing other pancakes. Repeat this process until all the batter is gone. Serve with a dollop of fat-free sour cream, low-sugar fruit jam, or your favorite sugar-free syrup, if desired.

Approx. 87 calories per pancake
3g protein, 2g total fat, 0.5g saturated fat, 0 trans fat,
15g carbohydrates, 3mg cholesterol, 130mg sodium, 2g fiber

Main Dishes

SPICY SOLE

MAKES 4 SERVINGS

Spicy Pistachio Pesto (page 486)
8 (3-ounce) fillets of sole
Salt and freshly ground pepper to taste
1 cup water
1 cup dry white vermouth
1 tablespoon fresh lemon juice

Make pesto sauce and set aside. Season fillets with salt and pepper and roll up, securing with toothpicks. Set aside. Bring water, vermouth, and lemon juice to a simmer; add rolled fillets, cover, and poach for about 7 minutes until flesh turns white and fish is cooked through. Remove rolled fillets from skillet with a slotted spoon. Serve plate immediately topped with Spicy Pistachio Pesto. Serve while hot.

Approx. 154 calories per 2 fillets
32g protein, 2g total fat, 0.6g saturated fat, 0 trans fat,
0 carbohydrates, 82mg cholesterol, 178mg sodium, 0 fiber

SPANISH PAELLA WITH SAFFRON RICE, SEAFOOD, AND CHICKEN

MAKES 8 SERVINGS

12 medium shrimp

7 hard-shelled clams

½ pound garlic-seasoned smoked pork sausage

2 pounds skinless, boneless chicken, cut into pieces

Dash of freshly ground pepper

¾ teaspoon garlic salt

½ cup extra-virgin olive oil

¼ pound lean boneless pork, cut into ½-inch cubes

½ cup chopped onion

½ medium red bell pepper, seeded and sliced

½ medium yellow bell pepper, seeded and sliced

1 large tomato, peeled and finely chopped

2 cloves fresh garlic, crushed

3 cups long-grain rice

½ teaspoon salt

¼ teaspoon ground saffron

6 cups water

1 cup frozen peas, thoroughly defrosted

Steam shrimp in a small amount of water until just pink, then set side. Scrub clams under running water, then steam in just enough water to cover them. When clams open, remove from water with a slotted spoon and set aside. Prick sausage with fork in several places, place in heavy skillet, and cover with cold water. Bring water to a boil and reduce heat to low. Simmer sausages, uncovered, for 15 minutes. Drain sausages well, slice into ¼-inch round pieces, and set aside. Rinse chicken, pat dry, and season with pepper and garlic salt. In a large skillet, heat ¼ cup olive oil, add chicken pieces, and fry until golden brown. Remove browned chicken from skillet and place on plate lined with paper towels. Add sausage pieces to skillet, quickly brown them, and then drain on plate lined with paper towels. Remove olive oil from skillet and dry skillet with paper towels. In the same skillet, heat ¼ cup fresh olive oil until hot. Add pork cubes and brown quickly. Add onion, red and yellow bell peppers, tomato, and garlic. Cook vegetables and meat, stirring constantly, until tender. Set aside. In a large pot, add rice, salt, saffron, and 6 cups of water; bring to a boil and cover, stirring occasionally, until rice is soft. Transfer rice, shrimp and remaining liquid, clams, sausage, chicken and pork cubes, and vegetables to an oven-safe casserole dish. Sprinkle peas over mixture, place pan on bottom rack of a 400-degree oven, and bake for 25–30 minutes or until liquid is absorbed. Do not stir. When paella is cooked, remove from oven, cover with clean kitchen towel, and let stand for 5 minutes. Serve immediately. NOTE: Oven should be preheated 30 minutes before paella is placed inside.

Approx. 523 calories per serving
38g protein, 13g total fat, 3g saturated fat, 0 trans fat,
61g carbohydrates, 117mg cholesterol, 819mg sodium, 3g fiber

SKEWERED MEDITERRANEAN GRILLED LAMB AND VEGETABLES

MAKES 4 SERVINGS

Juice from 2 lemons
⅓ cup extra-virgin olive oil
1 clove fresh garlic, minced
1 tablespoon chopped mint
Salt and freshly ground pepper to taste
1½ pounds lamb sirloin, cut into 1½-inch cubes
8 large bay leaves
8 fresh mushroom caps
8 small cherry tomatoes
1 large green bell pepper, seeded and cut into 1½-inch strips
2 small zucchini, cut into 1-inch cubes
4 medium onions, quartered

Mix together lemon juice, olive oil, garlic, mint, and salt and pepper to taste, and pour over lamb cubes in a resealable plastic baggie. Place in refrigerator and marinate overnight or for at least 8 hours. On 8 flat-bladed oiled skewers alternate meat, bay leaves, and vegetables. Grill over hot coals for about 15 minutes, turning skewers several times.

This dish goes well with a chopped salad of onions, cucumbers, tomatoes, and parsley. Use lemon juice for dressing.

Approx. 296 calories per serving
38g protein, 8g total fat, 3g saturated fat, 0 trans fat,
15g carbohydrates, 103mg cholesterol, 141mg sodium, 3g fiber

BAKED STUFFED TROUT

MAKES 4 SERVINGS

3 tablespoons extra-virgin olive oil
1 large onion, finely chopped
4 cloves fresh garlic, minced
⅔ cup plain bread crumbs
1 lemon, juiced and rind-grated
⅓ cup seedless dark raisins, chopped
½ cup pine nuts
2 tablespoons chopped fresh parsley
1 tablespoon chopped fresh dill
Salt and freshly ground pepper to taste
¼ cup egg substitute
4 (12-ounce) whole trout, scaled and gutted
Olive oil cooking spray
Lemon wedges for garnish

In a skillet, heat 2 tablespoons of olive oil, add onion and garlic, and cook until soft, then remove from heat. In a large bowl, mix bread crumbs, grated lemon rind, raisins, pine nuts, parsley, dill, and salt and pepper; add garlic mixture and egg and mix well together. Stuff each trout with mixture and place in a single layer on an oil-sprayed shallow baking pan. Make several diagonal slashes along the body of each fish and drizzle with lemon juice and remaining tablespoon of oil. Bake at 375 degrees for about 30–45 minutes or until fish flakes. Serve hot, garnished with lemon wedges.

Approx. 579 calories per serving
61g protein, 30g total fat, 5g saturated fat, 0 trans fat,
13g carbohydrates, 284mg cholesterol, 547mg sodium, 1g fiber

GREAT NORTHERN BEANS AND CHICKEN

MAKES 6 SERVINGS

2 (3-ounce) skinless, boneless chicken legs

2 (4-ounce) skinless, boneless chicken breasts

2 onions, chopped into large pieces

5 carrots, 1 sliced and others cut into large pieces

2 stalks celery, 1 sliced and other cut into large pieces

Olive oil cooking spray

2 cups canned low-sodium, fat-free chicken broth

4 cups canned Great Northern beans, drained and rinsed

2 tomatoes, peeled and chopped into large pieces

½ green bell pepper, chopped into large pieces

2 teaspoons fresh thyme

3 cloves fresh garlic, chopped

2 tablespoons chopped fresh parsley

Salt and freshly ground pepper to taste

Preheat the oven to 350 degrees. Rinse chicken under water and pat dry. Place chicken, half of the onions, 1 sliced carrot, and 1 sliced celery stalk in a saucepan. Add water to cover chicken, and cook over medium heat until chicken is tender. Strain and set aside. Lightly spray bottom and sides of a large casserole dish with cooking spray, and add chicken, 2 cups of broth, and beans. Add remaining carrot and celery pieces to casserole along with tomatoes, remaining onion, green bell pepper, thyme, garlic, parsley, and salt and pepper. Bake for 30–40 minutes, until mixture simmers. Serve while hot.

Approx. 352 calories per serving
34g protein, 7g total fat, 2g saturated fat, 0 trans fat,
39g carbohydrates, 82mg cholesterol, 267mg sodium, 2g fiber

BOUILLABAISSE

MAKES 4 SERVINGS

2 teaspoons extra-virgin olive oil

2 leeks, white and green parts, thinly sliced

3 cloves fresh garlic, minced

2 cups freshly chopped tomatoes

¼ cup dry white wine

1 tablespoon tomato paste

1 tablespoon freshly chopped parsley

½ teaspoon dried thyme

2 bay leaves

⅓ teaspoon crushed saffron

⅛ teaspoon fennel seeds

10 ounces fresh firm cod, cut into 1½-inch chunks

2 (6-ounce) fresh lobster tails, quartered

16 littleneck clams, scrubbed

3 ounces orzo, cooked and drained

In a large saucepan over medium-high heat, combine olive oil, leeks, and garlic; cook for about 3 minutes, stirring occasionally. Add tomatoes, 1½ cups of water, wine, tomato paste, parsley, thyme, bay leaves, saffron, and fennel seeds; stir to combine. Bring mixture to a boil, stirring occasionally. Add cod, lobster, and clams; return to boil. Reduce heat to low and simmer, covered, for 6–8 minutes. Fish and lobster should be cooked until done and clams until they open. Remove bay leaves. Spoon cooked orzo into 4 soup bowls; ladle Bouillabaisse over orzo and serve.

Approx. 278 calories per serving
29g protein, 5g total fat, 1g saturated fat, 0 trans fat,
26g carbohydrates, 71mg cholesterol, 268mg sodium, 2g fiber

SPICY BROCCOLI RABE WITH PENNE PASTA

MAKES 4 SERVINGS

2 pounds fresh broccoli rabe, cleaned, trimmed, and cut into 1-inch pieces
1 pound whole wheat penne pasta
3 tablespoons extra-virgin olive oil
5 cloves fresh garlic, thinly sliced
1 medium white onion, chopped
2 ounces anchovy fillets, drained
¼ teaspoon crushed red hot pepper flakes
Salt and freshly ground pepper to taste
Freshly grated Romano cheese for garnish (optional)

In a large saucepan, bring water and salt to a boil. Add broccoli rabe and cook about 5 minutes, until stems are tender. With a slotted spoon, transfer broccoli to a colander to drain. Return broccoli water to a boil and add pasta. Cook until tender and drain, reserving ¼ cup of pasta water. Return pasta to a saucepan and keep warm. In a large skillet, heat olive oil, then add garlic and onion; sauté for about 2 minutes, until golden. Add anchovies and hot pepper flakes, stirring for about 1 minute. Add broccoli rabe and cook another 5 minutes, until heated. To broccoli rabe mixture, add pasta and enough of reserved pasta liquid to lightly moisten; toss until well mixed. Add salt and pepper to taste. Garnish with Romano cheese. Serve warm.

Approx. 580 calories per serving
21g protein, 14g total fat, 2g saturated fat, 0 trans fat,
94g carbohydrates, 8mg cholesterol, 645mg sodium, 7g fiber

GRILLED CITRUS SALMON WITH GARLIC GREENS
MAKES 4 SERVINGS

¼ cup orange marmalade

2 tablespoons fresh lime juice

2 tablespoons fresh lemon juice

¼ cup low-sodium soy sauce

3 teaspoons grated orange rind

4 (3-ounce) salmon fillets

2 teaspoons extra-virgin olive oil

2 teaspoons minced fresh garlic

2 (10-ounce) bags fresh spinach

Scant amount of olive oil to rub on fish

Salt and freshly ground pepper to taste

1 teaspoon fresh garlic, mashed to rub on fish

1 heaping tablespoon capers, drained

1 tablespoon balsamic vinegar

4 scallions, white and light green parts, thinly sliced (2–3-inch lengths)

Whisk together marmalade, lime and lemon juices, soy sauce, and orange rind; pour mixture over fillets and marinate for 30 minutes in refrigerator. Prepare grill or preheat broiler. Heat olive oil in a heavy skillet over medium-high heat; add garlic and spinach, one bag at a time, and sauté, stirring often, until spinach is wilted (about 2 minutes). Reduce heat to very low, to keep warm. Combine olive oil, salt and pepper, mashed garlic, and capers. Rub mixture into both sides of salmon steaks. Grill the fish or broil 3–4 inches from flame for 2–2 ½ minutes on each side. Set fish aside. Remove spinach from heat and toss with vinegar; divide equally on 4 plates. Add grilled salmon fillet to bed of spinach on each plate and garnish with scallions. Serve.

Approx. 250 calories per serving
18g protein, 8g total fat, 1g saturated fat, 0 trans fat,
14g carbohydrates, 188mg cholesterol, 884mg sodium, 6g fiber

SICILIAN-STYLE LINGUINE WITH EGGPLANT AND ROASTED PEPPERS

MAKES 6 SERVINGS

2 large yellow bell peppers

1 small eggplant, peeled and cut into ½-inch cubes

2 tablespoons extra-virgin olive oil

2 tablespoons minced fresh oregano

2 tablespoons capers

4 teaspoons minced fresh garlic

1 (35-ounce) can peeled plum tomatoes

½ teaspoon crushed red hot pepper flakes

Salt and freshly ground pepper to taste

1 pound linguine

1 cup shredded fresh basil leaves

¾ cup grated Romano cheese

Preheat broiler. Cut bell peppers in half and remove seeds. Cut each half into strips and place on baking sheet, skin side up; broil until blackened. Set oven temperature to 400 degrees. Toss eggplant cubes with 1 tablespoon of olive oil, and place cubes in a single layer on a baking pan. Bake about 25 minutes, until very tender and browned, turning one time to bake evenly. Heat 1 tablespoon of olive oil in a large skillet over medium-high heat; add oregano, capers, and garlic, and sauté until garlic is lightly golden. Add eggplant, bell peppers, tomatoes and liquid, hot pepper flakes, and salt and pepper to taste. Cover, reduce heat, and simmer about 15 minutes, stirring occasionally. Cook pasta in boiling water, drain, and return it to the pot. Pour sauce over pasta, add basil, and gently toss. Sprinkle with Romano cheese and serve.

Approx. 336 calories per serving
13g protein, 10g total fat, 3g saturated fat, 0 trans fat,
50g carbohydrates, 15mg cholesterol, 461mg sodium, 6g fiber

PENNE WITH ROSEMARY AND BALSAMIC VINEGAR

MAKES 4 SERVINGS

8 ounces penne pasta

2 teaspoons extra-virgin olive oil

2 cups zucchini, cut into ½-inch cubes

3–4 cloves fresh garlic, minced

2 sprigs fresh rosemary, about 4–6 inches long

2 cups canned Italian peeled plum tomatoes, drained

1 tablespoon chopped fresh oregano

Salt and freshly ground pepper to taste

1 tablespoon balsamic vinegar

1 tablespoon + 1 teaspoon freshly grated Parmesan cheese

Bring water to a boil, add pasta, and cook pasta until *al dente*. Remove from heat, drain pasta, and return to pot, drizzling with scant amount of olive oil to keep pasta from sticking together. Set aside. In a large skillet, heat olive oil over medium-high heat. Sauté zucchini, garlic, and rosemary (about 4–5 minutes). Add tomatoes, oregano, and salt and pepper to taste. Decrease heat to a simmer and cook for about 10–12 minutes. Add vinegar and mix well. Place cooked pasta into a bowl, pour sauce over pasta, and toss to mix. Sprinkle with Parmesan cheese and serve.

Approx. 231 calories per serving
9g protein, 3g total fat, 0.6g saturated fat, 0 trans fat,
42g carbohydrates, 1mg cholesterol, 235mg sodium, 3g fiber

CHICKEN AND EGGPLANT

MAKES 8 SERVINGS

2 medium eggplants, peeled and cut into 1½-inch cubes

½ cup + 2 tablespoons extra-virgin olive oil, divided

3 pounds skinless, boneless chicken

2 large onions, chopped

4 cloves fresh garlic, chopped

1 teaspoon mixed spices

To make mixed spices combine:

2 teaspoons allspice

1 teaspoon ground cinnamon

1 teaspoon ground cloves

1 teaspoon fresh cilantro

1 teaspoon ground cumin

¼ teaspoon freshly ground pepper

4 large tomatoes, peeled, seeded, and chopped

2 teaspoons Thick Pomegranate Molasses (page 484)

3 tablespoons freshly squeezed lemon juice

Salt and freshly ground pepper to taste

2 tablespoons finely chopped fresh parsley

Salt eggplant pieces generously and let drain in a colander about 30 minutes (this rids eggplant of its bitter juices). After 30 minutes, rinse pieces under running cold water, gently squeeze pieces with hands to remove excess moisture, and pat dry with paper towels. In a large heavy skillet, heat ½ cup olive oil over medium heat. Add half of the eggplant pieces and sauté, turning frequently until golden brown. With a slotted spoon, transfer pieces to paper towels to drain and soak up excess oil. Repeat procedure with remaining eggplant, adding more olive oil if necessary. Pour olive oil from skillet, allow skillet to cool, and wipe clean. Rinse chicken pieces under cold water and pat dry with paper towels. Place chicken in skillet with 2 tablespoons of olive oil and sauté, turning to brown evenly on all sides. Transfer pieces to plate. Pour off all but 3 tablespoons of drippings from skillet. Add onions and sauté over medium heat, until golden brown. Add garlic and mixed spices and sauté about 30 seconds while stirring. Add tomatoes, Thick Pomegranate Molasses, lemon juice, and salt and pepper to taste. Return chicken and any juices from plate to skillet, spooning tomato mixture around pieces. Bring to a boil and reduce to low. Cover and simmer about 45 minutes or until chicken is tender. Stir in sautéed eggplant and parsley, cover, and simmer an additional 10 minutes. Adjust seasonings to taste. Serve with a side dish of pasta (optional).

Approx. 376 calories per serving
37g protein, 24g total fat, 4g saturated fat, 0 trans fat,
2g carbohydrates, 120mg cholesterol, 133mg sodium, 0.4g fiber

SPICY WHOLE WHEAT CAPELLINI WITH GARLIC
MAKES 4 SERVINGS

8 ounces whole wheat capellini pasta
¼ cup extra-virgin olive oil
4 cloves fresh garlic, chopped
1 teaspoon diced red hot pepper
Salt and freshly ground pepper to taste
Grated Pecorino or Parmesan cheese (optional)

Bring water to a boil, add pasta, and cook pasta until *al dente*. Remove from heat, drain pasta, and return to pot, drizzling with scant amount of olive oil to keep pasta from sticking together. Set aside. In a heavy skillet over medium heat, warm olive oil, then sauté garlic and hot pepper until tender (about 1–2 minutes). Add to pasta and toss. Add salt and pepper to taste and sprinkle with Parmesan cheese, if desired.

Approx. 299 calories per serving
8g protein, 16g total fat, 2g saturated fat, 0 trans fat,
35g carbohydrates, 4mg cholesterol, 0 sodium, 7g fiber

BROILED RED SNAPPER WITH GARLIC

MAKES 4 SERVINGS

1 whole red snapper (about 2–2 ½ pounds), scaled and gutted

3 tablespoons lemon juice

1 cup dry white wine

1 chili pepper, chopped

3 cloves fresh garlic, finely chopped

2 tablespoons extra-virgin olive oil

Salt and freshly ground pepper to taste

Olive oil cooking spray

2 tablespoons chopped fresh oregano

2 tablespoons chopped fresh parsley

Lemon wedges for garnish

Marinate cleaned fish for 1 hour in the refrigerator in a shallow pan with 1 tablespoon lemon juice, wine, chili pepper, and 1 clove garlic. Preheat broiler. Whisk together the remaining lemon juice, olive oil, and salt and pepper. Rub inside and outside of fish with mixture. Place fish on an oil-sprayed broiler pan and sprinkle with oregano. Broil fish for about 10 minutes, basting often with olive oil mixture and turning once, until golden brown. Meanwhile, mix together remaining garlic and parsley. Sprinkle the parsley mixture on top of cooked fish and serve hot, garnished with lemon wedges.

Approx. 185 calories per serving
25g protein, 11g total fat, 2g saturated fat, 0 trans fat,
0 carbohydrates, 46mg cholesterol, 81mg sodium, 0 fiber

PASTA WITH PINE NUTS AND SCALLOPS

MAKES 4 SERVINGS

8 ounces tagliatelle or *fettuccine*
4 tablespoons extra-virgin olive oil
3 cloves fresh garlic, finely chopped
1 leek, white part only, thinly sliced
10 pitted black olives, halved
¼ cup pine nuts
12 large sea scallops, halved
Salt and freshly ground pepper to taste
2 tablespoons chopped fresh basil
Parmesan cheese, finely grated, for garnish (optional)

Bring water to a boil, add pasta, and cook pasta until *al dente*. Remove from heat, drain pasta, and return to pot, drizzling with scant amount of olive oil to keep pasta from sticking together. Set aside. While pasta is cooking, heat olive oil in a skillet, add garlic and leek, and cook until soft but not brown. Add olives and pine nuts and sauté until pine nuts are lightly browned. Add scallops and cook until scallops are opaque. Add salt and pepper to taste. Add scallops and pan juices to pasta and toss. Sprinkle with basil and garnish with Parmesan cheese, if desired.

Approx. 409 calories per serving
17g protein, 23g total fat, 3g saturated fat, 0 trans fat,
41g carbohydrates, 45mg cholesterol, 139mg sodium, 1g fiber

SPICY SHRIMP WITH ANGEL HAIR PASTA

MAKES 4 SERVINGS

8 ounces angel hair pasta

1½ pounds medium shrimp, peeled and deveined

1 teaspoon low-calorie baking sweetener

¼ teaspoon salt

1 tablespoon chili powder

½ teaspoon ground cumin

½ teaspoon ground coriander

½ teaspoon dried oregano

1 tablespoon + 1 teaspoon extra-virgin olive oil

Lime wedges for garnish

Bring water to a boil, add pasta, and cook pasta until *al dente*. Remove from heat, drain pasta, and return to pot, drizzling with scant amount of olive oil to keep pasta from sticking together. Set aside. Sprinkle shrimp with sweetener and salt. Combine chili powder, cumin, coriander, and oregano, then lightly coat shrimp with spice mixture. Heat 1 tablespoon of olive oil in a large non-stick skillet over medium-high heat. Add half of the shrimp and sauté about 4 minutes, or until cooked. Remove cooked shrimp from pan and repeat procedure with 1 teaspoon olive oil and remaining shrimp. Divide cooked pasta into 4 servings, top with shrimp and pan sauce, and garnish with lime wedges. Serve immediately.

Approx. 320 calories per serving
28g protein, 5g total fat, 0.6g saturated fat, 0 trans fat,
28g carbohydrates, 161mg cholesterol, 759mg sodium, 5g fiber

FRUIT-GLAZED SALMON WITH COUSCOUS

MAKES 4 SERVINGS

¾ pound couscous

2 cups canned low-sodium, fat-free chicken broth, heated

½ cup apricot jam

3 tablespoons thinly sliced scallion

2 tablespoons prepared horseradish

1 tablespoon white wine vinegar

½ teaspoon salt (divided)

4 (6-ounce) salmon fillets, 1-inch thick, skinned

¼ teaspoon freshly ground pepper

2 teaspoons extra-virgin olive oil

Oil an oven-safe dish and place couscous in dish. Pour in chicken broth and let sit for 10 minutes until couscous is tender and liquid is absorbed. Cover dish and keep warm in a low-temperature oven until ready to serve. Meanwhile, combine apricot jam, scallion, horseradish, vinegar, and ¼ teaspoon of salt, and stir well with a whisk. Sprinkle salmon fillets with remaining salt and pepper. Heat olive oil in a large non-stick skillet over medium-high heat. Add salmon and cook for 3 minutes. Turn salmon and brush with half of apricot mixture. Wrap skillet handle with foil and bake salmon in skillet at 350 degrees for 5 minutes or until fish flakes. Remove from oven and brush salmon with remaining apricot mixture. Serve each fillet with couscous.

Approx. 396 calories per salmon fillet only
34g protein, 13g total fat, 2g saturated fat, 0 trans fat,
25g carbohydrates, 94mg cholesterol, 344mg sodium, 0 fiber

Approx. 198 calories per serving couscous only
7g protein, 0 total fat, 0 saturated fat, 0 trans fat,
40g carbohydrates, 0 cholesterol, 184mg sodium, 2g fiber

PASTA PRIMAVERA WITH SHRIMP

MAKES 4 SERVINGS

1 pound whole wheat penne pasta
½ cup canned low-sodium, fat-free chicken broth
Extra-virgin olive oil to drizzle + 2 teaspoons
2 dozen medium shrimp, cleaned, peeled, and deveined
1½ cups broccoli florets
1 medium red bell pepper, thinly sliced
1 cup halved button mushrooms
1 cup frozen peas
½ cup sliced scallions
4 cloves fresh garlic, minced
1 ounce (2 tablespoons) dry white wine
2 tablespoons freshly grated Parmesan cheese

Bring water to a boil, add pasta, and cook pasta until *al dente*. Remove from heat, drain pasta, and return to pot, drizzling with scant amount of olive oil to keep pasta from sticking together. Set aside. In a large non-stick skillet, heat ¼ cup broth, 2 teaspoons of olive oil, and shrimp; cook until shrimp are pink. With a slotted spoon remove shrimp and set aside. To skillet add remaining ¼ cup of broth, broccoli, red bell pepper, mushrooms, peas, scallions, and garlic. Cook, stirring frequently, for 4–5 minutes, until vegetables are tender and liquid is mostly absorbed. Stir in wine, simmer roughly 1 minute longer, and add shrimp to vegetable mixture. Place penne pasta in a large serving bowl and toss with remaining olive oil. Add vegetable mixture; toss to mix well. Sprinkle with Parmesan cheese.

Approx. 526 calories per serving
24g protein, 8g total fat, 1g saturated fat, 0 trans fat,
78g carbohydrates, 34mg cholesterol, 218mg sodium, 12g fiber

TURKISH MUSSEL STEW

MAKES 6–8 SERVINGS

1 cup dry white wine

1 cup water

6 dozen mussels, scrubbed and debearded (discard any open mussels)

2 tablespoons extra-virgin olive oil

1 medium onion, peeled and sliced

1 leek, white part only, sliced

6 cloves fresh garlic, coarsely chopped

4 large tomatoes, peeled and diced

2 large white potatoes, peeled, sliced about ¼-inch thick

2 medium carrots, cleaned and chunked

Pinch of saffron

2 bay leaves

Salt and freshly ground pepper to taste

¼ cup finely chopped fresh flat leaf parsley

In a large heavy saucepan combine wine, water, and mussels. Cover pan and steam mussels until they open (roughly about 7–10 minutes). Remove mussels from liquid and discard any that have not opened. Set mussel liquid aside. Remove mussels from shells and add a small amount of liquid to keep them moist. Strain remaining mussel liquid through cheesecloth and set aside. In a clean saucepan, add olive oil and gently sauté onion, leek, and garlic until tender, then add tomatoes and cook for another 1–2 minutes. Add potato slices, carrots, saffron, bay leaves, and strained mussel liquid; cover pan and cook over medium-low heat until vegetables are tender (about 30 minutes). Add mussels to mixture and continue cooking until all is heated thoroughly; add salt and pepper to taste. Remove from heat and stir in parsley. Serve while hot.

Approx. 236 calories per serving
14g protein, 9g total fat, 1g saturated fat, 0 trans fat,
20g carbohydrates, 28mg cholesterol, 297mg sodium, 1g fiber

PESTO STUFFED SHELLS

MAKES 4 SERVINGS

3 ounces (about 12) jumbo pasta shells
1 tablespoon extra-virgin olive oil
2 cloves fresh garlic, finely minced
1 cup thinly sliced button mushrooms
¼ teaspoon fresh thyme
1 cup red bell pepper, diced
½ cup yellow summer squash, diced
1 can (15 ounces) chickpeas, rinsed and drained
½ cup sliced leek, white and green parts
1 cup part-skim ricotta cheese
⅓ cup Basil Pesto Sauce (page 488) or market-fresh pesto sauce
Grated Parmesan cheese to taste, for garnish

Bring water to a boil, add pasta, and cook pasta until *al dente*. Remove from heat, drain pasta, and return to pot, drizzling with scant amount of olive oil to keep pasta from sticking together. Set aside. Heat olive oil in a large skillet over medium-high heat. Add garlic, mushrooms, and thyme, and sauté about 6 minutes. Add bell pepper and squash, then cook mixture until vegetables are crispy tender. Remove from heat; stir in chickpeas and leek. Add ricotta cheese and pesto sauce, then gently stir mixture. Spoon mixture evenly into cooked shells and garnish with Parmesan cheese, if desired.

Approx. 404 calories per serving
14g protein, 24g total fat, 6g saturated fat, 0 trans fat,
39g carbohydrates, 23mg cholesterol, 356mg sodium, 5g fiber

STEAMED SEA BASS

MAKES 6 SERVINGS

2 pounds sea bass (or grouper), 1-inch-thick whole fillets, if possible
2½ tablespoons extra-virgin olive oil
8 thin slices red onion
2 cloves fresh garlic, thinly sliced
10 medium fresh dill sprigs
8 lemon slices, ½-inch thick
1 tablespoon capers, rinsed and drained
Freshly ground pepper to taste
2 tablespoons dry white wine
Sea salt to taste

Cut parchment paper twice the size of fish and place on a baking sheet. Center fish on paper and drizzle with olive oil. Scatter onion slices, garlic, dill sprigs, and lemon slices on top of fish. Add capers and sprinkle with freshly ground pepper and a splash of wine. Wrap parchment paper around fish, folding top and tucking ends under fish to form a seal so steam cannot escape while baking. Bake in a 400-degree oven for 30 minutes. Check after 20 minutes for doneness; fish should be opaque in the center. If not, rewrap tightly and continue baking for an additional 10 minutes. To serve, place fish, still wrapped in parchment, on a platter. Open parchment when ready to serve; sprinkle on salt and serve immediately.

This dish goes well with rice, steamed vegetables, and/or couscous.

Approx. 205 calories per serving
28g protein, 7g total fat, 0.7g saturated fat, 0 trans fat,
4g carbohydrates, 62mg cholesterol, 103mg sodium, 0 fiber

GARLIC PASTA

MAKES 2 SERVINGS

4 ounces thin whole grain pasta
1 tablespoon extra-virgin olive oil
Garlic powder to taste
Salt and freshly ground pepper to taste

Cook and drain pasta according to package directions. Place well-drained hot pasta in a bowl and toss with olive oil, garlic powder, and salt and pepper to taste. Serve while hot.

Approx. 247 calories per serving
8g protein, 8g total fat, 1g saturated fat, 0 trans fat,
33g carbohydrates, 0 cholesterol, 18mg sodium, 4g fiber

TAHINI BAKED FLOUNDER

MAKES 4 SERVINGS

4 (3 ounce) fillets of flounder
2 tablespoons low-sodium soy sauce
2 tablespoons tahini paste
¼ cup fresh lemon juice
2 tablespoons extra-virgin olive oil
Freshly ground pepper to taste
2 oranges, peeled and sliced

Place fillets in a baking pan. Whisk together soy sauce, tahini paste, lemon juice, olive oil, and pepper. Pour mixture over fish and top fish with orange slices, cover and bake at 400 degrees for about 20–25 minutes or until fish flakes, then serve hot.

This dish goes well with steamed vegetables and rice.

Approx. 312 calories per serving
21g protein, 22g total fat, 3.2g saturated fat, 0 trans fat,
7.8g carbohydrates, 42mg cholesterol, 182mg sodium, 2g fiber

SPICY CHICKEN WITH COUSCOUS

MAKES 4 SERVINGS

¼ teaspoon ground cumin

¼ teaspoon ground turmeric

1 teaspoon ground cayenne

1 pound skinless, boneless chicken breasts, cut into 1-inch strips

1 teaspoon extra-virgin olive oil

5 cloves fresh garlic, finely minced

1 (16-ounce) can low-sodium, fat-free chicken broth

1 cup fresh peas

1 large white onion, diced

1 medium red bell pepper, diced

Salt and freshly ground pepper to taste

1 cup couscous

¼ cup chopped fresh cilantro, for garnish

Combine cumin, turmeric, and cayenne, and sprinkle evenly over chicken strips, then set aside. In a non-stick skillet, heat olive oil over medium-high heat until hot. Add chicken and garlic and cook about 3 minutes until chicken is lightly browned. Add broth, peas, onion, red bell pepper, and salt and pepper to taste to skillet; bring to boil, reduce heat, and simmer about 2–3 minutes, until chicken is cooked through. Stir in couscous, cover, and remove from heat. Let stand until liquid is absorbed. Garnish with cilantro.

Approx. 340 calories per serving
34g protein, 4g total fat, 0.6g saturated fat, 0 trans fat,
38g carbohydrates, 66mg cholesterol, 746mg sodium, 3g fiber

CITRUS SCALLOPS AND SHRIMP

MAKES 4 SERVINGS

3 cloves fresh garlic, finely minced

2½ tablespoons extra-virgin olive oil, divided

1½ pounds fresh arugula

½ pound large sea scallops, cut in halves

12 large shrimp, peeled and deveined

4 ounces fresh orange juice

Juice from ½ pink grapefruit

Juice from 1 lime

Juice from 1 lemon

1 teaspoon honey

½ teaspoon finely shredded orange zest

½ teaspoon finely shredded lime zest

Salt and freshly ground pepper to taste

2 scallions, sliced thin for garnish

In a large skillet over medium-high heat, sauté garlic in 1 tablespoon of olive oil for 1 minute; do not brown. Add arugula, cover, and cook 1 minute, until greens are wilted. In a separate skillet, over medium-high heat, heat remaining olive oil. Add scallops and shrimp and cook until scallops are opaque and shrimp pink, gently turning to keep from burning. Transfer scallops and shrimp to a heated plate, cover to keep warm, and set aside. Reserve skillet with seafood drippings and set aside. Combine orange juice, grapefruit juice, lime juice, lemon juice, honey, and orange and lime zest. Pour juice mixture into reserved seafood skillet and return skillet to medium heat. Stir the bottom and sides of pan to loosen any browned bits, incorporating them into juices. Bring to a boil and cook until liquid is reduced to half amount. Add salt and pepper to taste, cook for a few seconds, and remove from heat. Drain wilted arugula and divide between 4 plates, mounding in center. Divide scallops and shrimp into 4 portions and arrange on top of arugula. Pour juice glaze over seafood and garnish with scallions.

Approx. 309 calories per serving
34g protein, 11g total fat, 1g saturated fat, 0 trans fat,
26g carbohydrates, 45mg cholesterol, 276mg sodium, 2g fiber

ITALIAN POACHED SCALLOPS

MAKES 4 SERVINGS

1 cup fresh orange juice
1 pound fresh sea scallops
2 teaspoons grated orange peel
1 small ripe plum tomato, chopped
1 teaspoon chopped fresh marjoram
2 tablespoons low-fat sour cream
Salt and freshly ground pepper to taste

In a large non-stick skillet over medium heat, bring orange juice to a boil. Reduce heat and add scallops and orange peel. Cover and simmer 5 minutes or until scallops are opaque and tender. Remove scallops from heat and transfer to a plate; cover to keep warm. Add tomato and marjoram to orange juice sauce and simmer for roughly 2 minutes until liquid reduces to half of original amount. Stir in sour cream and cook until sauce thickens. Add salt and pepper to taste. Return scallops to skillet, mix with sauce, and heat through. Serve immediately with risotto and/ or vegetables.

Approx. 148 calories per serving
16g protein, 2g total fat, 0.5g saturated fat, 0 trans fat,
11g carbohydrates, 34mg cholesterol, 380mg sodium, 1g fiber

LIGHTLY BREADED GRILLED GROUPER

MAKES 4 SERVINGS

½ cup ripe pitted Kalamata olives

¼ cup plain bread crumbs

1 tablespoon capers, rinsed and drained

1 teaspoon extra-virgin olive oil

1 teaspoon lemon juice

1 clove fresh garlic

4 (4-ounce) grouper fillets

4–8 lime wedges for garnish

Heat grill to high heat; place oil-rubbed fish-grilling pan on grill rack to heat. In a food processor, process olives, bread crumbs, capers, olive oil, lemon juice, and garlic until smooth. Brush each side of fillets with olive oil mixture and place fillets on hot grill pan. Grill fillets, uncovered, for 5 minutes. Before turning fillets over, brush with olive oil mixture, then turn and grill for 5 additional minutes or until fillets flake easily. Remove fillets from grill, place on platter, and serve immediately, garnished with lime wedges.

This dish goes well with seasoned rice or couscous.

Approx. 159 calories per serving
24g protein, 4g total fat, <0.4g saturated fat, 0 trans fat,
4g carbohydrates, 45mg cholesterol, 388mg sodium, 0 fiber

SPICY STUFFED TILAPIA

MAKES 4 SERVINGS

4 (4-ounce) tilapia fillets
2 cups prepared crabmeat stuffing mix (¼ cup per fillet)
5 ounces fresh spinach leaves, rinsed and drained
1 tablespoon extra-virgin olive oil
½ teaspoon fresh crushed garlic
Sea salt and freshly ground pepper to taste
¼ cup dry-roasted pistachios, crushed
Red hot pepper sauce to drizzle

Rinse tilapia fillets under cold water and pat dry. Divide stuffing mix between 4 fillets, placing mix on the center of each fillet. Fold fillets over and secure with wooden skewers. Spread spinach on a baking sheet. Place stuffed fillets on bed of spinach. Drizzle fillets with olive oil, scatter with garlic, and season with sea salt and pepper to taste. Scatter pistachios evenly over fillets and drizzle hot pepper sauce over top. Bake at 350 degrees for 20–30 minutes or until fish flakes easily. Serve immediately.

Approx. 243 calories per serving
18g protein, 11g total fat, 5g saturated fat, 0 trans fat,
3.5g carbohydrates, 104mg cholesterol, 558mg sodium, 1g fiber

BAKED TILAPIA

MAKES 2 SERVINGS

4 (4-ounce) tilapia fillets

2 tablespoons extra-virgin olive oil

3 cloves fresh garlic, minced

2 scallions, white and green parts, chopped

½ cup fresh chopped parsley

Salt and freshly ground pepper to taste

Fresh spinach leaves

6 grape tomatoes, halved, for garnish

Juice from 2 lemons

1 lemon, quartered for garnish

Rinse fillets under cold water and pat dry. Place fillets in a baking dish. In mixing bowl combine olive oil, garlic, scallions, and parsley; pour over fish, cover, and refrigerate for 30 minutes. Sprinkle with salt and pepper and bake at 350 degrees for 15 minutes or until fish flakes easily. Divide cleaned spinach on 2 plates. Remove fish from oven, and place 2 fillets on top of spinach on each plate. Garnish each plate with tomato halves. Squeeze juice from lemons over fillets, garnish with lemon wedges, and serve.

Approx. 138 calories per serving (2 fillets per serving)
15g protein, 8g total fat, 1g saturated fat, 0 trans fat,
3g carbohydrates, 43mg cholesterol, 46mg sodium, 0 fiber

SPICY RIGATONI WITH MUSSELS
MAKES 6 SERVINGS

1 pound rigatoni pasta

½ cup dry white wine

2 pounds mussels, scrubbed and debearded (discard any open mussels)

2 tablespoons extra-virgin olive oil

2 cloves fresh garlic, minced

1½ cups cherry tomatoes, halved

1 teaspoon red hot pepper, diced (optional)

Salt and freshly ground pepper to taste

10–12 arugula leaves, chopped

Bring water to a boil, add pasta, and cook pasta until *al dente*. Remove from heat, drain pasta, and return to pot, drizzling with scant amount of olive oil to keep pasta from sticking together. Set aside. In another pot over high heat, add wine and mussels. Cook until mussels open. Discard any that do not open. Remove cooked mussels from liquid. Set aside. Sieve mussel liquid, reserve liquid only. Shell mussels except for 12 mussels (to be used for garnish). In large skillet heat olive oil, add garlic, and sauté. Add tomatoes and hot pepper and sauté for a few minutes. Add shelled mussels and 3–4 teaspoons of mussel liquid and season mixture with salt and pepper to taste. Place pasta in a large pasta server, fluff noodles with a fork, and toss with garlic–mussel mixture. Scatter arugula leaves over top, garnish with unshelled mussels, and serve.

Approx. 454 calories per serving
31g protein, 10g total fat, 1g saturated fat, 0 trans fat,
54g carbohydrates, 44mg cholesterol, 463mg sodium, 8g fiber

LINGUINE AND MIXED SEAFOOD

MAKES 4–6 SERVINGS

8 ounces natural clam juice

2 cups good dry white wine (not cooking wine)

¼ pound baby octopus, cleaned

¼ pound shrimp, peeled and deveined

¼ pound calamari, cleaned, cut into ¼-inch rings

20 mussels, scrubbed and debearded (discard any open mussels)

¼ pound bay scallops

3 tablespoons extra-virgin olive oil

3–4 cloves fresh garlic, minced

¼ teaspoon freshly chopped hot pepper

8 small ripe plum tomatoes, chopped into small chunks

Pinch of low-calorie baking sweetener

½ tablespoon chopped fresh parsley

½ tablespoon chopped fresh oregano

Salt and freshly ground pepper to taste

½ pound linguine

10–12 arugula leaves, chopped for garnish

10 pitted Kalamata black olives, halved, for garnish

In a large deep skillet, add clam juice, wine, octopus, shrimp, calamari, mussels, and scallops. Bring to boil, cover, and reduce heat to simmer, stirring occasionally, until calamari and squid are almost tender. Remove mussels and shell all but 9–12; set these aside for garnish and return shelled mussels to seafood skillet to keep warm. In a separate skillet, over medium heat, add olive oil and garlic and sauté until golden brown. Add hot pepper to garlic mixture, reduce heat to simmer, and cook for 1–2 additional minutes. Add tomatoes, sweetener, parsley, oregano, and salt and pepper to taste, and simmer another 3–4 minutes. Cover to keep warm and set aside. Bring water to a boil, add pasta, and cook pasta until *al dente*. Remove from heat, drain pasta, and return to pot, drizzling with scant amount of olive oil to keep pasta from sticking together. Set aside. With a slotted spoon remove seafood from skillet and strain remaining liquid through sieve or cheesecloth. Return seafood and 1 cup of strained liquid to skillet; add pasta and tomato mixture and toss all ingredients. Spoon entire pasta and seafood dish into a large pasta bowl, garnish with arugula, olives, and remaining unshelled mussels, and serve.

Approx. 375 calories per serving

21g protein, 8g total fat, 1g saturated fat, 0 trans fat,

34g carbohydrates, 98mg cholesterol, 235mg sodium, 2g fiber

LAMB AND BLACK OLIVES
MAKES 4–6 SERVINGS

2 tablespoons extra-virgin olive oil
3 cloves fresh garlic, crushed
1–2 sprigs fresh parsley
2 pounds ground lean lamb
2 tomatoes, peeled and chopped
½ teaspoon dried rosemary
12 pitted black olives, halved
1 cup dry white wine

Heat olive oil in a large skillet; add garlic and parsley, and sauté until golden brown. Add lamb, continuing to cook, and stir often until lamb is browned. Add tomatoes, rosemary, olives, and wine. Stir, cover, and cook 3–5 minutes or until lamb is cooked through and most of liquid has evaporated. Serve with rice.

Approx. 461 calories per serving
62g protein, 21g total fat, 6g saturated fat, 0 trans fat,
4g carbohydrates, 203mg cholesterol, 262mg sodium, 0.5g fiber

BLACKENED SWORDFISH
MAKES 4 SERVINGS

2 tablespoons olive oil
1 tablespoon freshly squeezed lemon juice
4 (6-ounce) swordfish steaks
1 tablespoon Creole seasoning mix of choice, divided
Lemon wedges

Preheat a cast-iron skillet in a 450-degree oven. Combine olive oil and lemon juice in a shallow bowl. Dip each steak into lemon mixture to coat and season both sides of each steak with ¼ tablespoon Creole seasoning. Place steaks on preheated skillet and cook for about 2 minutes. Turn steaks over and continue to cook until seasoning blackens and fish flakes easily. Do not burn steaks. Remove steaks from heat and serve immediately with lemon wedges.

Approx. 270 calories per serving
34g protein, 14g total fat, 3g saturated fat, 0 trans fat,
0 carbohydrates, 65mg cholesterol, 150mg sodium, 0 fiber

RIGATONI WITH GROUND LAMB
MAKES 6–8 SERVINGS

1 pound ground lean lamb
1 whole onion, minced
½ teaspoon crushed red hot pepper flakes
1½ cups frozen peas
2 tablespoons Spicy Garlicky Pesto Sauce (page 484)
Salt and freshly ground pepper to taste
1 pound whole grain rigatoni pasta
2–3 tablespoons fresh chopped mint, for garnish

In a heavy-bottomed saucepan cook lamb, onion, and hot pepper flakes for about 8 minutes, until lamb is cooked, stirring occasionally to break up meat. Add peas and cook for another 2–4 minutes. Add Spicy Garlicky Pesto Sauce and salt and pepper to taste, mix well, and set aside; keep warm. Cook rigatoni in boiling water until *al dente*, drain pasta, and toss with lamb pesto sauce. Garnish with mint.

Approx. 340 calories per serving
20g protein, 7.5g total fat, 1.5g saturated fat, 0 trans fat,
45g carbohydrates, 38mg cholesterol, 64mg sodium, 1g fiber

BOW TIE PASTA WITH EGGPLANT AND BLACK OLIVES
MAKES 6–8 SERVINGS

1 pound bow tie pasta

1 small eggplant, peeled and cut into 1–2-inch strips

Salt to taste

3 tablespoons extra-virgin olive oil

1 medium onion, chopped

Pinch of crushed red hot pepper flakes

6 cloves fresh garlic, minced

½ teaspoon dried oregano

4 tablespoons freshly chopped basil

12 pitted black olives, Nicoise or Kalamata, chopped

Salt and freshly ground pepper to taste

4 ounces crumbled feta cheese for garnish

Chopped fresh parsley for garnish

Bring water to a boil, add pasta, and cook pasta until *al dente*. Remove from heat, drain pasta, and return to pot, drizzling with scant amount of olive oil to keep pasta from sticking together. Set aside. Salt eggplant strips and microwave to reduce water content in eggplant. Squeeze each piece between paper towels to remove excess water. Heat olive oil over medium heat and sauté onion and hot pepper flakes for 1–2 minutes. Add eggplant, garlic, and oregano and sauté until eggplant is lightly browned. Add basil, olives, and salt and pepper to taste. Transfer pasta to a serving bowl and toss with eggplant mixture. Serve garnished with feta cheese and parsley.

Approx. 308 calories per serving
10g protein, 10g total fat, 3g saturated fat, 0 trans fat,
52g carbohydrates, 13mg cholesterol, 256mg sodium, 2g fiber

PASTA WITH RED CLAM SAUCE
MAKES 6–8 SERVINGS

1 pound whole grain angel hair pasta

1 cup dry white wine

4 ounces bottled clam juice

3 cloves fresh garlic, finely chopped

¼ teaspoon dried basil

48 small hard-shell clams, cleaned (discard any open clams)

2 tablespoons extra-virgin olive oil

½ white onion, chopped

1 pound whole tomatoes, peeled, seeded, and chopped

¼ teaspoon dried oregano

Salt and freshly ground pepper to taste

1 teaspoon chopped fresh parsley for garnish

Bring water to a boil, add pasta, and cook pasta until *al dente*. Remove from heat, drain pasta, and return to pot, drizzling with scant amount of olive oil to keep pasta from sticking together. Set aside. In a large skillet heat wine and clam juice, add 1 clove chopped garlic, basil, and clams in their shells, cover, and steam until shells open. Remove clams from liquid and discard any unopened clams. Strain liquid through strainer to remove grit and set liquid aside. Reserve 16 clams in their shells for garnish, then remove remaining clams from shells and return them to strained liquid. In a separate skillet, heat olive oil, add onion and remaining garlic, and sauté until golden. Add tomatoes, oregano, and salt and pepper to garlic mixture and cook for 8 minutes. Add shelled clams with strained liquid to tomato mixture and heat through for another 2–3 minutes, stirring to blend tastes. Pour clam sauce over pasta, toss, and garnish with reserved unshelled clams and parsley.

Approx. 284 calories per serving

23g protein, 6g total fat, 0.6g saturated fat, 0 trans fat,

47g carbohydrates, 46mg cholesterol, 82mg sodium, 6g fiber

PASTA WITH CLAMS, WINE, AND RED HOT PEPPERS
MAKES 6–8 SERVINGS

1 pound whole grain spaghetti

1 cup dry white wine

4 ounces bottled clam juice

48 small hard-shell clams, cleaned (discard any open clams)

2 tablespoons extra-virgin olive oil

3 cloves fresh garlic, finely chopped

1 small hot chili pepper, minced

4 tablespoons finely chopped fresh parsley

Salt and freshly ground pepper to taste

Bring water to a boil, add pasta, and cook pasta until *al dente*. Remove from heat, drain pasta, and return to pot, drizzling with scant amount of olive oil to keep pasta from sticking together. Set aside. In a large skillet, heat wine and clam juice, add clams in their shells, cover, and steam until shells open. Remove clams from liquid and discard any unopened clams. Strain liquid through strainer to remove grit and set aside. Reserve 16 clams in their shells for garnish; remove remaining clams from shells and return them to strained liquid. Set aside reserved unshelled clams. In a large skillet heat olive oil, garlic, chili pepper, and parsley, bring to a sizzle, and add shelled clams with strained juice, and salt and pepper to taste; stir and heat through. Pour sauce over pasta, toss, and garnish with reserved unshelled clams.

Approx. 308 calories per serving
28g protein, 7g total fat, 0.7g saturated fat, 0 trans fat,
49g carbohydrates, 51mg cholesterol, 86mg sodium, 7g fiber

WHOLE WHEAT SPAGHETTI WITH ANCHOVY
AND GARLIC SAUCE

MAKES 6–8 SERVINGS

1 pound whole wheat spaghetti
6 tablespoons extra-virgin olive oil + oil from anchovies
6 large cloves fresh garlic, pressed
2-ounce tin of anchovy fillets packed in oil, drained and chopped
Crushed red hot pepper flakes to taste
6–8 pitted black olives, chopped
2 tablespoons finely chopped fresh parsley
Freshly ground pepper to taste
Romano cheese, finely grated (optional)

Bring water to a boil, add pasta, and cook pasta until *al dente*. Remove from heat, drain pasta, and return to pot, drizzling with scant amount of olive oil to keep pasta from sticking together. Set aside. Combine both oils and garlic in a skillet over medium heat and cook about 1–2 minutes. Add anchovies, breaking into small pieces and stirring to blend well with other ingredients. Cook about 30 seconds and remove from heat. Fold in hot pepper flakes, olives, and parsley. Place pasta in a large serving bowl, add anchovy sauce, and toss to mix. Add pepper to taste, sprinkle with a small amount of grated Romano cheese, if desired, and serve.

Approx. 347 calories per serving
14g protein, 16g total fat, 1g saturated fat, 0 trans fat,
39g carbohydrates, 11mg cholesterol, 244mg sodium, 6g fiber

FETTUCCINE WITH SUNDRIED TOMATOES AND GOAT CHEESE
MAKES 6–8 SERVINGS

4 tablespoons chopped sundried tomatoes (in olive oil)

1 cup sliced scallions

4 cloves fresh garlic, minced

1 medium red bell pepper, thinly sliced

½ cup dry vermouth

¼ cup chopped fresh basil

10 pitted Kalamata olives

1 tablespoon capers, rinsed and drained

2 teaspoons dried oregano

1 pound whole wheat fettuccine, cooked and drained

6 ounces crumbled low-fat goat cheese

Drain oil from tomatoes and reserve oil; set tomatoes aside. In a large skillet, heat oil from tomatoes over medium heat. Add scallions and garlic to oil and sauté until soft. Add red bell pepper and ¼ cup of vermouth to garlic mixture. Cook peppers until crispy tender or until vermouth is almost evaporated. Reduce heat to simmer, and add tomatoes, remaining ¼ cup of vermouth, basil, olives, capers, and oregano. Simmer, stirring often to incorporate flavors (about 5–8 minutes), then reduce to very low heat to keep warm. Cook pasta to desired consistency (*al dente* would be best) and drain. Place pasta in a large bowl and toss with goat cheese until well blended. Add tomato mixture and toss again until well mixed. Serve.

Approx. 269 calories per serving
12g protein, 6g total fat, 2g saturated fat, 0 trans fat,
44g carbohydrates, 4mg cholesterol, 323mg sodium, 7g fiber

FLORENTINE ROASTED PORK

MAKES 6–8 SERVINGS

4 pounds lean loin pork

4 cloves fresh garlic, sliced thin

½ teaspoon dried rosemary

4 cloves fresh garlic, whole

5–6 tablespoons water

6–8 tablespoons hearty red wine (do not use a cooking wine)

Salt and freshly ground pepper to taste

If the skin of the loin has not already been scored, cut lines into skin about ⅛ inch apart. Cut through the flesh to the bone on one side and insert the garlic slices and rosemary. Press the whole garlic cloves into the scored skin of the loin and place loin into a roasting pan in a 350-degree oven with water and wine. Sprinkle loin generously with salt and pepper and roast for 2–2½ hours or until meat is very tender but still moist, basting occasionally. Serve with a variety of your favorite vegetables.

Approx. 352 calories per serving

47g protein, 17g total fat, 5.6g saturated fat, 0 trans fat,

0 carbohydrates, 136mg cholesterol, 144mg sodium, 0 fiber

CHICKEN WITH POMEGRANATE SAUCE

MAKES 6–8 SERVINGS

4 pounds skinless, boneless chicken breast, cut into small pieces

2 teaspoons paprika

Salt and freshly ground pepper to taste

¼ cup extra-virgin olive oil

4 cloves fresh garlic, minced

2 medium yellow onions, chopped

¼ cup chopped fresh parsley

1 small hot banana pepper, finely chopped

3 tablespoons Thick Pomegranate Molasses (page 484)

3–4 cups canned chunky tomatoes, undrained

Wash chicken, remove fat, and cut into small pieces. Sprinkle with paprika and salt and pepper. Heat olive oil in a saucepan, add chicken pieces, and stir-fry for about 2–3 minutes. Add garlic and stir-fry for another 2–3 minutes. Add onions, parsley, hot banana pepper, Thick Pomegranate Molasses, and tomatoes with liquid; cover and bring to boil. Cook over medium-low heat for about 30 minutes until chicken is tender. Serve with rice.

Approx. 364 calories per serving
50g protein, 14g total fat, 3g saturated fat, 0 trans fat,
8g carbohydrates, 160mg cholesterol, 401mg sodium, 1g fiber

CHICKEN PICCATA

MAKES 4 SERVINGS

4 (3-ounce) skinless, boneless chicken breast fillets, lightly pounded
Salt and freshly ground pepper to taste (optional)
2 teaspoons extra-virgin olive oil, divided
3 cloves fresh garlic, minced
1 cup canned low-sodium, fat-free chicken broth
2 tablespoons dry white wine
4 teaspoons lemon juice
1 tablespoon all-purpose flour
2 tablespoons chopped fresh parsley
1 tablespoon capers
Lemon wedges for garnish

Rinse chicken breast fillets under cold water and pat dry, then place breasts between layers of wax paper and lightly pound fillets with a meat mallet. Lightly sprinkle each fillet with salt and pepper, if desired. Heat 1 teaspoon of olive oil in a large heavy skillet over medium heat, add chicken fillets, and cook until fillets are lightly browned and centers cooked (juice will run clear). Transfer fillets to a serving platter and put in a low-temperature oven to keep warm. Add remaining teaspoon of olive oil and garlic to same skillet and cook for 30 seconds to soften. Combine chicken broth, wine, lemon juice, and flour in skillet. Stir to blend and continue stirring until mixture thickens. Add parsley and capers to sauce. Remove chicken from oven, place each fillet on a plate, and spoon mixture over fillets. Garnish with lemon wedges. Serve with cooked spinach linguine or pasta of choice.

Approx. 223 calories per serving
21g protein, 11g total fat, 2g saturated fat, 0 trans fat,
4g carbohydrates, 48mg cholesterol, 380mg sodium, <0.5g fiber

BROILED TUNA AND TOMATO

MAKES 4 SERVINGS

4 (3-ounce) tuna fillets
4 tablespoons extra-virgin olive oil
2 large cloves fresh garlic, minced
1 tablespoon chopped fresh parsley
Salt and freshly ground pepper to taste
1½ teaspoons white wine vinegar
8 (½-inch) slices fresh tomato
Fresh Italian parsley, chopped, for garnish

Rinse fillets, pat dry, and set aside. Combine in a covered container 2 tablespoons olive oil, garlic, parsley, and salt and pepper. Add fillets, turning to coat well. Marinate fillets at room temperature for 2 hours. In another bowl, combine remaining olive oil, vinegar, and salt and pepper, if desired. Arrange sliced tomatoes in a flat container in one layer and pour oil mixture over tomatoes; marinate at room temperature for 2 hours. Heat broiler, place tuna on grilling pan about 4 inches below heat, and broil each side of fillets for about 2–3 minutes. Arrange 2 slices of tomato on each plate; add tuna fillets to top of tomatoes and garnish with parsley. Serve while hot.

Approx. 224 calories per serving
20g protein, 18g total fat, 2.8g saturated fat, 0 trans fat,
2g carbohydrates, 38mg cholesterol, 35mg sodium, 0 fiber

SHRIMP IN SPICY BLACK BEAN SAUCE

MAKES 4–6 SERVINGS

2 jumbo cloves fresh garlic, minced

2 tablespoons + 2 teaspoons extra-virgin olive oil, divided

3 teaspoons chili powder

3 teaspoons ground cumin

2 cups canned black beans, rinsed and drained

1½ cups canned low-sodium, fat-free chicken broth

24 jumbo shrimp, peeled and deveined

Salt and freshly ground pepper to taste

Fresh parsley, chopped for garnish

Sauté all but 2 teaspoons of garlic in 1 tablespoon of olive oil until almost browned. Add chili powder and cumin and sauté for another minute. Add beans to garlic mixture, stirring frequently, and cook for another 3–4 minutes. Stir in chicken broth and transfer mixture to a food processor or blender. Puree mixture and return to skillet. Simmer sauce for 5 minutes, stirring often. Set aside, but keep warm. Rinse shrimp and pat dry; season with salt and pepper. Heat remaining olive oil and sauté shrimp with remaining garlic. Cook until shrimp are lightly browned outside and cooked through inside, turning often. Remove shrimp from olive oil with a slotted spoon and set aside. Warm sauce and pour onto serving platter. Arrange shrimp on top of sauce and garnish with parsley. Serve immediately, with rice, if desired.

Approx. 211 calories per serving
19g protein, 9g total fat, 1g saturated fat, 0 trans fat,
16g carbohydrates, 112mg cholesterol, 555mg sodium, 5g fiber

LEMONY CHICKEN AND VEGETABLES

MAKES 4 SERVINGS

3 tablespoons juice from fresh lemon halves + extra halves for garnish

1 tablespoon fresh grated lemon peel

2 tablespoons extra-virgin olive oil

¼ teaspoon salt (optional)

¼ teaspoon freshly ground pepper

4 cloves fresh garlic, freshly crushed

1 teaspoon paprika

1½ pounds skinless, boneless dark meat chicken

¾ pound yellow squash, quartered lengthwise

¾ pound zucchini, quartered lengthwise

¼ cup chopped fresh chives

Whisk together lemon juice, lemon peel, olive oil, salt, and pepper. Reserve 2 tablespoons of mixture in a separate cup. Add garlic and paprika to original mixture and pour over chicken; marinate in a covered container in the refrigerator for 3–4 hours. When chicken is marinated, heat grill to medium-high heat. Remove chicken from marinade and place on grill along with squash, zucchini, and juiced lemon halves. Close grill top and cook for 10–12 minutes or until juices from chicken run clear when pierced. Turn chicken 1 time while grilling. Cook squash, zucchini, and lemon halves until tender and brown. Remove chicken from grill and cut into 1-inch-wide pieces. Cut squash and zucchini pieces in half. Place chicken and vegetables on a platter and pour reserved marinade over vegetables; sprinkle with chives. Garnish platter with grilled lemon halves and serve.

Approx. 255 calories per serving
29g protein, 15g total fat, 3g saturated fat, 0 trans fat,
8g carbohydrates, 105mg cholesterol, 254mg sodium, 2g fiber

HORSERADISH-ENCRUSTED SALMON

MAKES 2 SERVINGS

Olive oil cooking spray
2 (6-ounce) salmon fillets, skin intact
⅓ cup plain dried bread crumbs
1 tablespoon low-fat sour cream
2 tablespoons prepared fresh horseradish
2 tablespoons chopped fresh dill
Aged balsamic vinegar to drizzle (optional)

Lightly spray a shallow baking pan with cooking oil. Rinse fillets under cold water, pat dry with paper towels, and place skin side down in baking pan. In a food processor, combine bread crumbs, sour cream, horseradish, and dill. Pulse ingredients on low speed into a thick paste. Divide into 2 portions and top each fillet with mixture. Place fillets in oven and bake at 350 degrees until fillets flake easily and topping crusts to a golden brown (about 12–15 minutes). Serve hot and drizzle with a small amount of balsamic vinegar, if desired.

Approx. 292 calories per serving
35g protein, 11g total fat, 2g saturated fat, 0 trans fat,
7g carbohydrates, 95mg cholesterol, 195mg sodium, 0 fiber

SALMON CAKES WITH SOUR CREAM DILL SAUCE
MAKES 8 SERVINGS

2 (14.75-ounce) cans of salmon

2 tablespoons extra-virgin olive oil, divided

¾ cup chopped scallions

3 cloves fresh garlic, minced

½ teaspoon crushed red hot pepper flakes

2 eggs

½ tablespoon lime juice

3 tablespoons cornstarch

Salt and freshly ground pepper to taste

1 cup fat-free or low-fat sour cream (optional)

4 tablespoons finely chopped fresh dill (optional)

Drain and separate salmon; set aside. In a heavy-bottomed skillet over medium-low heat, add 2 teaspoons olive oil, scallions, garlic, and hot pepper flakes. Sauté until scallions are soft, then set aside. In a bowl whisk together eggs, lime juice, cornstarch, and salt and pepper. Add egg mixture to scallion mixture and gently fold in salmon. Form salmon mixture into 8 cakes and refrigerate for about 30 minutes. Pour remaining olive oil into a large skillet over medium-low heat and add chilled salmon cakes. Slowly sauté cakes for about 2–3 minutes on each side until heated through. Mix sour cream and dill together and serve each salmon cake garnished with a tablespoon of sour cream and dill sauce, if desired.

Approx. 251 calories per serving
24g protein, 15g total fat, 3g saturated fat, 0 trans fat,
3g carbohydrates, 134mg cholesterol, 397mg sodium, <0.5g fiber

ENCRUSTED RED SNAPPER AND DILL SAUCE

MAKES 4 SERVINGS

4 (5–6-ounce) red snapper fillets
Olive oil cooking spray
4 tablespoons fresh lemon juice
Freshly ground pepper to taste
4 tablespoons prepared spicy brown mustard
2 plum tomatoes, deseeded and chopped
½ medium green bell pepper, finely chopped
2 cloves fresh garlic, chopped
2 tablespoons freshly chopped parsley
½ cup plain bread crumbs
2 tablespoons melted trans fat–free canola/olive oil spread

For Dill Sauce:

2 tablespoons extra-virgin olive oil
2 tablespoons chopped shallots
1 tablespoon chopped fresh garlic
2 ounces dry white wine (not cooking wine)
2 tablespoons light cream cheese
2 tablespoons fat-free cream cheese
3 tablespoons trans fat–free canola/olive oil spread
4 tablespoons freshly chopped dill
Salt to taste (optional)
Generous dash of white pepper

Rinse fillets under cold water and pat dry with paper towels. Place fillets on a non-stick baking sheet lightly coated with cooking oil spray. Drizzle lemon juice over fillets and season with pepper to taste. Spread 1 tablespoon of mustard on each fillet. Combine tomatoes, green bell pepper, garlic, parsley, and bread crumbs; stir to mix well. Cover each fillet with vegetable bread crumb mixture and drizzle top of mixture with melted canola/olive oil spread. Bake for about 15 minutes at 350 degrees or until fillets flake easily and topping is lightly golden brown and crusty.

Dill Sauce:

Heat olive oil in a non-stick skillet over medium heat and sauté shallots and garlic until soft. Add wine and simmer on low heat, stirring often until mixture becomes slightly syrupy. Slowly fold in both cream cheeses and canola/olive oil spread, constantly stirring until melted. Add in dill and salt and white pepper. Reduce heat to very low to keep warm until ready to serve. Drizzle sauce over and around sides of fillets.

Approx. 288 calories per serving without sauce
37g protein, 8g total fat, 2g saturated fat, 0 trans fat,
13g carbohydrates, 60mg cholesterol, 446mg sodium, 1g fiber

Approx. 359 calories per serving with sauce
38g protein, 15.5g total fat, 3.5g saturated fat, 0 trans fat,
13.5g carbohydrates, 63mg cholesterol, 523.5mg sodium, 0 fiber

ORANGE HORSERADISH-ENCRUSTED SCALLOPS

MAKES 4 SERVINGS

Olive oil cooking spray
1½ pounds sea scallops
⅓ cup plain dried bread crumbs
2 tablespoons prepared fresh horseradish
2 tablespoons freshly grated orange peel
1 tablespoon extra-virgin olive oil
Arugula leaves for garnish (optional)

Lightly spray the inside of a shallow oven-safe casserole dish with cooking oil. Place scallops in the casserole dish in a single layer. In a food processor, combine bread crumbs, horseradish, orange peel, and olive oil. Pulse ingredients on low speed into a thick paste. Spread mixture over the top of scallops and bake in a 350-degree oven until scallops are opaque and topping is a crusty golden brown (about 12–15 minutes). Divide into 4 portions and serve hot on a bed of arugula leaves, if desired.

Approx. 180 calories per serving (about 8 scallops)
28g protein, 5g total fat, <0.5g saturated fat, 0 trans fat,
7g carbohydrates, 50mg cholesterol, 406mg sodium, <0.5g fiber

STEAMED DUNGENESS CRAB

MAKES 2 SERVINGS

4 whole crab leg clusters (about 1½ pounds per cluster, fresh or frozen), large claws, cracked
4 large cloves fresh garlic, halved
Scant sprinkle of garlic salt (optional)
Water, enough to almost cover clusters
4 lemon wedges
Melted trans fat–free canola/olive oil spread for dipping (optional)

Place clusters in a large aluminum (turkey-sized) baking pan. Add garlic and garlic salt to taste, if desired. Cover clusters with water and cover pan tightly with foil. Bake covered at 450 degrees until water begins to steam. Allow to steam for about 5 minutes, reduce heat to 250 degrees, and allow clusters to bathe in seasoned water about 15–20 minutes longer. Remove from oven, serve warm with lemon wedges and melted canola/olive oil spread, if desired.

Approx. 280 calories per serving
3g protein, 3g total fat, <0.5g saturated fat, 0 trans fat,
2g carbohydrates, 194mg cholesterol, 962mg sodium, 0 fiber

GRILLED WHOLE RAINBOW TROUT AND CHIVE SAUCE

MAKES 4 SERVINGS

4 (7–8-ounce) whole boneless trout with skin intact, cleaned and dressed
Garlic powder to taste
Freshly ground pepper to taste
Sea salt to taste (optional)
Olive oil cooking spray
⅓ cup light sour cream
½ tablespoon water
4 teaspoons lime juice
⅛ teaspoon salt (optional)
⅛ teaspoon white pepper
3 tablespoons freshly chopped chives
Fresh spinach, sautéed (optional)

Turn on outdoor grill to high and close grill lid. Rinse trout under cold water and pat dry with paper towels. Season trout with garlic powder, pepper, and salt, if desired. Spray a cast-iron skillet with cooking oil and place skillet on grill. When skillet is hot, add fish. Turn trout over once to brown both sides and cook until meat flakes easily. While fish is browning, combine sour cream, water, and lime juice in a small saucepan. Heat on low, stirring constantly, until blended, then add salt, pepper, and chives. Remove sauce from direct heat, but keep warm. When trout is ready, place each trout on a bed of sautéed spinach and spoon ⅛ cup of chive mixture over each trout. Serve immediately, while hot.

Approx. 309 calories per serving
50g protein, 10g total fat, 3.6g saturated fat, 0 trans fat,
2g carbohydrates, 138mg cholesterol, 239mg sodium, 0 fiber

BLACKENED TUNA STEAKS WITH MUSTARD GINGER SAUCE

MAKES 4 SERVINGS

½ cup light orange juice

4 cloves fresh garlic, chopped

1 teaspoon finely grated ginger

3 tablespoons low-sodium soy sauce

2 tablespoons sherry

1 tablespoon Dijon mustard

1 tablespoon honey

4 (6-ounce) tuna steaks, about 1–1½ inches thick

1 lemon, quartered, for garnish

In a small bowl combine orange juice, garlic, ginger, soy sauce, sherry, mustard, and honey. Whisk for about 1 minute to blend marinade, then reserve and refrigerate ⅛ cup of marinade for basting tuna steaks during cooking. Rinse fish under cold water and pat dry with paper towels. Place fish in a single layer in a container and pour balance of marinade over fish. Put a tight-fitting lid on container and turn container over several times to allow marinade to coat all sides of fish. Refrigerate fish in marinade for 1–2 hours, if possible, or for at least 30 minutes. When fish has marinated long enough, turn on outdoor grill to high and close grill lid. Spray a cast-iron skillet with cooking oil and place skillet on grill. When skillet is very hot, remove fish from marinade container and place on hot skillet. Blacken fish on one side before turning over. Before turning, brush tops of fish generously with half of the reserved marinade. Turn over fish to blacken the other side and brush blackened side with the remainder of reserved marinade. Test centers and flakiness for desired doneness. Remove from heat, garnish with lemon wedges, and serve immediately.

Approx. 205 calories per serving
35g protein, 6g total fat, 1g saturated fat, 0 trans fat,
0 carbohydrates, 96mg cholesterol, 100mg sodium, 0 fiber

STUFFED SESAME CHICKEN BREASTS

MAKES 4 SERVINGS

4 (4–5-ounce) skinless, boneless chicken breasts

Salt and freshly ground pepper to taste

1 tablespoon dried tarragon or 4 sprigs fresh tarragon

½ red bell pepper, deseeded and thinly sliced

½ green bell pepper, deseeded and thinly sliced

4 tablespoons lime juice

¼ small red chili pepper, finely minced (optional)

¼ cup sesame seeds

Extra-virgin olive oil to drizzle

4 fresh tarragon sprigs for garnish

Rinse breasts under cold water and pat dry with paper towels. With a sharp knife, split open one side of breasts to create a pocket. Season inside of breasts with salt and pepper, as desired, and tarragon (¼ tablespoon of dried tarragon per breast or 1 full sprig stuffed inside the pocket of each breast). Insert slices of both red and green bell peppers into each breast pocket and then close, securing with a toothpick. Combine lime juice and chili pepper; set aside. Sprinkle each breast with a generous amount of sesame seeds and place breasts in a single layer on a nonstick baking sheet. Drizzle tops of breasts with lime/chili mixture and bake at 400 degrees for about 30 minutes or until chicken is tender and cooked through. Set oven to broil and lightly drizzle olive oil over the top of each breast. Place baking sheet under broiler and broil chicken breasts until sesame seeds are golden brown. Serve garnished with fresh sprigs of tarragon.

Approx. 237 calories per serving
37g protein, 8g total fat, 1g saturated fat, 0 trans fat,
4g carbohydrates, 96mg cholesterol, 85mg sodium, 1g fiber

BROILED MANGO CHICKEN BREAST FILLETS

MAKES 4 SERVINGS

4 (4–5-ounce) skinless, boneless chicken breast fillets

Salt and freshly ground pepper to taste

4 large bay leaves, crumbled

2 teaspoons finely chopped fresh garlic

6 large pitted black olives, halved

3 tablespoons of dry cream sherry

1 tablespoon extra-virgin olive oil

2 ripe but firm mangos, peeled and cut into wedges

Rinse fillets under cold water and pat dry with paper towels. Place fillets in a single layer in a shallow baking dish. Sprinkle tops of fillets with salt and pepper, as desired. Scatter crumbled bay leaves, garlic, and olives over fillets. In a small bowl combine sherry and olive oil. Whisk to blend and drizzle over fillets. Scatter mango wedges over and around fillets. Place baking dish in oven and bake at 350 degrees for about 8–10 minutes or until juices run clear when fillets are pierced with a fork. Set oven to broil. Transfer baking dish to top rack about 4 inches under heat and broil tops of fillets until lightly browned. Serve hot, drizzled with juices from baking dish and topped with pieces of mangos.

Approx. 297 calories per serving
36g protein, 8g total fat, 1g saturated fat, 0 trans fat,
18g carbohydrates, 96mg cholesterol, 86mg sodium, 1g fiber

BROILED SPICY TURKEY BURGERS

MAKES 4 PATTIES

1 pound freshly ground turkey breast
2 cloves fresh garlic, finely chopped
3 scallions, finely chopped
½ cup fresh spinach, chopped
½ cup Italian-seasoned bread crumbs
½ teaspoon red hot pepper sauce
½ teaspoon Worcestershire sauce
2 whole wheat pita loaves cut in half with pockets opened
Alfa sprouts, sliced tomato, lettuce, mustard, etc., as desired, for garnish

Turn on oven broiler. In a large bowl, combine ground turkey, garlic, scallions, spinach, bread crumbs, hot pepper sauce, and Worcestershire sauce. Stir to mix thoroughly and form into 4 equal-size patties. Place patties on a broiler pan and place in oven about 4 inches under broiler. Broil burgers on each side for roughly 6 minutes, turning only once. Cook until centers are no longer pink. Remove from oven. Place each burger inside a pita pocket and garnish as desired.

Approx. 219 calories per patty
22g protein, 9g total fat, 3g saturated fat, 0 trans fat,
10g carbohydrates, 84mg cholesterol, 229mg sodium, <1g fiber

WHOLE WHEAT PENNE WITH SHRIMP AND BROCCOLI

MAKES 4 SERVINGS

8 ounces whole wheat penne

⅓ cup canned low-sodium, fat-free chicken broth

4 cloves fresh garlic, finely chopped

½ pound broccoli florets, cut into smaller florets

½ green bell pepper, diced

½ red bell pepper, diced

¼ cup diced scallions, white and green parts

¼ teaspoon crushed red hot pepper flakes

16 ounces pre-cooked baby shrimp

½ cup Simple Tomato Pasta Sauce (page 492) or market-fresh tomato pasta sauce

½ cup chopped fresh basil

Salt and freshly ground pepper to taste

Grated Parmesan cheese for garnish (optional)

Bring water to a boil, add pasta, and cook pasta until *al dente*. Remove from heat, drain pasta, and return to pot, drizzling with scant amount of olive oil to keep pasta from sticking together. Set aside. While pasta is cooking, heat chicken broth in a large skillet, and add garlic, broccoli, green and red bell peppers, and scallions. Cover and cook vegetables over medium-low heat until crispy tender. Reduce heat to low and add hot pepper flakes and shrimp; stir to incorporate into vegetables and cook for about 2–3 minutes. Add pasta sauce and cook for an additional 2–3 minutes, stirring to mix well. Add penne and basil to sauce and season with salt and pepper to taste. Toss to coat pasta with sauce. Serve with a sprinkle of grated Parmesan cheese, if desired.

Approx. 315 calories per serving
20g protein, 3g total fat, 0.5g saturated fat, 0 trans fat,
42g carbohydrates, 75mg cholesterol, 605mg sodium, 5g fiber

BAKED FLOUNDER WITH CAPERS AND BABY SHRIMP

MAKES 4 SERVINGS

Olive oil cooking spray
8 (4-ounce) fillets of flounder
Scant amount of dried oregano
Scant amount of dried basil
Salt and freshly ground pepper to taste
20–24 cherry tomatoes, halved
4 teaspoons small capers, rinsed and drained
1 cup pre-cooked baby shrimp (defrosted and well drained)
6 tablespoons freshly grated Parmesan cheese
Scant amount of extra-virgin olive oil to drizzle
1 lemon, cut into 4 wedges for garnish

Lightly spray a shallow baking pan with cooking oil. Rinse fillets under cold water and pat dry. Place fillets in a single layer in baking pan, and add oregano, basil, and salt and pepper to taste. Scatter tomatoes, capers, and shrimp over fillets. Bake for about 8–10 minutes at 400 degrees. Remove from oven and turn oven to broil. Top fish with Parmesan cheese, drizzle olive oil over fish, and return to oven about 4 inches under broiler. Broil for about 15–20 seconds or until cheese lightly browns. Remove from oven and serve immediately, garnished with lemon wedges.

Approx. 272 calories per serving
53g protein, 5g total fat, 2g saturated fat, 0 trans fat,
<0.3g carbohydrates, 140mg cholesterol, 565mg sodium, 0 fiber

GRILLED TILAPIA

MAKES 4 SERVINGS

8 (4–5-ounce) tilapia fillets
Salt and freshly ground pepper to taste
Hot red pepper sauce to taste
Juice from 1 fresh lemon
Extra-virgin olive oil cooking spray
Fresh raw spinach for garnish

Rinse fillets under cold water and pat dry with paper towels. Place fillets on a large platter in a single layer, add salt and pepper to taste. Drizzle fillets with hot pepper sauce and fresh lemon juice. Refrigerate fillets for at least 30 minutes. Turn on outdoor grill and set to high heat. Spray a cast-iron skillet or grilling sheet lightly with olive oil spray, place on grill, and close grill top. Allow grill and skillet to reach 350–450 degrees. When skillet is hot enough, place fillets on skillet, seasoned side down, and close grill lid. Allow fillets to grill for about 4–5 minutes and then turn fillets over and allow other side to grill another 4–5 minutes or until fish turns opaque white. Remove from grill and serve hot on a bed of fresh spinach.

Approx. 200 calories per 2 fillets
42g protein, 5g total fat, 1g saturated fat, 0 trans fat,
2g carbohydrates, 110mg cholesterol, 120mg sodium, 0 fiber

BROILED GARLIC LAMB CHOPS

MAKES 4 SERVINGS

8 (4–5-ounce) lamb chops
4 cloves fresh garlic, finely chopped
½ tablespoon dried rosemary
Garlic salt to taste, if desired
3 tablespoons Dijon mustard
Juice from 1 lemon
1 tablespoon honey
2 tablespoons extra-virgin olive oil
¼ teaspoon red wine vinegar
Freshly ground pepper to taste
Fresh mint leaves for garnish

Set oven to broil. Rinse chops under cold water and pat dry with paper towels. Place them in a single layer on a broiling pan; set aside. Combine garlic and rosemary in a small bowl and mix. Vigorously rub garlic/rosemary mixture into both sides of chops, sprinkle with garlic salt, if desired, and place chops about 4 inches under broiler. Broil to desired doneness. While chops are broiling, mix together mustard, lemon juice, honey, olive oil, vinegar, and pepper to taste, and blend well to incorporate ingredients. Remove chops from oven and place 2 chops on each serving plate. Spoon mustard mixture over chops, garnish each serving with mint leaf, and serve immediately.

Approx. 574 calories per serving (2 chops)
68g protein, 24g total fat, 9g saturated fat, 0 trans fat,
6g carbohydrates, 216mg cholesterol, 192mg sodium, 0 fiber

TOMATO AND ANCHOVY SAUCE WITH PASTA
MAKES 6–8 SERVINGS

4 cloves fresh garlic, finely chopped

3 tablespoons extra-virgin olive oil

10 anchovy fillets in olive oil

1 tablespoon finely chopped fresh parsley

1 pound fresh tomatoes, peeled and chopped

Salt and freshly ground pepper to taste

1 pound whole grain pasta

¼ cup plain bread crumbs

¼ cup grated Romano cheese

Fresh parsley sprigs for garnish

In a large skillet over medium-high heat, sauté garlic in olive oil until golden brown. Add in anchovy fillets and oil from anchovies. Crumble fillets into fine pieces to dissolve in oil. Add parsley, tomatoes, and salt and pepper to anchovy mixture and simmer for about 20–25 minutes. In boiling water, cook pasta to your liking and drain well. Lightly toss pasta with sauce and place on platter. In a separate bowl mix together bread crumbs and Romano cheese. Top pasta with cheese mixture, garnish with parsley sprigs, and serve while hot.

Approx. 282 calories per serving
9g protein, 7g total fat, 2g saturated fat, 0 trans fat,
45g carbohydrates, 9mg cholesterol, 350mg sodium, 6g fiber

STEAMED MUSSELS WITH GARLIC AND DRY VERMOUTH

MAKES 2 SERVINGS

2 pounds fresh mussels, scrubbed and debearded (discard any open mussels)

1 tablespoon extra-virgin olive oil

3 cloves fresh garlic, minced

1 medium shallot, minced

1½ cups dry vermouth

1 cup canned low-sodium, fat-free chicken broth

Salt and freshly ground pepper to taste

1 tablespoon fresh lemon juice

Melted trans fat–free canola/olive oil spread (optional)

Lemon wedges for garnish

Keep cleaned mussels immersed in cold water until ready to steam. In a large skillet, heat olive oil and sauté garlic and shallot until tender, but do not brown. Add vermouth and chicken broth to skillet and stir to blend well with garlic mixture. With a slotted spoon, remove mussels from water and add to vermouth mixture. Add salt and pepper to taste, if desired. Cover skillet and increase heat to medium-high; steam mussels until all have opened, about 10 minutes. Reduce heat to very low to keep mussels warm until ready to serve, discarding any mussels that have not opened. To serve, remove mussels from skillet with a slotted spoon to individual serving bowls. Drizzle mussels with lemon juice and melted canola/olive oil spread, if desired. Garnish with lemon wedges and serve while hot.

Approx. 390 calories per serving (roughly 20–30 mussels)
54g protein, 10g total fat, 2g saturated fat, 0 trans fats,
17g carbohydrates, 127mg cholesterol, 1296mg sodium, 0 fiber

MEATLESS LASAGNA
MAKES 6–8 SERVINGS

1 pound whole grain lasagna noodles
3 cups sliced white mushrooms (about a 10-ounce box)
2½ tablespoons chopped fresh oregano
2½ teaspoons extra-virgin olive oil
2 large tomatoes (about 1½ pounds)
10 large pitted black olives, coarsely chopped
6 cloves fresh garlic, chopped
Salt and freshly ground pepper to taste
2 cups part-skim ricotta cheese
1 ounce grated Romano cheese
Freshly chopped fresh basil for garnish

Cook pasta per package instructions. Meanwhile, in a large skillet over medium-high heat, combine mushrooms, oregano, and olive oil. Sauté until mushrooms are tender; set aside. In a food processor or blender, process tomatoes until finely chopped. Add tomatoes and their juices, olives, garlic, and salt and pepper to mushroom mixture and simmer covered for about 10 minutes. Drain pasta. In a large oven-safe casserole dish, spread a thin layer of tomato and mushroom mixture, a layer of noodles, layer of ricotta cheese, followed by another layer of tomato and mushroom mixture, etc., until all of the ingredients are used. Finish with ricotta cheese. Top last layer of ricotta cheese with grated Romano cheese, followed by chopped basil for garnish. Place lasagna in oven and bake for about 15–20 minutes or until heated through. Remove from oven and serve while hot.

Approx. 318 calories per serving
9g protein, 1g total fat, <0.5g saturated fat, 0 trans fat,
40g carbohydrates, 0 cholesterol, 10mg sodium, 7g fiber

BLACK BEAN SEAFOOD BURGERS

MAKES 6 PATTIES

1 cup bulgur

1 cup hot water

1 tablespoon extra-virgin olive oil

2 tablespoons freshly chopped garlic

2 tablespoons freshly chopped white onion

Pinch of ground mixed pepper

1 cup fresh bay scallops

1 cup pre-cooked baby shrimp

1 can chopped clams, well drained

3 tablespoons chopped, deseeded plum tomatoes

¼ small hot pepper, finely chopped (optional)

1 cup canned black beans, well drained

½ cup egg substitute

Olive oil cooking spray

Hot sauce (optional)

Salt and freshly ground pepper to taste

Lettuce leaves and slices of tomato for garnish

Place bulgur in a bowl, add hot water and cover, set aside until water has been absorbed (about 10 minutes). Heat olive oil in a large skillet; add garlic and onion and sauté for about 2–3 minutes. Add a pinch of mixed pepper. Add scallops and sauté until opaque in color. Add shrimp, clams, tomatoes, hot pepper and beans; reduce heat to simmer, stir to blend flavors, and cook for another 3–4 minutes. Remove from heat and drain off any excess liquid. Transfer bean mixture to a large bowl, add bulgur and eggs, and stir to mix ingredients. Lightly spray a baking pan with cooking spray. Divide bean mixture into 6 portions and form into patties. Mixture will feel loose but will come together while baking. Place patties on baking sheet, sprinkle with hot sauce, and salt and pepper to taste, and place into a 400-degree oven to bake for about 10–15 minutes. Set oven to broil and lightly brown tops of patties. Remove from oven and serve with lettuce leaves and slices of tomato.

Approx. 196 calories per patty
17g protein, 4g total fat, <0.5g saturated fat, 0 trans fat,
27g carbohydrates, 32mg cholesterol, 317mg sodium, 3g fiber

MOM'S TURKEY BURGERS

MAKES 4 PATTIES

1 pound freshly ground turkey breast
4 cloves fresh garlic, chopped
¼ cup egg substitute or 1 whole egg
1 can (14 ounces) petite cut diced tomatoes with jalapeño peppers, well drained
¼ cup plain bread crumbs
Salt and freshly ground pepper to taste

Preheat oven to broil. In a large mixing bowl, combine turkey, garlic, egg, well-drained tomatoes (put tomatoes in a colander and press down on them with a heavy spoon to drain off as much liquid as possible), bread crumbs, and salt and pepper. Mix well to combine ingredients and form into 4 patties. Place patties on a baking sheet about 4 inches below broiler. Broil each side 3–4 minutes or until tops are crusty and juices run clear when pierced with a fork. Garnish as desired.

Approx. 283 calories per patty
23g protein, 17g total fat, 5g saturated fat, 0 trans fat,
0 carbohydrates, 85mg cholesterol, 75mg sodium, 0 fiber

FETTUCCINE WITH SMOKED SALMON AND BASIL PESTO
MAKES 4 SERVINGS

8 ounces whole grain fettuccine pasta

Extra-virgin olive oil to drizzle

¼ cup fresh Basil Pesto Sauce (page 488) or *market-fresh pesto*

10 pitted black olives, halved

½ tablespoon capers, rinsed well and drained

6 ounces nova smoked salmon (cut into thin strips)

1 tablespoon freshly grated Romano cheese

4 sprigs fresh basil leaves for garnish

Bring water to a boil, add pasta, and cook pasta until *al dente*. Remove from heat, drain pasta, and return to pot, drizzling with scant amount of olive oil to keep pasta from sticking together. Set aside. Meanwhile, warm pesto sauce in a saucepan under low heat, add olives and capers, remove from heat, and add salmon. In a large serving bowl, toss pasta with salmon mixture. Divide into 4 portions and serve each with ¼ tablespoon of Romano cheese, garnished with a fresh basil sprig.

Approx. 323 calories per serving
15g protein, 10g total fat, 2g saturated fat, 0 trans fat,
44g carbohydrates, 14mg cholesterol, 540mg sodium, <1g fiber

BROILED HALIBUT STEAKS WITH TOMATO PESTO

MAKES 4 SERVINGS

4 (6-ounce) halibut steaks
Olive oil cooking spray
Salt and freshly ground pepper to taste
4 tablespoons market-fresh tomato pesto
4 lemon wedges for garnish

Preheat oven to broil. Rinse steaks under cold water and pat dry with paper towels. Lightly spray a broiler pan with cooking spray and place steaks on pan. Season steaks with salt and pepper to taste and place pan under broiler about 4 inches from heat. Cook 4–5 minutes per side or until steaks are opaque in color. Warm pesto in a small saucepan over low heat, stirring constantly. Place steaks on individual plates and top each steak with 1 tablespoon of pesto. Garnish with lemon wedge.

Approx. 261 calories per serving
46g protein, 6g total fat, <1g saturated fat, 0 trans fat,
2g carbohydrates, 69mg cholesterol, 275mg sodium, 0 fiber

CODFISH IN SUNDRIED TOMATO PESTO SAUCE

MAKES 4 SERVINGS

4 medium tomatoes, chopped

4 cloves fresh garlic, chopped

¼ cup market-fresh sundried tomato pesto

1 tablespoon Sambuca

2 tablespoons chopped sundried tomatoes, drained

1 teaspoon capers, drained and well rinsed

10 Kalamata olives, pitted and halved

4 (6-ounce) fillets of cod

⅔ cup dry vermouth

1 bay leaf

¼ teaspoon peppercorns

Salt and freshly ground pepper to taste

4 lemon wedges for garnish

4 fresh parsley sprigs for garnish

In a large heavy skillet, add tomatoes, garlic, pesto, Sambuca, sundried tomatoes, capers, and olives. Cook mixture over medium-low heat. Stir often to marry flavors. Reduce heat to low to keep sauce warm. In a separate skillet, add cod, vermouth, bay leaf, peppercorns, and salt and pepper to taste. Bring to a boil and reduce heat to simmer; cover and simmer for 10–12 minutes or until fish is opaque in color and flakes easily. Meanwhile, warm a platter in the oven at 175 degrees. When fish is ready, transfer to warm platter and return platter to oven to keep fish warm. Drain liquid from fish skillet through a strainer, add strained liquid to tomato pesto sauce, and simmer for 2–3 minutes. Remove fish from oven and spoon sauce over fish; garnish with lemon wedges and parsley sprigs. Serve immediately.

Approx. 214 calories per serving

39g protein, 3.8g total fat, 0.3g saturated fat, 0 trans fat,

10g carbohydrates, 54mg cholesterol, 441mg sodium, 2g fiber

TROUT ALMANDINE

MAKES 4 SERVINGS

4 (4-ounce) trout fillets
1½ tablespoons trans fat–free canola/olive oil spread, melted
3 tablespoons fresh lemon juice
½ teaspoon dried thyme
1 tablespoon finely chopped white onion
Salt to taste
Paprika to sprinkle
3 tablespoons finely chopped fresh parsley
¼ cup sliced raw almonds
Canola oil cooking spray
4 lemon wedges for garnish

Rinse fillets under cold water and pat dry with paper towels. Combine melted canola/olive oil spread, lemon juice, thyme, onion, and salt in a small mixing bowl and whisk to blend flavors. Place fillets in a single layer in an oven-safe casserole dish and pour mixture over fish. Allow mixture to get under fillets as well. Top each fillet with paprika and parsley. Bake at 375 degrees for 12–15 minutes or until fish flakes easily and is opaque in color. Turn oven to broil. Top fish with almonds and spray with a scant amount of cooking spray. Place fillets about 4 inches under broiler and broil fillets for 2–3 minutes or until almonds are lightly toasted. Remove from broiler and serve immediately with lemon wedges.

Approx. 184 calories per serving
24g protein, 10g total fat, 1g saturated fat, 0 trans fat,
2g carbohydrates, 60mg cholesterol, 51mg sodium, 1g fiber

BROILED SCALLOPS WITH ORANGE GINGER SAUCE

MAKES 4 SERVINGS

Olive oil cooking spray
1½ pounds sea scallops
Salt and freshly ground pepper to taste
¼ of a fresh lime
Juice from 3 fresh oranges
¼ cup light mayonnaise
2 tablespoons prepared fresh horseradish
¼ teaspoon honey
¼ teaspoon ground ginger
1 tablespoon extra-virgin olive oil
Generous pinch of all-purpose flour

Spray a large oven-safe casserole dish with cooking spray. Place scallops in a single layer in casserole dish. Sprinkle scallops with salt and pepper to taste. Squeeze juice from ¼ of a fresh lime over scallops. Place casserole dish about 4 inches under broiler and broil scallops until opaque; turn scallops over after 3 minutes and broil other side until also opaque in color. Remove from oven, set aside, and set oven to bake at 175 degrees. Combine orange juice, mayonnaise, horseradish, honey, ginger, olive oil, and salt and pepper in a small saucepan. Whisk to blend on low heat to a simmer. When sauce begins to simmer, whisk in flour. Cook for 1–2 minutes, whisking constantly until sauce is smooth. Add sauce to scallops and return to a slightly warm oven of 175 degrees for 3–4 minutes to allow sauce to thicken and marry flavors with scallops. Serve hot.

Approx. 210 calories per serving
29g protein, 6g total fat, 0.1g saturated fat, 0 trans fat,
13g carbohydrates, 57mg cholesterol, 389mg sodium, 0 fiber

CRAB PATTY BURGERS

MAKES 4 PATTIES

1 pound crabmeat, well drained
¼ cup diced celery
1 tablespoon chopped green bell pepper
1 tablespoon chopped white onion
1 teaspoon Worcestershire sauce
1 teaspoon hot red pepper sauce (optional)
½ teaspoon salt (optional)
Dash of Old Bay seasoning
1 cup light mayonnaise
½ cup grated cheddar cheese
Scant amount of canola oil cooking spray
Lemon wedges for garnish

Mix all ingredients in a large bowl, except lemon wedges. Form into 4 patties and place on broiling sheet lightly sprayed with cooking oil. Place under broiler and broil for about 2 minutes or until patties are lightly browned. Garnish with lemon wedges and serve.

Approx. 375 calories per patty
27g protein, 26g total fat, 5g saturated fat, 0 trans fat,
5g carbohydrates, 136mg cholesterol, 875mg sodium, 0.2g fiber

PAN-GRILLED GROUND PORK BURGERS

MAKES 4 PATTIES

Canola oil cooking spray

1½ pounds fresh lean ground pork

4 scallions, white and green parts, chopped

½ teaspoon garlic powder

½ teaspoon paprika

¼ teaspoon cayenne

Freshly ground pepper to taste

1 tablespoon chopped capers

Raw onion and stone-ground mustard for garnish (optional)

Lightly spray a stovetop ridged grill pan with cooking oil. Turn stovetop to high heat and preheat pan. Mix pork, scallions, spices, and capers together. Divide into 4 patties. When grill pan is very hot, place patties in pan, reduce heat to medium-high, and grill each side for about 4–5 minutes or until juices run clear, flipping patties only once. When completely cooked, serve garnished with sliced raw onion and stone-ground mustard, if desired.

Approx. 220 calories per patty

30g protein, 11g total fat, 4g saturated fat, 0 trans fat,

0 carbohydrates, 85mg cholesterol, 148mg sodium, 0 fiber

MUSSELS IN SPICY RED SAUCE

MAKES 2 SERVINGS

4 cloves fresh garlic, chopped

1 small onion, chopped

½ tablespoon extra-virgin olive oil

1 (28-ounce) can seasoned diced tomatoes, undrained

½ cup dry vermouth or other dry white wine

2 tablespoons canned low-sodium, low-fat chicken stock (optional)

1 teaspoon dried oregano

½ teaspoon Tabasco sauce, or to taste

Salt and freshly ground pepper to taste

1 large shallot, chopped

1 cup water

1 cup dry vermouth

40 small mussels in shells, scrubbed and debearded (about 1½–2 pounds)

Crusty bread (optional)

In a large skillet, sauté garlic and onion in olive oil until soft; do not brown. Add tomatoes and juice, ½ cup vermouth, chicken stock, oregano, Tabasco, and salt and pepper to taste. Stir to blend flavors, bring to a boil, cover, reduce heat to low, and simmer for 15–20 minutes, stirring occasionally. Reduce heat to very low to keep sauce warm. In a large skillet, add shallot, water, 1 cup vermouth, and mussels. Cover skillet and bring to a boil. Reduce heat to simmer and cook until mussels open (5–8 minutes). Discard any mussels that do not open. With a slotted spoon, remove cooked mussels from steam pan and add to sauce. Remove 1 cup of steam broth with shallots included and add to sauce and mussels. Stir sauce to blend in broth and to cover mussels with sauce. Cover skillet and allow mixture to remain on low heat to keep warm for another 5–10 minutes while flavors marry. Divide mussels and sauce into 2 portions, and serve warm with crusty bread to sop up the sauce.

Approx. 240 calories per serving
16g protein, 6g total fat, 0.7g saturated fat, 0 trans fat,
20g carbohydrates, 35mg cholesterol, 770mg sodium, 2g fiber

BAKED OR GRILLED MUSSELS

MAKES 2 SERVINGS

1 large shallot, chopped

1 cup water

1 cup dry vermouth

40 small (about 2 pounds) mussels in shells, scrubbed and debearded

Extra-virgin olive oil to drizzle

2 cloves fresh garlic, finely chopped

2 tablespoons chopped fresh parsley

½ cup plain bread crumbs

Salt and freshly ground pepper to taste

Lemon wedges for garnish

Tabasco sauce (optional)

Crusty bread (optional)

In a large skillet, add shallot, water, vermouth, and mussels. Cover skillet and bring to boil. Reduce heat to simmer and cook until mussels open, about 5–8 minutes; discard any mussels that do not open. Remove mussels with a slotted spoon to a baking tray. Drizzle opened shells with a small amount of olive oil, sprinkle with chopped garlic, parsley, bread crumbs, and salt and pepper to taste. Bake at 350 degrees for about 8–10 minutes or until bread crumbs are golden brown, or grill on a medium-high heat grill (grilling may take a little longer). Divide into 2 portions and serve with lemon wedges, Tabasco sauce, and crusty bread, if desired.

Approx. 126 calories per serving
14g protein, 2g total fat, 0.5g saturated fat, 0 trans fat,
12g carbohydrates, 35mg cholesterol, 336mg sodium, 0 fiber

CHICKEN AND FETA

MAKES 4 SERVINGS

1 cup plain low-fat Greek yogurt
1 tablespoon freshly squeezed lemon juice
½ tablespoon chopped fresh oregano
½ tablespoon chopped fresh rosemary
¼ teaspoon freshly ground pepper
2 large cloves fresh garlic, minced
4 (4-ounce) skinless, boneless chicken breasts
Olive oil cooking spray
⅓ cup crumbled feta cheese
1 tablespoon chopped fresh parsley for garnish

Combine first 6 ingredients in a resealable plastic baggie. Add chicken and toss to coat. Refrigerate marinated chicken for at least 30 minutes. Preheat oven to broil. Remove chicken from bag, reserving marinade. Place chicken on a broiler pan coated with cooking spray. Place pan 6 inches below heat and broil for about 7–8 minutes. Turn chicken, then add reserved marinade to chicken, and top with feta cheese. Continue to broil chicken for an additional 7 minutes or until chicken is cooked through. Remove from oven, sprinkle with parsley, and serve.

Approx. 259 calories per serving
41g protein, 7g total fat, 4g saturated fat, 0 trans fat,
2g carbohydrates, 109mg cholesterol, 608mg sodium, 0 fiber

GRILLED GROUPER

MAKES 4 SERVINGS

¼ cup freshly squeezed lime juice
2 tablespoons chopped fresh cilantro, divided
2 teaspoons olive oil
4 (4-ounce) grouper fillets
¼ teaspoon salt
¼ teaspoon freshly ground pepper
Olive oil cooking spray

Combine lime juice, cilantro, and olive oil in a shallow dish. Add fish fillets to marinade, turning fish to coat well. Cover dish and refrigerate for 30 minutes, turning fish over once after 15 minutes. Remove fish from marinade and discard marinade. Season fish with salt and pepper. Place fish in a cooking spray–coated fish rack and grill in an uncovered grill over a medium-high heat. Grill fish on both sides for about 10 minutes each or until fish flakes easily when tested with a fork. Serve immediately.

Approx. 180 calories per serving
33g protein, 3g total fat, 1g saturated fat, 0 trans fat,
1g carbohydrates, 82mg cholesterol, 105mg sodium, 0 fiber

CRUSTED CHICKEN BREASTS

MAKES 4 SERVINGS

4 (4-ounce) skinless, boneless chicken breasts, pounded to ½-inch thickness
2 tablespoons light mayonnaise
Salt and freshly ground pepper to taste
½ cup grated Pecorino cheese

Preheat oven to 500 degrees. Line a baking sheet with foil and stand a roasting rack inside sheet. With a spatula, lightly coat chicken with mayonnaise, season with salt and pepper to taste, and sprinkle with Pecorino cheese. Place chicken on rack and bake for roughly 5 minutes. Switch oven to broil. Broil chicken until cooked through and cheese is golden brown.

Approx. 246 calories per serving
40g protein, 5g total fat, 3g saturated fat, 0 trans fat,
1g carbohydrates, 111mg cholesterol, 421mg sodium, 0 fiber

FETTUCCINI WITH PROVOLONE CHEESE AND BLACK OLIVE PASTE

MAKES 4 SERVINGS

8 ounces fettuccini
1 tablespoon olive oil
5 tablespoons Black Olive Paste (page 480)
Freshly ground pepper to taste
1½ tablespoons pine nuts
4 ounces provolone cheese, finely grated

Preheat broiler. Cook and drain pasta according to package instructions. Combine drained pasta, olive oil, olive paste, and ground pepper in an oven-safe casserole dish. Spread out evenly. Scatter nuts over pasta and sprinkle on provolone cheese. Place casserole about 6 inches under broiler and heat until cheese is crisp and golden. Serve warm.

Approx. 338 calories per serving
12g protein, 12g total fat, 3g saturated fat, 0 trans fat,
42g carbohydrates, 9mg cholesterol, 519mg sodium, 2g fiber

MUSHROOM AND RICOTTA CANNELLONI

MAKES 4 SERVINGS

½ ounce dried shiitake mushrooms

4½ cups finely chopped cremini mushrooms

2 tablespoons trans fat–free canola/olive oil spread

1 cup low-fat ricotta cheese

2½ teaspoons dried thyme

1 tablespoon lemon zest

3 teaspoons Red Pesto Sauce (page 479)

Salt and freshly ground pepper to taste

8 cannelloni tubes

1 (16-ounce) container fresh marinara sauce

½ cup shaved Parmesan cheese

Soak dried mushrooms in a bowl of boiled water for 15 minutes; then drain and finely chop. In a skillet over medium heat, combine shiitake and cremini mushrooms and canola/olive oil spread and cook until mushrooms are soft and browned and liquid is absorbed. With a slotted spoon, transfer mushrooms to paper towels to drain. In a bowl, combine ricotta cheese with mushrooms. Add in thyme, lemon zest, pesto sauce, and salt and pepper to taste. Mix well and refrigerate for 2 hours. Preheat oven to 400 degrees. Cook cannelloni as per package directions and drain. Fill tubes with mushroom mixture. Place filled tubes in a lightly oiled, shallow casserole dish in a single layer. Pour marinara sauce over pasta and sprinkle with Parmesan cheese, then bake for about 30 minutes until sauce is bubbling and pasta is a golden brown.

Approx. 287 calories per serving
15g protein, 9g total fat, 3g saturated fat, 0 trans fat,
7g carbohydrates, 27mg cholesterol, 310mg sodium, 1g fiber

CRAB CAKES

MAKES 8 SERVINGS

1 pound shelled crabmeat

¼ cup fat-free half-and-half

3 tablespoons light mayonnaise

1 egg, beaten

¼ teaspoon cayenne pepper

1 teaspoon dry mustard

1 tablespoon Worcestershire sauce

2 cups bread crumbs

2 scallions, sliced

4 tablespoons olive oil

Paprika to sprinkle

Pick through the crabmeat to remove any bits of shell. In a small bowl, combine the crabmeat with half-and-half, mayonnaise, egg, cayenne pepper, mustard, and Worcestershire sauce. Stir to blend. Add in bread crumbs and scallions, mix into a sticky consistency, and then shape into patties. Place patties on baking sheet lined with waxed paper and chill for 1 hour in refrigerator. Heat olive oil in a large skillet over medium-high heat. Cook patties for 6–7 minutes, then flip patties over, sprinkle tops with paprika, and cook for 5–6 minutes or until cooked through. Serve warm.

Approx. 108 calories per serving
5g protein, 9g total fat, 1g saturated fat, 0 trans fat,
0 carbohydrates, 58mg cholesterol, 227mg sodium, 0 fiber

SAUTÉED MIXED FISH OVER GARLIC COUSCOUS

MAKES 6 SERVINGS

1 pound codfish, cut into 1-inch pieces
½ pound raw shrimp, peeled, deveined, and coarsely chopped
½ pound bay scallops
4 scallions, sliced
½ cup chopped fresh chives
½ cup chopped fresh parsley
3 tablespoons bread crumbs
1 tablespoon Dijon mustard
1 tablespoon light mayonnaise
2 eggs, beaten
Salt and freshly ground pepper to taste
2 tablespoons olive oil
Hot sauce to taste (optional)
2 (5.4-ounce) boxes garlic-flavored couscous

In a large bowl, combine codfish, shrimp, scallops, scallions, chives, parsley, bread crumbs, mustard, mayonnaise, eggs, and salt and pepper to taste. Using a large spoon, mix ingredients. In a large skillet, heat olive oil over medium heat. Add fish mixture and cook, stirring often, until fish is cooked through and lightly browned. Sprinkle with hot sauce, if desired. Reduce heat to very low and cover to keep warm. Prepare couscous as per package instructions. Divide fish into 6 portions and serve over couscous.

Approx. 172 calories per serving
30g protein, 6g total fat, 0 saturated fat, 0 trans fat,
43g carbohydrates, 157mg cholesterol, 323mg sodium, 1g fiber

GNOCCHI WITH SHRIMP AND ASPARAGUS

MAKES 4 SERVINGS

1 (16-ounce) package vacuum-packed gnocchi

1 tablespoon olive oil

½ cup sliced shallots

4 cups sliced asparagus (about 1 pound)

¾ cup canned low-sodium, fat-free chicken broth

1 pound large raw shrimp, peeled, deveined, tails off, coarsely chopped

Salt and freshly ground pepper to taste

2 tablespoons freshly squeezed lemon juice

⅓ cup grated Parmesan cheese

Bring 2 cups water to a boil in a large pot. Add gnocchi and cook for 4 minutes or until done (gnocchi will rise to surface). Remove gnocchi with a slotted spoon, place in a bowl, and set aside. In a large skillet, add olive oil and shallots. Cook over medium heat, stirring, until shallots begin to brown, about 1–2 minutes. Stir in asparagus and broth. Cover and cook until asparagus is crispy tender, about 3–4 minutes. Add shrimp and salt and pepper to taste, then cover and let simmer until shrimp is pink and almost cooked through. Add gnocchi to shrimp mixture along with lemon juice and cook, stirring, until heated through, about 2 minutes. Remove from heat, sprinkle with Parmesan cheese, and let stand until cheese is melted, about 1–2 minutes, and serve.

Approx. 358 calories per serving
29g protein, 7g total fat, 2g saturated fat, 0 trans fat,
40g carbohydrates, 179mg cholesterol, 814mg sodium, 2g fiber

PORK MARSALA

MAKES 4 SERVINGS

6 thin-cut (about ½-inch) boneless pork chops, cut into ¼-inch pieces

Salt and freshly ground pepper to taste

¼ cup all-purpose flour, divided

3 tablespoons trans fat–free canola/olive oil spread, divided

1 tablespoon olive oil

8 ounces button mushrooms, quartered

1 small white onion, finely chopped

¾ cup sweet Marsala wine

½ cup canned low-sodium, fat-free chicken broth

2 teaspoons freshly squeezed lemon juice

1 tablespoon chopped fresh parsley

Pasta of choice

Rinse chops under cold water and pat dry with paper towels. In a small bowl, combine salt and pepper with 3 tablespoons flour. Lightly dredge pork chops in flour mixture, shaking off any excess flour. Melt 2 tablespoons canola/olive oil spread and olive oil in a large skillet over medium-high heat. Add chops and cook until browned, about 2 minutes per side. Transfer to a plate, cover with foil, and set aside. Melt remaining spread in the same skillet and add mushrooms, onion, and salt and pepper to taste. Cook for about 8 minutes until mushrooms are soft and browned. Add in remaining flour, stirring to incorporate, about 1 minute. Whisk in Marsala and broth and cook until slightly thickened, roughly 2 minutes. Add pork pieces, juices from plate, lemon juice, and parsley, and let simmer until ingredients are heated through and flavors have melded. Serve over cooked pasta.

Approx. 336 calories per serving
18g protein, 20g total fat, 5g saturated fat, 0 trans fat,
6g carbohydrates, 51mg cholesterol, 331mg sodium, 0 fiber

CHICKEN AND PENNE PASTA IN A GARLIC SAUCE

MAKES 6 SERVINGS

8 cloves fresh garlic, minced

¼ teaspoon crushed red hot pepper flakes (more or less to taste)

6 tablespoons olive oil

4 skinless, boneless chicken breasts (roughly 1½ pounds)

Salt and freshly ground pepper to taste

1 pound whole wheat penne pasta

1 (5-ounce) bag baby spinach

½ cup chopped fresh basil

6 tablespoons freshly squeezed lemon juice

1 cup grated Parmesan cheese

In a small skillet, combine garlic, hot pepper flakes, and olive oil, cook over medium heat until garlic is fragrant and browned. Set aside. Rinse chicken under cold water and pat dry with paper towels. Sprinkle with salt and pepper. In a large skillet add 1 tablespoon of garlic-oil mixture and heat over medium-high heat until olive oil begins to smoke. Add chicken and cook about 5 minutes per side until well-browned and cooked through. Remove from skillet, allow to cool slightly before cutting breasts into thin slices, and set aside. Cook pasta according to package instructions. Drain pasta, reserving ½ cup of pasta liquid. Return pasta to pot and stir in chicken, spinach, basil, lemon juice, Parmesan cheese, and remaining garlic-oil mixture. Add reserved pasta water, as desired, to thin sauce. Serve.

Approx. 583 calories per serving
40g protein, 22g total fat, 5g saturated fat, 0 trans fat
58g carbohydrates, 80mg cholesterol, 440mg sodium, 4g fiber

CHICKEN AND WILD RICE WITH GARDEN VEGETABLES
MAKES 4 SERVINGS

For Marinade (discard after use):

1½ cups balsamic vinegar

½ cup canola or olive oil

½ cup honey

⅓ cup chopped fresh oregano

⅓ cup chopped fresh sage

½ teaspoon ground cumin

4 skinless, boneless chicken breasts (about 1½ pounds)

4 tablespoons trans fat–free canola/olive oil spread

2 cups canned low-sodium, fat-free chicken broth

1 cup long grain wild rice

½ cup fresh or frozen peas

½ cup fresh or frozen corn

½ cup diced celery

3 scallions, thinly sliced

Salt and freshly ground pepper to taste

Marinade:

In a large, resealable plastic baggie, combine vinegar, oil, honey, oregano, sage, cumin, and chicken breasts. Turn to coat chicken with ingredients and refrigerate for at least 3 hours. When chicken has marinated, remove with tongs, allowing excess marinade to drip off. Transfer to a plate and discard remaining marinade.

In a large skillet, melt canola/olive oil spread over medium-high heat. Add chicken and cook until browned on both sides and well done (juices will run clear when cooked through). Transfer to a warmed plate and cover with foil. In the same skillet, pour in broth, scraping up loose chicken pieces and drippings to blend with broth. Add in rice, peas, corn, celery, and scallions. Bring to a boil, then reduce heat to a simmer. Stir to mix ingredients, then cover and cook until liquid is absorbed and rice is tender. Slice chicken and serve over rice and vegetable mixture. Add salt and pepper to taste if needed.

Approx. 518 calories per serving
35g protein, 14g total fat, 3g saturated fat, 0 trans fat,
59g carbohydrates, 65mg cholesterol, 320mg sodium, 5g fiber

LEMONY PASTA WITH GOAT CHEESE AND SPINACH

MAKES 4 SERVINGS

¾ pounds ziti pasta
6 ounces fresh goat cheese
10 cups fresh baby spinach
3 cups fresh parsley, chopped
2 cups fresh cilantro, chopped
1 tablespoon grated lemon zest
1 tablespoon freshly squeezed lemon juice
½ cup pine nuts for garnish

In a large pot, cook pasta according to package instructions. Drain and reserve 2 cups pasta liquid. In the same empty pot, combine 1 cup cooked pasta and goat cheese and heat over medium heat. Add the remaining cooked pasta, spinach, parsley, cilantro, and lemon zest and juice. Stir, adding remaining reserved pasta water a little at a time to create a light sauce that coats pasta. Transfer to 4 plates, sprinkle with pine nuts, and serve.

Approx. 305 calories per serving
13g protein, 23g total fat, 9g saturated fat, 0 trans fat,
5g carbohydrates, 32mg cholesterol, 210mg sodium, 1g fiber

ROASTED SEAFOOD MEDLEY

MAKES 6 SERVINGS

For the Lobster:

2 tablespoons olive oil, divided

1½ tablespoons fresh garlic paste blend

2 teaspoons minced fresh parsley

Juice from ½ of a lemon

3 large frozen uncooked lobster tails, thawed and cut lengthwise in half

Butter spray (optional)

Salt and freshly ground pepper to taste

Paprika to sprinkle

For the Shrimp and Scallops:

4 tablespoons olive oil

8 teaspoons minced shallots

4 teaspoons minced fresh parsley

¼ teaspoon lemon zest

Salt and freshly ground pepper to taste

6 uncooked jumbo shrimp (about 12 ounces), peeled, deveined, and butterflied

6 very large sea scallops

For the Crab:

2 pounds cooked large Alaskan King crab legs, cut lengthwise in half

4 tablespoons water

¼ cup trans fat–free canola/olive oil spread, melted

2 tablespoons freshly squeezed lemon juice

Lemon wedges

Fresh Italian parsley sprigs

Preheat oven to 450 degrees. Brush 2 large roasting pans with 1 tablespoon olive oil each. Mix together garlic paste, 2 teaspoons minced parsley, and juice from half a lemon in a small bowl. Arrange lobster tails, cut side up, in 1 roasting pan. Brush tails with garlic mixture, spray each tail with butter spray, if desired, and sprinkle with salt and pepper and a generous amount of paprika. Roast until flesh is opaque in center, about 15 minutes.

Meanwhile, in another small bowl, combine 4 tablespoons olive oil, minced shallots, 4 teaspoons minced parsley, lemon zest, and salt and pepper to taste. Mix well to blend. Set aside. In the second roasting pan, combine shrimp and scallops in a single layer. Using a spoon, stir often while drizzling half of the lemon zest–shallot mixture over shrimp and scallops, reserving half of mixture for crab legs. Place second roaster in oven next to lobster pan. Roast shrimp and scallops until opaque and cooked through.

When lobster is roasted, transfer to a large platter and cover with foil to keep warm. Arrange crab legs in lobster roaster, drizzle with remaining lemon zest–shallot mixture and with water. Roast just until legs are heated through, about 5 minutes. Add shrimp, scallops, and crab legs to lobster platter. Scrape drippings from both roasters into a small bowl, then add in melted canola/olive oil spread and lemon juice. Whisk to blend and drizzle mixture over tops of seafood. Garnish with lemon wedges and parsley sprigs and serve.

Approx. 433 calories per serving
32g protein, 27g total fat, 3g saturated fat, 0 trans fat,
2g carbohydrates, 207mg cholesterol, 532mg sodium, 0 fiber

PORK CHOPS AND SAGE

MAKES 4 SERVINGS

2 tablespoons all-purpose flour
1 tablespoon chopped fresh sage
Salt and freshly ground pepper to taste
4 (96-ounce) bone-in pork chops, excess fat removed
2 tablespoons olive oil
2 tablespoons trans fat–free canola/olive oil spread
2 tablespoons white wine, for deglazing

Combine flour, sage, and salt and pepper to taste on a large, low-rimmed plate. Dust both sides of each pork chop with the flour mixture. Combine olive oil and canola/olive oil spread in a large skillet and heat over medium-high heat. Add pork chops and cook for 6–7 minutes on each side or until thoroughly cooked; reduce heat to a simmer. With a slotted large spatula, transfer pork chops to a warmed plate. Add wine to skillet and scrape up pieces from bottom of pan to create a deglazed sauce. Pour deglazed sauce over pork chops and serve.

Approx. 345 calories per serving
37g protein, 20g total fat, 5g saturated fat, 0 trans fat,
0 carbohydrates, 107mg cholesterol, 162mg sodium, 0 fiber

EASY TURKEY MEATLOAF
MAKES 8 SERVINGS

1 tablespoon olive oil

3 cloves fresh garlic, chopped

1½ cups chopped white onion

½ cup chopped carrot

½ cup chopped celery

Salt to taste

½ teaspoon freshly ground pepper

1½ teaspoons Worcestershire sauce

⅓ cup canned low-sodium, fat-free chicken broth

3 ounces tomato paste

2 large eggs, beaten

¾ cup Italian style bread crumbs

1¾ pounds ground turkey

Olive oil cooking spray

Preheat oven to 375 degrees. Heat olive oil in a medium skillet over medium-high heat. Add garlic and onion and sauté until soft and fragrant. Add carrot, celery, and salt and pepper, then cook until vegetables are soft. Stir in Worcestershire sauce, broth, tomato paste, and eggs. Allow to slightly cool. Transfer mixture to a bowl and fold in bread crumbs and ground turkey. Mix ingredients well. Spray the inside of a 9x13 inch loaf pan with cooking oil. Transfer turkey mixture to loaf pan and spread out evenly. Bake for 1 hour or until meat thermometer inserted into center reads 170 degrees. Remove from oven and let stand for 5 minutes before serving.

Approx. 224 calories per serving
20g protein, 12g total fat, 2g saturated fat, 0 trans fat,
8g carbohydrates, 132mg cholesterol, 309mg sodium, 1g fiber

TURKEY TETRAZZINI

MAKES 8 SERVINGS

Olive oil cooking spray
1 pound spaghetti
½ cup trans fat–free canola/olive oil spread
½ cup all-purpose flour
3 cups canned low-sodium, fat-free chicken broth
2 cups low-fat milk
8 ounces frozen peas
1½ cups grated Parmesan cheese, divided
4 cups chopped cooked turkey meat
Paprika to sprinkle

Preheat oven to 350 degrees. Lightly spray the inside of an oven-safe casserole dish with cooking oil. Bring a large pot of water to a rapid boil and cook pasta as per package instructions. Drain pasta and transfer to casserole dish. In a sauce-pan, melt canola/olive oil spread over medium heat. Stir in flour until smooth. Add broth, milk, and peas. Cook and stir until it comes to a boil. Stir in 1¼ cups Parmesan cheese and remove mixture from heat. Add in turkey meat, stir, and pour mixture over pasta. Toss to mix and sprinkle top with remaining cheese and paprika. Transfer to oven and bake for 1 hour, until top is lightly browned.

Approx. 550 calories per serving
37g protein, 29g total fat, 8g saturated fat, 0 trans fat,
107g carbohydrates, 17mg cholesterol, 393mg sodium, 2g fiber

GRILLED COD

MAKES 4 SERVINGS

1½ pounds fresh codfish

Olive oil cooking spray

Salt to taste

¼ teaspoon freshly ground pepper

⅛ teaspoon garlic powder

2 tablespoons trans fat–free canola/olive oil spread

2 tablespoons freshly squeezed lemon juice

Lemon wedges

Heat grill to medium-high heat. Place a rimmed baking sheet on grill. Spray both sides of fish with cooking oil and sprinkle fish with salt, pepper, and garlic powder. Place fish on baking sheet and grill, turning once, until opaque (about 3–5 minutes per side depending on thickness). In a small microwavable bowl, combine canola/olive oil spread and lemon juice and melt in microwave. Drizzle fish with mixture and serve with lemon wedges.

Approx. 189 calories per serving
30g protein, 6g total fat, 2g saturated fat, 0 trans fat,
0 carbohydrates, 63mg cholesterol, 170mg sodium, 0 fiber

CHICKEN CACCIATORE

MAKES 4 SERVINGS

4 chicken thighs

2 chicken breasts, with skin and bones and halved

Salt and freshly ground pepper to taste

1 cup all-purpose flour

3 tablespoons olive oil

1 green bell pepper, seeded and sliced

1 red bell pepper, seeded and sliced

1 onion, chopped

1 carrot, finely chopped

1 celery stalk, finely chopped

3 cloves fresh garlic, finely chopped

⅔ cup white wine

1 (28-ounce) can chopped tomatoes, undrained

3 tablespoons capers

1½ teaspoons dried oregano

Rinse chicken and pat dry with paper towels. Combine salt and pepper with flour in a bowl and lightly dredge chicken in flour mixture. Heat olive oil in a large skillet over medium-high heat. Add chicken and sauté for about 5 minutes per side. Remove from skillet and set aside. In the same skillet, combine green and red bell peppers, onion, carrot, celery, and garlic and sauté until tender. Add wine and let simmer until reduced by half, about 5 minutes. Add tomatoes and juices, capers, oregano, and salt and pepper to taste. Return chicken to skillet, cover, and let simmer for roughly 30 minutes, stirring often, until chicken is completely cooked through. Divide into 4 portions and serve.

Approx. 455 calories per serving
29g protein, 13g total fat, 4g saturated fat, 0 trans fat,
31g carbohydrates, 86mg cholesterol, 445mg sodium, 2g fiber

PASTA WITH SALMON SAUCE

MAKES 4 SERVINGS

8 ounces spaghetti pasta
Extra-virgin olive oil to drizzle
½ cup reduced-fat feta cheese
1 tablespoon chopped fresh parsley for garnish

For Salmon Sauce:

1½ cups fat-free half-and-half
⅔ cup whiskey
6 ounces smoked salmon, cut into thin strips
Generous pinch of cayenne pepper
Salt and freshly ground pepper to taste

Cook pasta according to package instructions. Drain and drizzle with a scant amount of olive oil. Toss pasta and set aside.

Sauce:

In a small saucepan, combine half-and-half and whiskey and bring to a simmer. Do not boil. Add salmon, cayenne, and salt and pepper to taste. Transfer pasta to a large pasta bowl, pour in sauce, and toss to coat. Sprinkle on feta cheese and parsley and serve immediately.

Approx. 388 calories per serving
18g protein, 5g total fat, 2g saturated fat, 0 trans fat,
49g carbohydrates, 17mg cholesterol, 568mg sodium, 2g fiber

MUSTARD AND SMOKED PAPRIKA BAKED CHICKEN

MAKES 4 SERVINGS

1½ pounds skinless, bone-in chicken

4 tablespoons trans fat–free canola/olive oil spread, melted

4 tablespoons Dijon mustard

2 tablespoons freshly squeezed lemon juice

2 teaspoons light brown sugar

1 teaspoon smoked paprika

1 teaspoon dried basil

½ teaspoon dried parsley

Salt and freshly ground pepper to taste

Preheat oven to 400 degrees. Arrange chicken pieces in an oven-safe casserole dish. In a bowl, combine canola/olive oil spread, mustard, lemon juice, sugar, paprika, basil, parsley, and salt and pepper to taste. Brush half of the mixture over tops of chicken and bake at 400 degrees for 15 minutes. Remove casserole from oven, carefully turn chicken over, and coat surface with remaining mustard mixture. Return chicken to oven to bake for additional 15 minutes. Test for doneness by piercing thick part of chicken with the tines of a fork; juices should run clear.

Approx. 229 calories per serving
40g protein, 5g total fat, 2g saturated fat, 0 trans fat,
2g carbohydrates, 100mg cholesterol, 349mg sodium, 1g fiber

PENNE WITH PANCETTA AND MUSHROOMS

MAKES 4 SERVINGS

1½ cups canned sodium-free, fat-free beef broth

1 cup dry red wine

2 tablespoons olive oil, divided

1 tablespoon minced fresh garlic

10 ounces assorted mixed mushrooms, cut into large pieces

Salt and freshly ground pepper to taste

4 ounces thinly sliced pancetta, coarsely chopped

2 tablespoons trans fat–free canola/olive oil spread

¼ teaspoon dry Italian seasoning mix

10 ounces penne pasta

½ cup finely grated Parmesan cheese + more for garnish

In a medium saucepan, bring broth and wine to a boil over medium-high heat. Cook until reduced to roughly 1 cup, about 20 minutes. Meanwhile, heat 1 table-spoon olive oil in a large skillet over medium-high heat. Add garlic and sauté until fragrant and soft. Add mushrooms and salt and pepper. Sauté mushrooms until tender. Transfer mushrooms to a plate and add remaining olive oil and pancetta pieces to pan. Sauté until pancetta starts to brown. Add wine reduction, canola/olive oil spread, and Italian seasoning and let simmer until liquid thickens slightly, about 3–5 minutes. Add mushrooms to mixture and season with salt and pepper to taste.

Cook pasta as per package instructions. Drain and reserve ½ cup pasta liquid. Stir pasta and ½ cup Parmesan cheese into mushroom mixture and cook over medium heat, adding reserved pasta water a little at a time if mixture is dry. Cook until sauce thickens and clings to pasta. Transfer to large pasta bowl and serve with a sprinkling of Parmesan cheese.

Approx. 471 calories per serving
18g protein, 16g total fat, 3g saturated fat, 0 trans fat,
56g carbohydrates, 11mg cholesterol, 368mg sodium, 2g fiber

WHITE BEANS AND WILD MUSHROOMS WITH CHICKEN

MAKES 4–6 SERVINGS

2 tablespoons olive oil

4 cloves fresh garlic, minced

6 cups, halved assorted mushrooms (such as cremini, oyster, shiitake, button)

1 cup canned low-sodium, fat-free chicken broth

2 (15.5-ounce) cans white beans, drained and rinsed

2 tablespoons fresh garlic paste blend

Crushed red hot pepper flakes to taste

Salt and freshly ground pepper to taste

2 tablespoons porcini-infused olive oil

4 (4-ounce) skinless, boneless chicken breasts, cut to bite-sized pieces

4 tablespoons chopped fresh parsley

Grated Parmesan cheese (optional)

In a large skillet, heat olive oil over medium-high heat. Add garlic and sauté until fragrant. Add mushrooms and cook until softened. Add broth, beans, garlic paste, hot pepper flakes, and salt and pepper to taste. Stir to incorporate ingredients and reduce heat to a simmer. Let simmer uncovered, stirring occasionally, until juices thicken. While bean mixture simmers, heat porcini olive oil in a separate skillet over medium-high heat and cook chicken until cooked through and lightly browned. Add salt and pepper to taste. Add chicken and juices to bean mixture and continue to let simmer, stirring occasionally. Add parsley and continue to let simmer for 5 more minutes or until juices have thickened. Serve hot with a sprinkling of Parmesan cheese, if desired.

Approx. 210 calories per serving
9g protein, 13g total fat, 3g saturated fat, 0 trans fat,
22g carbohydrates, 63mg cholesterol, 513mg sodium, 6g fiber

PASTA FRESCA WITH FRESH CRAB AND LEMON

MAKES 2 SERVINGS

5 tablespoons olive oil, divided

2 cloves fresh garlic, minced

1 cup grape tomatoes, halved

1 red jalapeño pepper, seeded and thinly sliced

Salt to taste

2 tablespoons chopped fresh basil + more for garnish

1 tablespoon trans fat–free canola/olive oil spread

1 small shallot, finely chopped

10 ounces cooked and shelled jumbo lump crabmeat

4 tablespoons white wine or vermouth

1 (9-ounce) package of fresh linguine pasta

½ of a fresh lemon to squeeze

Finely grated Parmesan cheese for garnish

In a large skillet, heat 4 tablespoons of olive oil over medium-high heat. Add garlic and sauté until fragrant and starts to sizzle. Add tomatoes and cook for a few minutes until they begin to break down. Reduce heat to a simmer and add jalapeño slices, salt, and 2 tablespoons chopped basil. Stir mixture and cook for another 2 minutes. Transfer tomato mixture to a small bowl and set aside. In the same skillet, heat canola/olive oil spread with remaining olive oil over medium-high heat. Add shallot and sauté until lightly browned. Add crabmeat, gently sautéing until crabmeat begins to brown. Add wine to crab mixture, gently scraping loose bits of crabmeat and other bits from sides and bottom of pan. Return reserved tomato mixture to crabmeat mixture and gently stir to combine, reducing heat to very low to keep sauce warm.

Cook fresh pasta as per package instructions and drain. Add pasta to tomato mixture and toss to coat. Divide pasta into 2 portions and top with remaining chopped basil. Squeeze fresh lemon juice over each serving and sprinkle with Parmesan cheese. Serve immediately.

Approx. 300 calories per serving
72g protein, 13g total fat, 2g saturated fat, 0 trans fat,
23g carbohydrates, 132mg cholesterol, 370mg sodium, 1g fiber

ROASTED SALMON WITH WILTED SPINACH

MAKES 4 SERVINGS

½ tablespoon brown sugar

½ tablespoon smoked paprika

½ teaspoon Saigon cinnamon

½ teaspoon orange zest

¼ teaspoon salt or to taste

4 (4-ounce) salmon fillets, skinless

2 teaspoons olive oil

3 teaspoons fresh minced garlic

1 (9-ounce) bag fresh spinach

Preheat oven and a shallow heavy-bottomed roasting pan to 400 degrees. In a small bowl, combine sugar, paprika, cinnamon, orange zest, and salt. Rub both sides of fillets evenly with spice mix and place fillets on roaster. Roast for roughly 10 minutes, turning once after about 5 minutes or until fish flakes easily with a fork. While fish is roasting, add olive oil to a skillet over medium heat, then add garlic and sauté until fragrant. Add a few bunches of spinach at a time, until all is wilted. When fillets are cooked, divide spinach onto 4 plates, top each with a salmon fillet, and serve.

Approx. 292 calories per serving
26g protein, 19g total fat, 3g saturated fat, 0 trans fat,
4g carbohydrates, 70mg cholesterol, 106mg sodium, 1g fiber

STUFFED ZUCCHINI WITH VEGETABLES AND SWEET ITALIAN SAUSAGE

MAKES 6 SERVINGS

6 large zucchini squash

2 tablespoons olive oil + more to drizzle

Salt and freshly ground pepper to taste

2 cups torn stale bread, crust removed

2 cups fat-free milk

2 cloves fresh garlic, minced

1 small onion, finely chopped

1 yellow bell pepper, finely minced

½ pound ground turkey sausage

½ cup grated Parmesan cheese

1 teaspoon dry Italian seasoning mix

2 tablespoons chopped fresh parsley

Preheat oven to 375 degrees. Cut zucchini in half lengthwise. With a melon spoon, scoop out the zucchini flesh to form a cavity. Reserve flesh and set aside. Cut off a slice from the bottom of each zucchini piece to allow squash to lie flat in the bottom of a casserole dish. Drizzle each piece with olive oil, season with salt and pepper to taste, and set aside.

Place the torn bread in a bowl and add milk. Allow bread to soften in liquid for 10 minutes. Heat 2 tablespoons olive oil in a large skillet over medium-high heat. Add garlic, onion, and yellow bell pepper and sauté until soft. Add reserved chopped zucchini flesh and continue to cook until soft, about 5 minutes. In a large bowl, combine sausage, sautéed vegetables, Parmesan cheese, Italian seasoning, and parsley. Squeeze milk from bread and add bread to mixture. Using your hands, mix ingredients to blend. Stuff the cavity of each zucchini with a generous amount of stuffing mixture. Place casserole dish with stuffed zucchini on the middle rack of oven and bake for 20–30 minutes until sausage is cooked through and browned.

Approx. 213 calories per serving
16g protein, 11g total fat, 3g saturated fat, 0 trans fat,
15g carbohydrates, 76mg cholesterol, 236mg sodium, 4g fiber

HONEY MUSTARD SHRIMP

MAKES 4 SERVINGS

1 tablespoon olive oil

2 cloves fresh garlic, minced

¾ canned cup low-sodium, fat-free chicken broth

1 pound raw medium shrimp (about 30–32 shrimp), peeled and deveined

¼ cup fresh honey mustard salad dressing, store bought

½ teaspoon garlic powder

Salt and freshly ground pepper to taste

In a large skillet, heat olive oil and add garlic. Sauté until garlic is soft. Add broth and shrimp and cook until shrimp becomes pink and cooked through. Reduce heat to very low to keep shrimp warm. In a saucepan, warm the honey mustard dressing with garlic powder and salt and pepper. Drain liquid from shrimp and add warmed mustard mixture to shrimp, then return to very low heat while stirring to coat shrimp and incorporate flavors, about 5 minutes. Serve immediately.

Approx. 202 calories per serving
23g protein, 8g total fat, 1g saturated fat, 0 trans fat,
8g carbohydrates, 172mg cholesterol, 270mg sodium, 0 fiber

PEPPERED FILLET OF SOLE

MAKES 4 SERVINGS

1 tablespoon olive oil

1 tablespoon trans fat–free canola/olive oil spread

2 cups sliced button mushrooms

1 medium shallot, finely chopped

4 (4-ounce) sole fillets

1 teaspoon lemon pepper seasoning

1 teaspoon paprika

Cayenne pepper to taste

1 medium tomato, chopped

2 scallions, thinly sliced

In a large skillet over medium heat, melt olive oil and canola/olive oil spread. Add mushrooms and shallot and sauté until soft. Place fillets over mushroom mixture. Sprinkle each fillet with lemon pepper seasoning, paprika, and cayenne. Cover skillet and cook over medium heat until fish flakes easily. Divide into 4 portions and sprinkle each serving with tomatoes and scallions. Serve while hot.

Approx. 203 calories per serving
31g protein, 8g total fat, 2g saturated fat, 0 trans fat,
0 carbohydrates, 86mg cholesterol, 158mg sodium, <0.5g fiber

BROILED SPICY RAINBOW TROUT

MAKES 4 SERVINGS

For Fish:

4 (6-ounce) fillets (about ½-inch thickness)

2 teaspoons olive oil

1 tablespoon spice seasoning (below)

2 tablespoons chopped fresh parsley

1 scallion, chopped

Lemon wedges for garnish

For the Seasoning:

1¼ teaspoons freshly ground pepper

2 teaspoons salt or to taste

¼ teaspoon cayenne pepper

1 tablespoon paprika

1 teaspoon chili pepper

1 teaspoon dried oregano

1 teaspoon dry mustard

Preheat broiler. Rinse fillets under cold water and pat dry. Lightly oil fillets on both sides with a basting brush.

Make seasoning by combining ground pepper, salt, cayenne, paprika, chili pepper, oregano, and mustard in a bowl. Sprinkle both sides of fillets with seasoning and place skin-side down in a broiler pan. Place pan 4–6 inches below broiler and broil fillets for 4–5 minutes or until fish flakes easily. Serve fillets sprinkled with parsley, scallion, and lemon wedges.

Approx. 324 calories per serving
34g protein, 17g total fats, 2g saturated fats, 0 trans fats,
1g carbohydrates, 100mg cholesterol, 66mg sodium, 1g fiber

BROILED CHICKEN AND BARLEY WITH VEGETABLES

MAKES 4 SERVINGS

¼ cup freshly squeezed lemon juice

1 teaspoon olive oil

2 cloves fresh garlic, minced

½ teaspoon dried oregano

¼ teaspoon dried basil

4 (4-ounce) skinless, boneless chicken breasts

1½ cups canned low-sodium, fat-free chicken broth

2 cups quick barley

1 teaspoon olive oil

1 medium carrot, chopped

¾ cup chopped fresh mushrooms

½ cup chopped green bell pepper

¼ cup chopped onion

Salt and freshly ground pepper to taste

In a large, resealable plastic baggie, combine the first 5 ingredients. Seal bag and shake well to blend ingredients. Add chicken, reseal bag, and toss again until chicken is well coated. Refrigerate to marinate for at least 1 hour. In a large saucepan, bring broth to a boil. Stir in barley. Reduce heat, then cover and let simmer for 10–12 minutes or until tender. In a non-stick skillet, heat olive oil over medium-high heat. Add carrot, mushrooms, green bell pepper, onion, and salt and pepper to taste. Sauté until pepper and onion are tender. Stir vegetables into barley and keep warm. Preheat broiler. Place marinated chicken on a broiler pan about 4–6 inches from heat. Broil chicken until juices run clear, about 4–8 minutes or until meat thermometer reads 170 degrees. Serve chicken fillets over barley mixture.

Approx. 410 calories per serving
32g protein, 13g total fat, 1g saturated fat, 0 trans fat,
44g carbohydrates, 65mg cholesterol, 195mg sodium, 6g fiber

SCALLOPS WITH BRAISED APPLES

MAKES 4 SERVINGS

1 large Granny Smith apple, cored, peeled, and cut to ¼-inch cubes
¼ cup unsweetened apple juice
2 tablespoons freshly squeezed lemon juice
2 tablespoons olive oil
1 pound sea scallops (about 12 scallops)
Salt and freshly ground pepper to taste
1 tablespoon trans fat–free canola/olive oil spread
¼ cup pea shoots

In a small bowl, combine cubed apples and both juices. Set aside. In a large skillet, heat olive oil over medium-high heat. Add scallops, seasoned with salt and pepper to taste, and cook until golden brown and just cooked through. Transfer to a warming plate. Add canola/olive oil spread to the same skillet. Melt the spread while scraping up browned bits of scallops from the bottom of the skillet. Add reserved apple mixture to skillet and cook, stirring often until juice is thickened and apple cubes are tender. Spoon apple sauce over warmed scallops, top with pea shoots, and serve.

Approx. 213 calories per serving
25g protein, 11g total fat, 2g saturated fat, 0 trans fat,
9g carbohydrates, 35mg cholesterol, 197mg sodium, 1g fiber

ORECCHIETTE WITH SPINACH, KALE, TOASTED BREAD CRUMBS, AND PINE NUTS IN A RED SAUCE

MAKES 4 SERVINGS

½ pound whole wheat orecchiette pasta

⅓ cup pine nuts

2 tablespoons olive oil

¼ cup finely chopped white onion

2 tablespoons finely chopped fresh garlic

1 cup panko bread crumbs

¼ cup canned low-sodium, fat-free chicken broth

1 cup fresh spinach leaves

1 cup fresh kale, leaves only, torn into bite-sized pieces

Salt and freshly ground pepper to taste

24 ounces fresh, store-bought marinara sauce

Grated Parmesan cheese for garnish

Cook pasta according to package instructions. Drain pasta and set aside. In a large skillet over medium heat, toast pine nuts until golden brown, stirring often. Once toasted, remove from skillet and set aside. In the same skillet, add olive oil, onion, and garlic, and cook until soft and fragrant. Add bread crumbs and continue to cook, stirring mixture often until crumbs are browned. Remove from heat and toss with toasted pine nuts. Set aside. In a separate skillet, add broth, spinach, and kale. Season with salt and pepper to taste. Cook and stir often until spinach and kale soften and wilt. Add spinach-kale mixture to garlic-onion mixture and toss. In a saucepan over medium heat, warm marinara sauce. Add drained pasta and heated marinara to spinach-kale mixture and toss well to coat pasta. Sprinkle with Parmesan cheese and serve.

Approx. 488 calories per serving
12g protein, 24g total fat, 3g saturated fat, 0 trans fat,
61g carbohydrates, 0 cholesterol, 448mg sodium, 4g fiber

GARLIC SALMON LINGUINI
MAKES 6 SERVINGS

1 pound fresh salmon fillet, skinless
Blackening seasoning of choice
2 tablespoons olive oil
4 cloves fresh garlic, minced
¾ cup canned low-sodium, fat-free chicken broth
⅛ teaspoon cayenne pepper (optional)
Salt and freshly ground pepper to taste
¼ cup minced fresh parsley
2 (9-ounce) packages fresh linguini

Preheat oven to 450 degrees. While oven reaches temperature, place a cast-iron skillet in oven to heat. Season fillet on both sides with desired amount of blackening seasoning. When oven and pan have reached desired heat, place fillet in skillet and cook until fillet is opaque halfway through, about 3 minutes depending on thickness. Turn fillet over and cook remaining side until fish flakes easily. While fish is cooking, add olive oil to a separate skillet and heat on stove over medium-high heat. When olive oil is hot, add garlic and cook until fragrant. Reduce heat and add chicken broth. Keep warm until salmon is cooked. Cut cooked fillet into bite-sized pieces and add to chicken broth. Season with cayenne, if desired, and salt and pepper to taste. Add minced parsley and allow flavor to warm and blend. Cook pasta according to package instructions. Drain pasta and add salmon mixture to noodles, tossing pasta well to coat.

Approx. 209 calories per serving
18g protein, 9g total fat, 1g saturated fat, 0 trans fat,
15g carbohydrates, 56mg cholesterol, 67mg sodium, 1g fiber

BONELESS CHICKEN CUTLETS

MAKES 4 SERVINGS

¾ cup all-purpose flour

½ cup liquid eggs

½ cup unseasoned bread crumbs

¼ cup freshly grated Parmesan cheese

1 tablespoon mustard powder

4 (4-ounce) skinless, boneless chicken cutlets

4 tablespoons olive oil

Salt and freshly ground pepper to taste

Lemon wedges

Set out 3 shallow bowls. Place flour in one bowl, eggs in the second bowl, and mix together the bread crumbs, Parmesan cheese, and mustard powder in the third bowl. Dredge cutlets with flour, gently shaking cutlets to remove the excess. Then dip chicken into the eggs, coating both sides, again allow cutlets to drip off any excess egg back into bowl. Finally, coat cutlets with bread crumb mixture. Heat olive oil in a large cast-iron skillet over medium-high heat. Cook cutlets (about 4 minutes on each side) until golden brown and cooked through. Juices should run clear. Place cooked chicken on a paper towel–lined plate to absorb any excess oil. Season with salt and pepper to taste and serve with wedges of lemon.

Approx. 375 calories per serving
30g protein, 18g total fat, 3g saturated fat, 0 trans fat,
10g carbohydrates, 70mg cholesterol, 430mg sodium, 1g fiber

PAN-ROASTED SALMON FILLETS
MAKES 4 SERVINGS

1 tablespoon olive oil
4 (6-ounce) salmon fillets, with skin on
Salt and freshly ground pepper to taste
2 teaspoons low-sodium fish seasoning of choice
Dill sauce (optional)

Preheat oven to 350 degrees. In a large cast-iron skillet, heat olive oil over medium heat. Season skin-side of fillets with salt and pepper to taste. When olive oil is hot, place fillets in pan, skin-side down, and cook until skin is crispy, about 5 minutes. Sprinkle tops of fillets with fish seasoning. Transfer fillets (do not turn fillets over) in the skillet to the oven and roast until opaque in the center, about 4–5 minutes. Serve with a side of dill sauce, if desired.

Approx. 244 calories per serving
34g protein, 14g total fat, 2g saturated fat, 0 trans fat,
0 carbohydrates, 94mg cholesterol, 75mg sodium, 0 fiber

BAKED CHILEAN SEA BASS
MAKES 4 SERVINGS

Olive oil cooking spray
4 (6-ounce) Chilean sea bass fillets
Salt and freshly ground pepper to taste
Cayenne pepper to taste

Preheat oven to broil. Spray a shallow baking pan with cooking oil. Place sea bass on pan and sprinkle with salt and pepper and cayenne to taste. Lightly spray tops of fish with cooking oil and broil until lightly browned. Turn fish over and broil other side a few minutes longer until browned. Turn off broiler and set oven to bake at 425 degrees. Continue to bake fish for an additional 15–20 minutes, depending on thickness of fish, until it flakes easily. Serve immediately.

Approx. 164 calories per serving
32g protein, 4g total fat, 0 saturated fat, 0 trans fat,
0 carbohydrates, 70mg cholesterol, 110mg sodium, 0 fiber

SPINACH AND SWISS CHEESE QUICHE

MAKES 8 SERVINGS

1 (9-inch) unbaked whole wheat pie crust
5 large eggs or 1¼ cups liquid eggs
¾ cup low-fat or 2% milk
½ teaspoon salt or to taste
¼ teaspoon freshly ground pepper
½ cup thawed frozen spinach (about ½ of a 10-ounce bag), squeezed to reduce moisture
1 cup shredded low-fat Swiss cheese (about 4 ounces)

Preheat oven to 375 degrees. Place pie crust in a pie dish and crimp the edges. In a bowl, whisk together the eggs, milk, and salt and pepper. Spread spinach evenly in the bottom of the crust and pour egg mixture over the top of the spinach. Sprinkle with Swiss cheese and bake at 375 degrees for roughly 15 minutes. Reduce heat to 325 degrees and continue to bake for an additional 20 minutes or until egg mixture has puffed and crust is browned. Remove from oven and allow pie to stand for 5 minutes before slicing.

Approx. 186 calories per serving
9g protein, 9g total fat, 6g saturated fat, 0 trans fat,
15g carbohydrates, 27mg cholesterol, 486mg sodium, 2g fiber

ROASTED CORNISH HENS

MAKES 4 SERVINGS

¼ teaspoon dried sage
¼ teaspoon dried thyme
Salt and freshly ground pepper to taste
4 Rock Cornish hens (1–1¼ pounds each), rinsed and dried
1½ tablespoons trans fat–free canola/olive oil spread, melted
½ cup dry white wine or dry unsweetened vermouth

Preheat oven to 375 degrees. Combine sage, thyme, and salt and pepper in a small bowl and stir to mix. Divide salt mixture in half, season insides of hens with half of the mixture, and tie the legs of each hen together. Place hens on a rack in a shallow roasting pan. Sprinkle the remaining salt mixture over each hen. Drizzle melted canola/olive oil spread and wine over the tops of the hens and place hens in oven to roast for roughly 20–25 minutes or until a meat thermometer inserted in the thigh reaches 170 degrees. Remove from oven and tent hens with foil for about 10 minutes before serving.

Approx. 408 calories per serving
58g protein, 14g total fat, 3g saturated fat, 0 trans fat,
0 carbohydrates, 264mg cholesterol, 564g sodium, 0 fiber

POMODORA SAUCE AND GRILLED CHICKEN

MAKES 4 SERVINGS

½ cup slivered almonds
4 (6-ounce) skinless, boneless chicken breasts
Freshly grated Parmesan cheese for garnish

For Pomodora Sauce:

¼ cup olive oil
1 large red bell pepper, chopped
1 medium-large yellow onion, chopped
6 teaspoons minced fresh garlic
1 (14.5-ounce) can petite diced tomatoes, well drained
3 tablespoons chopped fresh basil leaves
1 tablespoon red wine vinegar

Preheat oven to 350 degrees. Place almonds on heavy tinfoil and bake until golden brown. Remove from oven.

Grill chicken breasts as desired. When cooked, place each breast on a platter and cover with pomodora sauce. Sprinkle on almond slivers and Parmesan cheese and serve.

Sauce:

In a large skillet over high heat, warm olive oil. Add red bell pepper, onion, and garlic and cook until onion pieces are tender and liquid is evaporated, stirring frequently. Add in tomatoes, basil, and vinegar. Cook until heated through. Reduce heat to very low to keep sauce warm.

Approx. 299 calories per serving
48g protein, 16g total fat, 1g saturated fat, 0 trans fat,
11g carbohydrates, 144mg cholesterol, 288mg sodium, 1g fiber

EASY BAKED EGGPLANT PARMESAN

MAKES 4 SERVINGS

½ cup liquid eggs

¼ cup bread crumbs

1 large eggplant, with skin on and sliced lengthwise into 8 slices (about ½-inch thickness each)

Olive oil cooking spray

Garlic salt to sprinkle (optional)

1 cup shredded low-fat mozzarella cheese

1 (14.5-ounce) can diced tomatoes with basil, garlic, and oregano, drained

1 (8-ounce) can tomato sauce with basil, garlic, and oregano

Chopped fresh parsley for garnish

Grated Parmesan cheese for garnish

Preheat oven to 425 degrees. Place eggs in a large, shallow dipping bowl. Place bread crumbs in another large, shallow bowl. Dip each slice of eggplant into eggs and then into bread crumbs, coating both sides of each piece. Place pieces on lightly oil-sprayed baking sheet. If desired, lightly sprinkle each slice with garlic salt. Bake eggplant until slices are tender and lightly browned, roughly 5 minutes on each side. Sprinkle tops of one side of the eggplant with shredded mozzarella cheese and bake for 1 minute longer until cheese softens and browns slightly. While eggplant is baking, combine tomatoes and sauce in a saucepan and heat on medium-low heat to let simmer until slightly thickened, about 10 minutes. Divide tomato mixture into 4 shallow serving plates and top each plate with 2 slices eggplant. Sprinkle each serving with parsley and Parmesan cheese and serve.

Approx. 196 calories per serving
13g protein, 5g total fat, 3g saturated fat, 0 trans fat,
23g carbohydrates, 15mg cholesterol, 616mg sodium, 6g fiber

SPICY MEDITERRANEAN PASTA

MAKES 4 SERVINGS

3 tablespoons olive oil
6 cloves fresh garlic, finely chopped
1 (14.5-ounce) can diced tomatoes with basil, garlic, and oregano, undrained
1 (15-ounce) can cannellini beans, drained and rinsed
2 tablespoons balsamic vinegar
Crushed red hot pepper flakes to taste
1 (13.25-ounce) box whole grain medium pasta shells
2 medium heads fresh broccoli, florets only
Salt and freshly ground pepper to taste
Freshly grated Parmesan cheese (optional)

In a large skillet, heat olive oil over medium heat. Add garlic and cook until fragrant. Add tomatoes with juices, beans, vinegar, and hot pepper flakes. Cook for about 5–8 minutes, stirring often. Set aside and keep warm. Cook pasta according to package directions. Add broccoli florets to cooking pasta during the last 8 minutes of cooking time. Drain pasta, reserving 1 cup of cooking liquid. Return pasta and broccoli florets to pot and add tomato mixture. Sprinkle with desired salt and pepper and toss to incorporate sauce. If pasta is too dry, add small amounts of reserved pasta liquid until desired consistency. Sprinkle top with Parmesan cheese and serve.

Approx. 503 calories per serving
20g protein, 10g total fat, 1g saturated fat, 0 trans fat,
89g carbohydrates, 0 cholesterol, 521mg sodium, 6g fiber

WHITE BEANS AND SMOKED PAPRIKA SHRIMP
MAKES 4–6 SERVINGS

4 tablespoons olive oil, divided, + more to drizzle

6 cloves fresh garlic, minced and divided

3 dried red chilies

2 bay leaves, best to use fresh leaves if possible

1 (28-ounce) can diced tomatoes, fully drained

2 tablespoons tomato paste

2 (15-ounce) cans cannellini beans, rinsed and drained

1 cup canned low-sodium, fat-free chicken broth

1 pound large raw shrimp, peeled and deveined

1 teaspoon smoked paprika

Garlic salt and freshly ground pepper to taste

2 tablespoons chopped flat leaf parsley for garnish

4 slices toasted crusty bread (optional)

Preheat broiler. Heat 2 teaspoons of olive oil in a heavy-bottomed skillet over medium heat. Add 3 cloves garlic, chilies, and bay leaves. Cook, stirring continuously, until fragrant, about 2–3 minutes. Add diced tomatoes. With the back of a spoon, smash tomatoes until they are completely broken into a mash and cook for about 5 minutes. Add tomato paste, constantly stirring until sauce is a deep red, about 3–5 minutes. Stir in beans and broth, bring to a simmer, and cook until juices are slightly reduced and thickened, about 4–5 minutes. Transfer bean mixture to an oven-safe casserole dish. In a bowl, add remaining olive oil and garlic, shrimp, and paprika. Season with garlic salt and pepper to taste. Toss shrimp until evenly coated. Scatter shrimp over bean mixture in an even layer. Place casserole under broiler and broil until shrimp are golden and cooked through, about 3–5 minutes. Remove from heat and drizzle a scant amount of olive oil over shrimp and beans and garnish with chopped parsley. Serve with crusty bread, if desired.

Approx. 289 calories per serving
33g protein, 4g total fat, 1g saturated fat, 0 trans fat,
25g carbohydrates, 114mg cholesterol, 888mg sodium, 8g fiber

SAUTÉED SHRIMP AND MUSHROOM COUSCOUS

MAKES 4 SERVINGS

1½ cups canned low-sodium, fat-free chicken broth, divided

12 large button mushrooms, cleaned and quartered

6–8 scallions, white and green parts, chopped

3 tablespoons fresh garlic paste blend, divided

1 tablespoon porcini-infused olive oil

Salt and freshly ground pepper to taste

3 cloves fresh garlic, minced

24 large fresh or frozen shrimp, peeled, deveined, and defrosted if frozen

Crushed red hot pepper flakes to taste

2 tablespoons olive oil

¼ tablespoon dried parsley

⅛ teaspoon dried thyme

⅛ teaspoon dried rosemary

⅔ cup fine couscous

Grated Parmesan cheese to sprinkle (optional)

In a large skillet over medium heat, bring 1 cup broth, mushrooms, and scallions to a boil. Reduce heat to a simmer and add 2 tablespoons garlic paste, stirring to blend. Stir occasionally until mushrooms soften. Drizzle mixture with porcini oil, stir, and add salt and pepper to taste. Drain off liquid from mushroom mixture and reserve both liquid and mushrooms in separate bowls. Set both aside. In the same skillet, combine remaining broth, garlic, shrimp, and hot pepper flakes. Bring to a boil, reduce heat to medium, and cook shrimp until pink and cooked through. Remove from heat and set aside. In a saucepan, add reserved mushroom liquid plus water to equal 1½ cups. Add olive oil, remaining garlic paste, parsley, thyme, and rosemary. Bring to a rapid boil, then remove from heat. Add couscous, stir, cover, and allow to stand until liquid is absorbed, about 5 minutes. Fluff couscous with a fork and transfer to a large bowl. Add mushroom-scallion mixture and gently toss to mix. With a slotted spoon, transfer cooked shrimp to couscous-mushroom mixture and again toss to incorporate all ingredients. Add salt and pepper to taste, sprinkle top with Parmesan cheese, if desired, and serve.

Approx. 353 calories per serving
16g protein, 4g total fat, 0.5g saturated fat, 0 trans fat,
27g carbohydrates, 64mg cholesterol, 694mg sodium, 2g fiber

BAKED MEATBALLS
MAKES ROUGHLY 65 MEATBALLS

4 large eggs, beaten
½ cup low-fat milk
4 slices bread, torn into pieces
½ cup finely chopped white onion
3 cloves fresh garlic, finely chopped
¼ cup finely chopped green bell pepper
Salt and freshly ground pepper to taste
½ cup grated Parmesan cheese
1½ pounds lean ground beef
1½ pounds lean ground pork

Preheat oven to 375 degrees. In a large bowl, add eggs, milk, bread, onion, garlic, green bell pepper, salt and pepper, and Parmesan cheese. Mix together. Add both meats and mix well using your hands to blend mixture. Form meat mixture into balls and place on a rimmed baking sheet. Bake for 25–30 minutes.

Approx. 37 calories per meatball
4.5g protein, 3g total fat, <0.5g saturated fat, 0 trans fat,
0 carbohydrates, 29mg cholesterol, 34mg sodium, 0 fiber

LASAGNA MADE EASY

MAKES 12 SERVINGS

1½ pounds lean ground beef

1 pound ground Italian seasoned lean sausage

3 cloves fresh garlic, minced

1 large white onion, chopped

2 (14.5-ounce) cans whole tomatoes, undrained

2 (6-ounce) cans tomato paste

4 tablespoons dried parsley, divided

2 tablespoons dried basil

2 tablespoons dried oregano

¾ teaspoon fennel seed

Salt and freshly ground pepper to taste

3 cups low-fat cottage cheese

2 whole eggs, beaten

½ cup grated Parmesan cheese

1 (10-ounce) package lasagna noodles

1 pound sliced low-sodium mozzarella cheese

Combine beef, sausage, garlic, and onion in a large skillet and cook over medium-high heat until browned. Drain off half amount of fat. Add tomatoes, tomato paste, 2 tablespoons parsley, basil, oregano, fennel seed, and salt and pepper to taste. Let simmer for 40–45 minutes. While meat sauce simmers, mix together cottage cheese, eggs, Parmesan cheese, and remaining parsley in a small bowl. Stir and set aside. Cook lasagna noodles as per package directions. Arrange 4 cooked noodles in the bottom of a baking dish, overlapping noodles if needed. Spoon half of the cottage cheese mixture evenly over noodles and add a layer of mozzarella cheese. Spread less than half of meat sauce mixture over the top. Repeat procedure until all noodles have been used, ending with a layer of meat sauce. Sprinkle the top with Parmesan cheese and a layer of mozzarella cheese. Bake in a 350-degree oven for 20–30 minutes or until top is hot, bubbles, and is slightly browned.

Approx. 429 calories per serving
41g protein, 14g total fat, 6g saturated fat, 0 trans fat,
25g carbohydrates, 127mg cholesterol, 561mg sodium, 4g fiber

PAN-SEARED PARMESAN CHEESE SCALLOPS WITH RICE PILAF

MAKES 4 SERVINGS

1 tablespoon trans fat–free canola/olive oil spread

1 tablespoon olive oil

1½–2 pounds bay scallops

½ teaspoon garlic salt or to taste

½ teaspoon garlic powder

Freshly ground pepper to taste

⅛ cup grated Parmesan cheese

Generous pinch of paprika

2 tablespoons chopped fresh parsley

Choice of store-bought rice pilaf, cooked to package instructions

Freshly squeezed lemon juice to drizzle

Melt canola/olive oil spread and olive oil in a saucepan over medium-high heat. Add scallops and sprinkle with garlic salt, garlic powder, and pepper. Cook for 2 minutes on each side of the scallops. Add Parmesan cheese, paprika, and parsley. Remove from heat and pour over rice pilaf with a drizzling of fresh lemon juice.

Approx. 228 calories per serving
33g protein, 7g total fat, 2g saturated fat, 0 trans fat,
8g carbohydrates, 107mg cholesterol, 295mg sodium, 0 fiber

LEMON-PEPPER SALMON

MAKES 2 SERVINGS

Olive oil cooking spray
2 (4–5-ounce) salmon fillets, skinless
Lemon pepper seasoning to taste
1 lemon, cut in wedges for garnish

Preheat oven to 450 degrees. Lightly spray a cast-iron skillet with cooking oil and place in oven to heat. While oven is heating, rinse fillets and pat dry with paper towels. Season 1 side of each fillet with a generous amount of lemon pepper seasoning. When oven reaches desired temperature, place fillets seasoned side down on hot skillet and cook for roughly 10–15 minutes, turning once after about 6–7 minutes. Cook until fish flakes easily and serve with lemon wedges.

Approx. 259 calories per serving
28g protein, 15g total fat, 3g saturated fat, 0 trans fat,
0 carbohydrates, 84mg cholesterol, 84mg sodium, 0 fiber

SEARED GOLDEN SEA SCALLOPS

MAKES 4 SERVINGS

16 medium-large sea scallops (about 1¼ pounds dry scallops)
2 tablespoons canola/olive oil spread, melted
2 teaspoons minced fresh garlic
1 tablespoon finely chopped thyme
1 teaspoon salt or to taste
Freshly ground pepper to taste

In a medium bowl, marinate the scallops with olive oil, garlic, thyme, salt and pepper for 20–30 minutes. Drain off oil mixture from scallops and heat over medium-high heat. When fats begin to smoke, gently add scallops but do not let scallops touch one another. Sear the scallops for 1½ minutes on each side. Scallops should have a golden crust on each side but still be translucent in the center. Serve immediately.

Approx. 235 calories per serving
24g protein, 13g total fat, 2g saturated fat, 0 trans fat,
3g carbohydrates, 47mg cholesterol, 278mg sodium, 1g fiber

FUSILLI AND FRESH TOMATO

MAKES 6 SERVINGS

¾ cup extra-virgin olive oil (more, if desired)

1½ tablespoons balsamic vinegar

1½ tablespoons red wine vinegar

4½ pounds Italian plum tomatoes, halved, seeds removed, and flesh cut into bite-sized pieces

¾ cup packed fresh basil leaves, torn into pieces

1 pound dry fusilli pasta

Salt and freshly ground pepper to taste

Combine olive oil and both vinegars in a bowl and whisk to blend. In a separate bowl, hand crush tomato pieces to release juices, then add basil and vinegar mixture. Stir, cover bowl, and marinate at room temperature for at least 1 hour. Cook fusilli as per package directions. Drain and add to vinegar-tomato mixture. Allow pasta to sit and soak up vinegar-tomato mixture for 20–30 minutes. Stir often to allow pasta to absorb flavors of sauce. Add salt and pepper to taste and extra olive oil, if desired. Serve slightly warmed or at room temperature.

Approx. 540 calories per serving
11g protein, 29g total fat, 4g saturated fat, 0 trans fat,
60g carbohydrates, 0 cholesterol, 10mg sodium, 15g fiber

LIGHTLY PAN-FRIED CRUSTED TROUT WITH DILL SAUCE

MAKES 4 SERVINGS

¾ cup fine cornmeal

Salt and freshly ground pepper to taste

¾ cup plain low-fat yogurt, divided

4 boneless trout fillets (about 1 pound), rinsed and patted dry

2 tablespoons olive oil, divided

1 lemon, halved, one half to juice and the other wedged for garnish

⅓ cup chopped fresh dill

Place cornmeal in a shallow dish and season with salt and pepper. Spread 1 tablespoon of yogurt on the flesh side of each fillet. Press yogurt side of fillet into cornmeal mixture to coat flesh. In a heavy-bottomed skillet, heat 1 tablespoon of olive oil over medium-high heat. When olive oil is hot, add 2 fillets to pan, skin side down, and cook until skin is crispy and golden brown, about 3 minutes. Flip fillets and cook other side until golden brown, about another 3 minutes. Repeat with other 2 fillets, adding remaining olive oil and reducing heat if necessary. Transfer cooked fillets to warmed plates. Combine remaining yogurt, lemon juice, and dill in a small bowl. Serve a dapple of dill sauce and a lemon wedge with each fillet.

Approx. 340 calories per serving
27g protein, 16g total fat, 2g saturated fat, 0 trans fat,
30g carbohydrates, 69mg cholesterol, 99mg sodium, 2g fiber

WHOLE ROASTED BRANZINO WITH BUTTERY LEMON SAUCE

MAKES 4 SERVINGS

4 (1–1½-pound) whole branzino, cleaned, with head and tail intact
¼ cup olive oil, reserving some to drizzle
Salt and freshly ground pepper to taste
1 lemon, thinly sliced into 8 slices
4 fresh parsley sprigs

For Buttery Lemon Sauce:

¼ cup trans fat–free canola/olive oil spread
1 tablespoon chopped capers
1 tablespoon freshly squeezed lemon juice
1 tablespoon chopped fresh parsley

Preheat oven to 400 degrees. Rinse fish and pat dry. Score each fish lengthwise, down to bone, and then crosswise 2 times. Place fish on a lightly oiled baking sheet and brush inside and outside of each fish with olive oil. Sprinkle skin of fish with salt and pepper to taste. Stuff cavity of each fish with 2 lemon slices and 1 sprig parsley. Bake fish uncovered for 4 minutes. Gently turn over and cook for an additional 4 minutes. Reset oven to broil, drizzle tops of fish with olive oil, and cook for 3–5 minutes more or until skin blisters and fish flakes easily.

Sauce:

While fish is cooking, make sauce by melting canola/olive oil spread in a small pot over low heat. Add capers, lemon juice, and parsley. When fish is cooked and ready to serve, drizzle each fish with a small amount of lemon-caper sauce.

Approx. 322 calories per serving
31g protein, 29g total fat, 4g saturated fat, 0 trans fat,
0 carbohydrates, 67mg cholesterol, 187mg sodium, 0 fiber

SARDINES PASTA WITH LEMON AND GARLIC
MAKES 4 SERVINGS

6 cloves fresh garlic, minced

4 tablespoons olive oil, divided

1 cup bread crumbs + extra for garnish (optional)

8 ounces fresh fettuccine pasta

¼ cup freshly squeezed lemon juice

Salt and freshly ground pepper to taste

2 (3–4-ounce) cans boneless sardines in tomato sauce, broken into small pieces

½ cup chopped fresh parsley

¼ cup finely shredded Parmesan cheese

In a small non-stick skillet, sauté garlic in 2 tablespoons of olive oil until fragrant but not browned. Set aside. Heat remaining oil in a separate pan and add bread crumbs. Cook, stirring frequently, until crispy and golden brown. Cook and drain fresh pasta according to package directions. In a bowl, whisk together lemon juice, salt and pepper, and garlic. Add pasta, sardines with sauce, parsley, and Parmesan cheese. Toss gently and serve with bread crumbs sprinkled on top, if desired.

Approx. 362 calories per serving
19g protein, 18g total fat, 3g saturated fat, 0 trans fat,
57g carbohydrates, 36mg cholesterol, 687mg sodium, 3g fiber

RIGATONI IN A FRESH HERB SAUCE

MAKES 8 SERVINGS

3 tablespoons olive oil

2 medium carrots, minced

1 yellow onion, chopped

1 leek, white part only, diced

3 cloves fresh garlic, minced

½ cup red table wine

1 (35-ounce) can Roma tomatoes, undrained and crushed by hand

1 bay leaf

Salt and freshly ground pepper to taste

1 pound rigatoni

½ cup chopped fresh parsley

10 fresh basil leaves, chopped

1 tablespoon minced fresh oregano

2 tablespoons chopped black olives

⅓ cup coarsely grated Pecorino-Romano cheese

Heat olive oil in a large skillet over medium heat. Add carrots, onion, and leek and sauté for about 9 minutes or until soft. Add garlic and cook, stirring, until fragrant, about 1 minute. Add wine and cook, stirring, until reduced by half, about 5 minutes. Add tomatoes with juices and bay leaf. Season with salt and pepper to taste. Let simmer uncovered for 15–20 minutes. Meanwhile, cook pasta according to package directions. Remove bay leaf from sauce. Add parsley, basil, and oregano and let simmer for about 2 minutes longer. Add olives. Put drained pasta in a large serving bowl, add sauce, and toss gently. Top with Pecorino-Romano cheese.

Approx. 402 calories per serving
12g protein, 7g total fat, 2g saturated fat, 0 trans fat,
54g carbohydrates, 4mg cholesterol, 535mg sodium, 4g fiber

PASTA AND WHITE BEANS

MAKES 4 SERVINGS

3 cups whole grain penne pasta
2 (15-ounce) cans diced tomatoes with basil and oregano
3–4 cloves fresh garlic, minced
1 small white onion, diced
1 (15-ounce) can cannellini beans, rinsed and drained
1 (9-ounce) bag fresh spinach, cleaned and torn into pieces
1 (6-ounce) log fresh soft goat cheese, broken into small chunks
Crusty bread

Cook pasta according to package directions. In a large skillet, bring tomatoes, garlic, onion, and beans to a boil. Reduce heat to a low simmer and cook for roughly 10 minutes. Add spinach and continue to let simmer until leaves are wilted, stirring mixture occasionally. Drain cooked pasta and divide onto 4 plates. Top pasta with tomato-spinach mixture and scatter on chunks of goat cheese. Serve with hearty crusty bread.

Approx. 303 calories per serving
14g protein, 8g total fat, 3g saturated fat, 0 trans fat,
42g carbohydrates, 20mg cholesterol, 719mg sodium, 6g fiber

PARMESAN-CRUSTED FISH

MAKES 4 SERVINGS

Olive oil cooking spray
⅓ cup panko bread crumbs
¼ cup finely shredded Parmesan cheese
Salt and freshly ground pepper to taste
4 codfish fillets (about 1–1½ pounds)
¼ cup melted trans fat–free canola/olive oil spread
½ tablespoon fresh garlic paste blend

Preheat oven to 350 degrees. Lightly spray a baking sheet with cooking oil. In a large, shallow baking dish, mix together panko bread crumbs, Parmesan cheese, and salt and pepper to taste. Roll fillets in mixture to coat all sides. Blend together melted canola/olive oil spread and garlic paste in a small bowl. Place fillets on baking sheet and drizzle garlic-butter mixture over top of fillets. Bake uncovered for 4–6 minutes for each ½-inch thickness until crumbs are golden brown and fish flakes easily.

Approx. 283 calories per serving
32g protein, 14g total fat, 4g saturated fat, 0 trans fat,
4g carbohydrates, 69mg cholesterol, 320mg sodium, 0 fiber

SALMON WITH SMOKED PAPRIKA

MAKES 4 SERVINGS

¼ cup orange juice

1 tablespoon olive oil

1 teaspoon thyme

4 (4–5-ounce) salmon fillets, skinless

½ tablespoon smoked paprika

½ tablespoon brown sugar

½ teaspoon cinnamon

1 teaspoon orange zest

In a shallow dish, stir to mix orange juice, olive oil, and thyme. Add salmon, turning to coat fillets with juice mixture. Cover dish with plastic wrap and refrigerate. When fillets have marinated for at least 30 minutes, place a shallow cast-iron skillet on the top oven rack and preheat oven to 450 degrees. In a small pinch bowl, mix together paprika, brown sugar, cinnamon, and zest. When oven reaches desired heat, remove fillets from marinade and rub tops of fillets with paprika mixture. Place fillets in heated skillet and cook for 3–4 minutes. Turn fillets over once and continue cooking until fish flakes easily.

Approx. 202 calories per serving
22g protein, 11g total fat, 1g saturated fat, 0 trans fat
2g carbohydrates, 62mg cholesterol, 85mg sodium, <0.5mg fiber

BEANS AND MORE BEANS

MAKES 8 SERVINGS

2 tablespoons canola oil

4 cloves fresh garlic, chopped

1 large white onion, chopped

1 small green bell pepper, diced

1 jalapeño pepper, deseeded and diced

1 (28-ounce) can small red kidney beans, drained and rinsed

1 (15-ounce) can chickpeas, drained and rinsed

1 (15-ounce) can pinto beans, drained and rinsed

¼ cup quinoa

1 cup frozen yellow corn

½ cup diced carrot

½ cup diced celery

1 (28-ounce) can diced tomatoes with basil, garlic, and oregano

2 cups canned low-sodium, fat-free chicken broth

2 tablespoons chili powder or to taste

Salt and freshly ground pepper to taste

Whole grain crusty bread

In a large pot, heat olive oil, garlic, onion, and green bell pepper, and sauté until soft. Add the jalapeño and sauté for another 2–3 minutes. Add the remaining ingredients (except bread) and bring to a boil. Reduce heat to low, cover, and let simmer for 30–40 minutes, stirring occasionally, until quinoa grains are soft. Serve with crusty bread.

Approx. 276 calories per serving
15g protein, 4g total fat, <0.5g saturated fat, 0 trans fat,
80g carbohydrates, 0 cholesterol, 948mg sodium, 10g fiber

ORECCHIETTE PASTA AND ROASTED TOMATOES

MAKES 4 SERVINGS

1½ pounds cherry tomatoes

3 cloves fresh garlic, chopped

4 tablespoons capers, drained and rinsed

1½ tablespoons fresh oregano leaves, divided

3 tablespoons olive oil

Salt and freshly ground pepper to taste

1 pound orecchiette pasta (equals roughly 2½ cups cooked pasta per serving)

Grated Parmesan cheese (optional)

Preheat oven to 450 degrees. In a resealable plastic baggie, add tomatoes, garlic, capers, 1 tablespoon oregano, olive oil, and salt and pepper to taste. Toss until tomatoes are well coated. Spread out tomato mixture on a rimmed baking sheet and roast until tomatoes burst and begin to brown, about 25–30 minutes. Cook pasta according to package instructions and drain, reserving ½ cup pasta water. Return pasta and half of reserved water to pot and add tomato mixture. Cook on medium-high until sauce slightly thickens. If needed, add remaining water to create a sauce that covers pasta. Sprinkle with remaining oregano and Parmesan cheese, if desired, and serve.

Approx. 342 calories per serving

15g protein, 12g total fat, 1g saturated fat, 0 trans fat,

39g carbohydrates, 0 cholesterol, 8mg sodium, 6g fiber

PAN-SEARED HALIBUT WITH LEMON-CAPER SAUCE

MAKES 4 SERVINGS

4 (6-ounce) halibut steaks

Pinch of salt and freshly ground pepper (optional)

2 tablespoons olive oil, divided

1 tablespoon trans fat–free canola/olive oil spread

1 clove fresh garlic, finely minced

2 lemons, 1 to juice and zested to make ½ teaspoon lemon zest and 1 quartered for garnish

2 tablespoons freshly squeezed lemon juice

4 teaspoons capers, drained, rinsed, and chopped

4 tablespoons chopped fresh parsley

Rinse steaks under cold water and pat dry. Season one side of each steak with a pinch of salt and pepper, if desired. In a large, heavy-bottomed skillet, heat 1 tablespoon olive oil and canola/olive oil spread over medium-high heat. Cook halibut steaks in skillet until golden brown on both sides, about 7 minutes. Set aside but keep warm. Heat remaining olive oil in a small skillet, then add garlic, lemon zest and juice, and capers. Let simmer for 30–40 seconds. Add parsley and drizzle mixture over seared halibut steaks. Garnish with lemon wedges and serve immediately.

Approx. 272 calories per serving

35g protein, 14g total fat, 2g saturated fat, 0 trans fat,

0 carbohydrates, 54mg cholesterol, 152mg sodium, 0 fiber

PAN-SEARED LEMON-PEPPER TILAPIA

MAKES 2 SERVINGS

4 (3–4 ounces) tilapia fillets
Ground lemon pepper seasoning to taste
1 tablespoon extra-virgin olive oil
1 tablespoon trans fat–free canola/olive oil spread
1 lemon, quartered

Rinse fillets under cold water, pat dry with paper towels, and generously coat one side of each fillet with lemon pepper seasoning. In a large skillet, add olive oil and canola/olive oil spread over medium-high heat. Use a cooking brush to mix them together and spread evenly on bottom of skillet. When oil mixture is hot, reduce heat to medium and place fillets lemon-pepper side down in skillet to cook (about 3 minutes, depending on thickness of fillets). Generously sprinkle other side of each fillet with lemon pepper seasoning and turn fillets. Continue cooking until fish flakes. Remove fillets from heat and serve immediately. Garnish with lemon wedges.

Approx. 278 calories per serving (2 fillets)
46g protein, 11g total fat, 3g saturated fat, 0 trans fat,
0 carbohydrates, 114mg cholesterol, 158mg sodium, 0 fiber

PASTA WITH TOFU IN A SPICY MARINARA SAUCE
MAKES 4–6 SERVINGS

¼ cup canned low-sodium, fat-free chicken broth
1 large green bell pepper, seeded and cut into 1-inch pieces
1 large white onion, peeled and cut into 1-inch pieces
4–6 cloves fresh garlic, coarsely chopped
1 (28-ounce) can peeled Italian tomatoes, drained and halved
16 small black olives
1 (8-ounce) package extra-firm plain tofu, drained and cut into 1-inch pieces
1 (24-ounce) jar marinara sauce
Salt and freshly ground pepper to taste
Crushed red hot pepper flakes to taste (optional)
Cooked pasta of choice

In a large skillet, add broth, green bell pepper, onion, and garlic. Cook over medium heat until pepper pieces are tender. Reduce heat to low and add tomatoes, olives, tofu, marinara sauce, salt and pepper, and hot pepper flakes. Cover and allow to simmer on very low (about 10–15 minutes), stirring occasionally to mix ingredients and making sure tofu pieces are well covered with sauce. The longer the tofu lingers in the sauce and blends with other ingredients, the more flavorful it becomes. Serve over your favorite pasta.

Approx. 63 calories per serving (sauce only, does not included pasta of choice)
4g protein, 5g total fat, <0.5g saturated fat, 0 trans fat,
5g carbohydrates, 0 cholesterol, 292mg sodium, 1g fiber

SPINACH FETTUCCINE WITH BABY ARTICHOKES

MAKES 4 SERVINGS

8 ounces spinach fettuccine

9-ounce package baby artichokes, thawed

3 tablespoons extra-virgin olive oil

6 cloves fresh garlic, finely chopped

16 large raw shrimp, peeled and deveined

½ cup dry vermouth

2 large plum tomatoes, finely chopped

1 cup canned low-sodium, fat-free chicken broth

12 pitted black olives, halved

1½ tablespoons trans fat–free canola/olive oil spread

1 teaspoon fresh lemon peel, finely grated

Salt to taste (optional)

½ teaspoon ground nutmeg

1 tablespoon chopped fresh parsley

Lemon wedges for garnish

Cook pasta per box directions, then remove from heat, drain pasta, and return to pot, drizzling with scant amount of olive oil to keep pasta from sticking together. Set aside. Cut artichokes lengthwise, remove outer leaves, cut off bases, and trim off tops about ⅓ way down. Remove fuzzy choke inside, discard, and cut remaining choke in half again. Repeat procedure until all chokes are cleaned and quartered. In a large skillet, add 2 tablespoons of olive oil and garlic and sauté for 1 minute; add artichokes and cook for another 1–2 minutes. Add shrimp and vermouth; continue cooking, stirring often, until shrimp are pink. Add tomatoes, broth, olives, canola/olive oil spread, lemon peel, salt, nutmeg, and pasta. Toss to coat pasta with sauce. Heat mixture until warmed through. Stir in parsley and drizzle with remaining olive oil. Garnish with lemon wedges.

Approx. 437 calories per serving
17g protein, 17g total fat, 3g saturated fat, 0 trans fat,
51g carbohydrates, 43mg cholesterol, 195mg sodium, 2g fiber

ROSEMARY ROASTED CHICKEN BREASTS

MAKES 4 SERVINGS

4 chicken breasts with rib bones and skin (about 9–12 ounces each)
Salt and freshly ground pepper to taste
2 tablespoons trans fat–free canola/olive oil spread (room temperature)
3 teaspoons freshly minced rosemary leaves
3 cloves fresh garlic, finely chopped
1 teaspoon fresh lemon zest
Extra-virgin olive oil to drizzle

Rinse breasts under cold water and pat dry, then remove any excess fat. Sprinkle rib bone sides of breasts with salt and pepper to taste and place breasts rib side down on broiler pan. With a sharp pointed knife, insert blade into one end of skin and gradually slide blade under skin to create a pocket between skin and breast meat. In a small bowl combine canola/olive oil spread, rosemary, garlic, and lemon zest. Stir to blend flavors and textures. Divide into 4 portions. Use a small flat knife to stuff rosemary mixture into skin pockets of chicken breasts. With a finger, gently press on the skin to spread rosemary mixture over the breast meat inside the pockets (the skin pockets will allow the rosemary mixture and flavors to soak into the meat as the chicken bakes). Sprinkle the tops of each breast with freshly ground pepper and a drizzle of olive oil. Place broiler pan in oven on rack placed in center of oven and bake breasts for about 40–45 minutes at 450 degrees. Remove from oven and peel off skin before serving, if desired.

Approx. 233 calories per serving (with skin on)
29g protein, 12g total fat, 3.4g saturated fat, 0 trans fat,
0 carbohydrates, 83mg cholesterol, 109mg sodium, 0 fiber

CHICKEN AND SPICY HUMMUS

MAKES 4 SERVINGS

¼ cup olive oil

1 tablespoon finely chopped fresh garlic

½ teaspoon ground cumin

½ teaspoon freshly ground pepper

1½ pounds skinless, boneless chicken breast, cut into 2-inch cubes

1 red bell pepper, sliced lengthwise into 1-inch-wide strips

1 yellow banana pepper, sliced lengthwise into 1-inch-wide strips

1 red onion, cut into strips

Salt to taste

½ cup prepared spicy hummus (page 369)

4 lemon wedges for garnish

Pita wedges (optional)

Combine olive oil, garlic, cumin, black pepper, chicken, red and yellow peppers, onion, and salt in a resealable plastic baggie. Toss all ingredients until chicken is well coated with olive oil and seasonings. Line a broiler pan with tinfoil and spread chicken mixture out in a single layer. Place pan 4–6 inches under heat and broil ingredients for roughly 8–10 minutes, stirring once, until chicken is cooked through and veggies are lightly blackened. Divide hummus and chicken mixture each into 4 equal portions. Place hummus on plate and top with chicken mixture. Garnish plate with lemon wedge and serve with toasted pita wedges, if desired.

Approx. 435 calories per serving
43g protein, 22g total fat, 3g saturated fat, 0 trans fat,
17g carbohydrates, 96mg cholesterol, 281mg sodium, 2g fiber

TURKEY MEATBALLS WITH WHOLE GRAIN PASTA AND TOMATO SAUCE

MAKES 4 SERVINGS

1½ pounds lean ground turkey breast

½ cup finely diced onion

1⅓ cups finely diced celery

2 tablespoons finely diced green bell pepper

1 tablespoon dry Italian seasoning mix

4 cloves fresh garlic, finely chopped

3 cups bread crumbs

½ cup liquid egg substitute

Salt and freshly ground pepper to taste

Olive oil cooking spray

8 ounces cooked whole grain spaghetti

2 cups Simple Tomato Pasta Sauce (page 492) or market-fresh tomato pasta sauce

In a large bowl combine ground turkey, onion, celery, green bell pepper, Italian seasoning, garlic, bread crumbs, egg, and salt and pepper. Mix well to combine ingredients and form into 12 meatballs. Heat a large skillet sprayed with a small amount of cooking oil; reduce heat to medium-low and add meatballs. Cook turning often until meatballs are completely cooked and outsides lightly browned. Serve with pasta and sauce.

Approx. 279 calories per serving
10g protein, 7.5g total fat, 0.8g saturated fat, 0 trans fat,
55g carbohydrates, 11mg cholesterol, 8mg sodium, 1g fiber

CALAMARI IN SPICY RED SAUCE

MAKES 4–6 SERVINGS

3 cups low-sodium canned tomato sauce

1 (28-ounce) can peeled Italian tomatoes, broken into pieces

1 cup Chianti wine

2 tablespoons freshly squeezed lemon juice

1 tablespoon extra-virgin olive oil

3 cloves fresh garlic, chopped

1 small onion, chopped

1 teaspoon black pepper

Salt to taste (optional)

½ teaspoon cayenne pepper

6 fresh basil leaves, chopped

⅓ cup grated Romano cheese

2 pounds cleaned calamari, cut in ½-inch rings

In a large deep skillet, add tomato sauce, tomato pieces, wine, lemon juice, olive oil, garlic, onion, pepper, salt to taste, cayenne, basil, and Romano cheese. Simmer on medium-low heat for about 30 minutes to allow alcohol to burn off and infuse other ingredients with its flavor. Add calamari rings and continue to simmer for an additional 20–30 minutes, stirring occasionally. Calamari is cooked when it plumps and becomes opaque in color. Do not overcook calamari; it becomes tough. This goes well with cooked fettuccine.

Approx. 224 calories per serving
26g protein, 5g total fat, 0.7g saturated fat, 0 trans fat,
16g carbohydrates, 186mg cholesterol, 306mg sodium, 3g fiber

BLACK BEANS AND BROWN RICE
MAKES 4–6 SERVINGS

1½ cups dry black beans

5 cups water or canned low-sodium, fat-free chicken broth

2 bay leaves

1 teaspoon freshly ground black pepper

Salt to taste

2 cloves fresh garlic, chopped

1 medium onion, chopped

1 medium green bell pepper, chopped

½ teaspoon cayenne pepper

10 green Manzanilla olives, pitted and halved

1 tablespoon extra-virgin olive oil

½ cup Edmundo cooking wine or a dry white wine

3 cups cooked brown rice

Raw chopped onion for garnish

Wash beans under cold running water. Place beans, water or broth, and bay leaves in a large heavy-bottomed pot and bring to a boil. Boil for about 2–3 minutes. Remove from heat, cover, and soak beans for 1 hour. Add black pepper, salt to taste, garlic, onion, and bell pepper, bring to boil, then reduce heat to simmer, cover, and cook until beans are tender (about 1–1½ hours), adding extra water or broth, if needed. When beans are tender, add cayenne, olives, olive oil, and wine. Cook on simmer for roughly 20–30 minutes to allow alcohol to evaporate and flavors to marry. Serve over brown rice and garnish with raw chopped onion.

Approx. 350 calories per serving (with chicken broth)
17g protein, 6g total fat, 0.57g saturated fat, 0 trans fat,
57g carbohydrates, 2mg cholesterol, 250mg sodium, 8g fiber

Approx. 321 calories per serving (with water)
13g protein, 4g total fat, 0.57g saturated fat, 0 trans fat,
56g carbohydrates, <1mg cholesterol, 250mg sodium, 8g fiber

LENTIL STEW
MAKES 6–8 SERVINGS

1½ cups lentils

1 medium onion, chopped

4 cloves fresh garlic, chopped

1 tablespoon extra-virgin olive oil

5 cups canned low-sodium fat-free chicken broth

1 tablespoon Worcestershire sauce

1 (15-ounce) can diced tomatoes, undrained

1 bay leaf

½ teaspoon fresh thyme

½ teaspoon cayenne

¼ teaspoon freshly ground pepper

Salt to taste

2 large potatoes, peeled and chopped

4 medium carrots, chopped

1 (10-ounce) bag fresh spinach

Dollop low-fat sour cream for garnish (optional)

Multigrain crusty bread (optional)

Rinse lentils and set aside. In a large deep skillet, sauté onion and garlic in olive oil until tender but not browned. Add lentils, chicken broth, Worcestershire sauce, tomatoes, bay leaf, thyme, cayenne, pepper, and salt to taste. Bring to a boil, cover, and reduce to simmer for 20 minutes. Add potatoes, carrots, and spinach, and stir to incorporate all ingredients. Bring to a boil, cover, reduce to medium-high, and cook for 20–30 minutes or until lentils and vegetables are tender and most of the liquid has been absorbed. Remove bay leaf and serve stew garnished with a dollop of sour cream and a multigrain crusty bread, if desired.

Approx. 215 calories per serving
15g protein, 3.3g total fat, 0.3g saturated fat, 0 trans fat,
36g carbohydrates, 1mg cholesterol, 123mg sodium, 7g fiber

GRILLED BLACKENED SALMON

MAKES 4 SERVINGS

1 teaspoon sea salt

1 tablespoon paprika

1 teaspoon onion powder

1 teaspoon garlic powder

1 teaspoon cayenne pepper

1 teaspoon mixed pepper flakes

½ teaspoon dried thyme

½ teaspoon dried basil

⅛ cup olive oil

4 (6–7-ounce) salmon fillets

Place a dry cast-iron skillet on grill and heat to 400 degrees. Mix all seasonings together. Brush both sides of fillets with scant amount of olive oil and drench both sides in seasonings. Place fillets on hot skillet and blacken each side about 3–4 minutes or until blackened and fish flakes easily.

Approx. 426 calories per serving
34g protein, 19g total fat, 0.9g saturated fat, 0 trans fat,
3g carbohydrates, 130mg cholesterol, 240mg sodium, 0.7g fiber

ANGEL HAIR WITH FRESH MARINARA
MAKES 6–8 SERVINGS

16 ounces whole grain angel hair pasta

4 tablespoons extra-virgin olive oil

½ white onion, chopped

6 cloves fresh garlic, chopped

1 (28-ounce) can crushed Italian tomatoes

1 (6-ounce) can tomato paste

4–5 chopped fresh basil leaves

4 tablespoons freshly chopped parsley

1 teaspoon crushed red hot pepper flakes

Salt and freshly ground pepper to taste

½ cup white wine (optional)

Grated Parmesan cheese (optional)

Bring water to a boil, add pasta, and cook pasta until *al dente*. Remove from heat, drain pasta, and return to pot, drizzling with scant amount of olive oil to keep pasta from sticking together. Set aside. Heat olive oil in a heavy-bottomed skillet and sauté onion and garlic, but do not brown. Reduce heat to simmer. Add crushed tomatoes and tomato paste, basil, parsley, hot pepper flakes, salt and pepper, and wine, and simmer for 30–40 minutes, stirring occasionally. Serve sauce over pasta and sprinkle with Parmesan cheese, if desired.

Approx. 310 calories per serving
9.2g protein, 8.6g total fat, 0.8g saturated fat, 0 trans fat,
48g carbohydrates, 0 cholesterol, 246mg sodium, 6.6g fiber

LEMON SHRIMP PASTA

MAKES 4–6 SERVINGS

30–36 large shrimp, peeled and deveined

Juice from 4 fresh lemons

1 teaspoon lemon pepper seasoning

12 ounces bow tie pasta

1 tablespoon extra-virgin olive oil

4 cloves fresh garlic, chopped

4 scallions, white and green parts, sliced

10 black olives, pitted and coarsely chopped

⅛ teaspoon crushed red hot pepper flakes

1 teaspoon ground garlic powder

3 tablespoons trans fat–free canola/olive oil spread

Salt to taste (optional)

Grated Parmesan cheese for garnish (optional)

Place shrimp in a large resealable plastic baggie and add lemon juice and lemon pepper seasoning. Allow shrimp to marinate in refrigerator for at least 30 minutes. Bring water to a boil, add pasta, and cook pasta until *al dente*. Remove from heat, drain pasta, and return to pot, drizzling with scant amount of olive oil to keep pasta from sticking together. Set aside. In a large skillet add olive oil, garlic, and scallions, and sauté lightly until soft. Add black olives and hot pepper flakes, then set aside but keep warm. When shrimp has marinated, add shrimp, lemon juice, and garlic powder to scallion mixture. Bring to a low simmer and cook until shrimp are pink and cooked through. Add pasta, canola/olive oil spread, and salt to taste to shrimp mixture, and allow spread to melt while tossing pasta and lemon shrimp mixture to blend flavors. Serve hot with a sprinkle of Parmesan cheese, if desired.

Approx. 326 calories per serving
16g protein, 9.5g total fat, 1.7g saturated fat, 0 trans fat,
42.2g carbohydrates, 64.5mg cholesterol, 232mg sodium, 0.4g fiber

GRILLED WHOLE SEA BASS

MAKES 4 SERVINGS

2 (1½-pound) sea bass, dressed and gutted
2 sprigs fresh rosemary
½ of a fresh lemon, thinly sliced
Olive oil to drizzle
¼ teaspoon garlic powder
¼ teaspoon onion powder
Lemon pepper seasoning to taste

For Sauce:

1 teaspoon sea salt (optional)
2 teaspoons capers, drained
4 cloves fresh garlic, crushed
4 tablespoons water
3 sprigs fresh rosemary
2 fresh bay leaves
1 teaspoon lime juice
2 tablespoons extra-virgin olive oil
Freshly ground pepper to taste

Wash fish and pat dry with paper towel, then place 1 sprig of rosemary and ½ of lemon slices (divided) in the cavity of each fish. Drizzle a small amount of olive oil over each fish and sprinkle with garlic powder, onion powder, and lemon pepper seasoning. Grill for about 5 minutes on each side or until fish is cooked through. Drizzle with sauce and serve garnished with remaining lemon slices.

Sauce:

In a food processor add salt, capers, garlic, and water; process until smooth. In a bowl crush rosemary and bay leaves. Add crushed bay leaf mixture and lime juice to garlic mixture. Stir in olive oil and pepper, and mix to blend.

Approx. 388 calories per serving
63g protein, 17g total fat, 2.9g saturated fat, 0 trans fat,
0 carbohydrates, 140mg cholesterol, 801mg sodium, 0 fiber

VEAL SCALOPPINE

MAKES 4 SERVINGS

1 pound (16 ounces) boneless veal, trimmed of excess fat
Salt and freshly ground pepper to taste
Olive oil cooking spray

For Sauce:

¼ cup canned low-sodium, fat-free chicken broth

½ cup chopped white onion

4 cloves fresh garlic, finely chopped

1 (12-ounce) can diced Italian herb tomatoes

4 tablespoons dry white wine

½ teaspoon dried oregano

6 anchovies, drained and broken into pieces

1 tablespoon capers, drained

Divide veal into 4 pieces. Place pieces one at a time between 2 pieces of wax paper. Starting from center, pound pieces with a meat mallet, working your way toward the edges, until the meat is about ⅛ of an inch in thickness. Season lightly with salt and pepper and set aside. Repeat procedure with all remaining pieces. Spray a large heavy skillet with cooking oil and heat over medium-high heat. Add veal pieces to skillet and cook for 2–4 minutes, turning fillets over once, until they reach desired doneness. Place fillets on a platter and cover with sauce. Serve warm.

Sauce:

Put chicken broth in a medium saucepan, add onion and garlic, and cook until tender. Stir in tomatoes, wine, oregano, anchovies, and capers. Cover pan and bring to a quick boil; reduce to very low heat, then simmer uncovered for 5–10 minutes.

Approx. 202 calories per serving
26g protein, 3.3g total fat, 0.98g saturated fat, 0 trans fat,
13.7g carbohydrates, 96mg cholesterol, 768mg sodium, 2g fiber

SPICY EGGPLANT
MAKES 6–8 SERVINGS

4 tablespoons extra-virgin olive oil

1 (1-pound) eggplant, thinly sliced (about ⅛-inch thick)

½ cup liquid egg substitute

¼ cup all-purpose flour

2 tablespoons finely minced fresh garlic

Salt and freshly ground pepper to taste

Cholula hot sauce or other spicy red hot sauce to taste

1½ cups fresh marinara sauce

Heat 1 tablespoon of olive oil in heavy-bottomed skillet over medium-high heat. Dip eggplant slices in egg and then lightly into flour. Sprinkle slices with garlic and salt and pepper to taste. Cook, adding only as much olive oil as needed, until golden brown, and transfer to warmed plate. Repeat until all eggplant slices are cooked. Layer cooked eggplant in an oven-safe casserole dish and drizzle each layer with a small amount of hot sauce and fresh marinara sauce. Repeat layers until all eggplant is used. Do not overdo sauces! Keep in 175-degree oven until ready to serve.

Approx. 117 calories per serving
1g protein, 10g total fat, 2g saturated fat, 0 trans fat,
3g carbohydrates, 0 cholesterol, 212mg sodium, 1g fiber

Side Dishes

SAFFRON RICE
MAKES 4–6 SERVINGS

3–4 cups canned low-sodium, fat-free vegetable broth
1 tablespoon extra-virgin olive oil
4 tablespoons chopped shallots
2 cloves fresh garlic, minced
1 cup short-grain rice
1 cup dry white wine
¼ teaspoon crushed saffron threads
½ teaspoon dried thyme
Salt and freshly ground pepper to taste

Bring broth to a boil, then reduce heat to a low simmer. In a large skillet, heat olive oil, add shallots and garlic, and sauté until soft (about 5 minutes). Add rice and continue to sauté, stirring constantly to keep mixture from burning. Add wine, saffron, and thyme, stirring constantly, scraping in any brown bits from pan. When wine is absorbed, slowly add simmering broth, stirring constantly as broth is absorbed and rice has become tender (about 15–20 minutes). It's possible some of the broth will be left over. Add salt and pepper to taste.

Approx. 282 calories per serving
5g protein, 2g total fat, 0.34g saturated fat, 0 trans fat,
49g carbohydrates, 0 cholesterol, 87mg sodium, 2g fiber

ZESTY LEMON SWISS CHARD

MAKES 4–6 SERVINGS

1¼ pounds Swiss chard, cleaned and trimmed

2 tablespoons fresh lemon juice

1½ teaspoons extra-virgin olive oil

1 tablespoon lemon pepper seasoning

Salt to taste

½ cup golden raisins

2 tablespoons pine nuts

Shred Swiss chard into thin strips and place in a large bowl. Combine lemon juice, olive oil, lemon pepper seasoning, and salt; mix well with whisk. Drizzle mixture over chard and toss. Add raisins and pine nuts and toss. Let stand for 15 minutes before serving.

Approx. 120 calories per serving

2g protein, 5g total fat, 0.7g saturated fat, 0 trans fat,

21g carbohydrates, 0 cholesterol, 302mg sodium, 1g fiber

ORZO WITH FETA CHEESE AND BROCCOLI FLORETS

MAKES 8 SERVINGS

2 cups broccoli florets

3 cups canned low-sodium, fat-free chicken broth

8 ounces orzo (about 1 cup)

6 ounces feta cheese

In boiling water, cook broccoli florets until crispy tender. Drain, set aside, and keep warm. In a saucepan, bring chicken broth to a boil, reduce heat, add orzo, and cook until liquid is absorbed. Stir often to keep from burning. Fluff orzo with fork and add feta cheese, stirring to blend together. Transfer orzo to serving platter and top with broccoli florets.

Approx. 174 calories per serving

8g protein, 7g total fat, 3g saturated fat, 0 trans fat,

22g carbohydrates, 195mg cholesterol, 237mg sodium, 0 fiber

ROASTED PEPPERS
MAKES 4–6 SERVINGS

4 large red bell peppers
2 cloves fresh garlic, peeled and sliced
4 tablespoons extra-virgin olive oil
Salt and freshly ground pepper to taste

Clean peppers and pat dry. Place peppers on moderately hot grill or on a rack under a broiler 1–2 inches from heat, turning often until skin is charred and blistered. Charring of entire skin takes about 15–20 minutes. Remove from grill or broiler and place peppers aside to cool. When cool enough to handle, rub off blackened skins. Cut each pepper in half, remove stalk and seeds, and cut into ½-inch strips. Place strips in a bowl and add garlic, olive oil, and salt and pepper to taste. Toss and set aside for about 30 minutes before serving.

Approx. 108 calories per serving
1g protein, 10g total fat, 1g saturated fat, 0 trans fat,
7g carbohydrates, 0 cholesterol, 2mg sodium, 2g fiber

CLASSIC SPINACH AND PINE NUTS

MAKES 4 SERVINGS

¼ cup golden raisins

4 tablespoons pine nuts

2 tablespoons extra-virgin olive oil

4 cloves fresh garlic, chopped

1½ (10-ounce) bags fresh spinach, cleaned

Fresh lemon juice

Extra-virgin olive oil to taste

Salt and freshly ground pepper to taste

Place raisins in a bowl and cover with boiling water. Let stand for approximately 10 minutes, until raisins are plump; drain well. In a skillet over medium heat, toast pine nuts, stirring constantly for about 1–2 minutes. Remove from heat and set aside. In a large skillet, heat olive oil. Add garlic and sauté for 1–2 minutes, until golden. Add spinach a little at a time until it all becomes wilted (about 3–5 minutes), stirring constantly. Pour raisins over spinach and mix well. With a slotted spoon, transfer spinach to a serving dish, and sprinkle pine nuts over top. Serve immediately or, if serving at room temperature, add fresh lemon juice and olive oil and salt and pepper to taste.

Approx. 149 calories per serving
4g protein, 12g total fat, 2g saturated fat, 0 trans fat,
10g carbohydrates, 0 cholesterol, 41mg sodium, 2g fiber

CHILLED STUFFED PASTA SHELLS

MAKES 4 SERVINGS

1 cup (canned) hearts of palm, chopped and well drained

1 cup chopped zucchini

2 cloves fresh garlic, finely minced

8 large pitted black olives, chopped

2 tablespoons chopped fresh parsley

2 tablespoons + 2 teaspoons extra-virgin olive oil

4 teaspoons freshly squeezed lemon juice

Salt and freshly ground pepper to taste

12 jumbo pasta shells, cooked al dente and drained

4 cups mixed salad greens

Combine hearts of palm, zucchini, garlic, olives, and parsley in a large bowl. Whisk together olive oil, lemon juice, and salt and pepper for vinaigrette. To bowl of vegetables, add 2 tablespoons of vinaigrette; gently mix. Stuff shells with vegetable mixture, cover, and refrigerate until well chilled. Refrigerate remaining vinaigrette. To serve, divide greens into 4 equal portions, top each serving with 3 stuffed shells, and drizzle with remaining vinaigrette.

Approx. 210 calories per serving
5g protein, 11g total fat, 1.4g saturated fat, 0 trans fat,
24g carbohydrates, 0 cholesterol, 255mg sodium, 2g fiber

GREEK RICE

MAKES 4 SERVINGS

1 cup short-grain rice

2 cups canned low-sodium vegetable broth

1 tablespoon extra-virgin olive oil

2 teaspoons minced fresh garlic

2 tablespoons finely chopped onion

5 ounces fresh spinach, cleaned and chopped

¼ teaspoon dried oregano

Salt and freshly ground pepper to taste

¼ cup crumbled feta cheese

1 tablespoon lemon juice

Bring rice in vegetable broth to boil, cover tightly, reduce heat to simmer, and cook until liquid is absorbed. While rice is cooking, heat olive oil over medium-high heat and sauté garlic and onion until golden. Reduce heat to medium; add spinach a little at a time to allow spinach to wilt while mixing in garlic. When spinach is wilted, mix in oregano and salt and pepper to taste. Remove spinach mixture from heat, and add cooked rice, feta cheese, and lemon juice; toss well.

Approx. 255 calories per serving
12.5g protein, 5.7g total fat, 1.3g saturated fat, 0 trans fat,
22g carbohydrates, 5mg cholesterol, 146mg sodium, 1g fiber

GARLIC RICE

MAKES 4 SERVINGS

½ tablespoon extra-virgin olive oil

4 cloves fresh garlic, minced

1 cup basmati long-grain rice

2 cups canned low-sodium, fat-free chicken broth

¼ cup grated Parmesan cheese

2 tablespoons chopped fresh parsley

3 jumbo cloves roasted fresh garlic, cut into small pieces

Salt and freshly ground pepper to taste

Fresh chopped parsley or cilantro for garnish

In a skillet, heat olive oil and sauté fresh garlic until golden brown. Bring rice in chicken broth to a boil, cover tightly, reduce heat to simmer, and cook until liquid is absorbed. Remove rice from heat and add olive oil and sautéed garlic, Parmesan cheese, parsley, roasted garlic, and salt and pepper to taste; toss well. Garnish with parsley or cilantro and serve.

Approx. 194 calories per serving
5g protein, 3g total fat, 0.3g saturated fat, 0 trans fat,
38g carbohydrates, 0 cholesterol, 3mg sodium, 1g fiber

COUSCOUS, TOMATOES, AND BLACK BEANS

MAKES 4–6 SERVINGS

1½ cups canned low-sodium vegetable broth

1 cup couscous

1 tablespoon extra-virgin olive oil

2 cloves fresh garlic, minced

¼ cup fresh lemon juice

¼ teaspoon freshly ground pepper

1½ cups canned black beans, rinsed and drained

4 large plum tomatoes, chopped

½ cup red onion, finely chopped

Fresh parsley, finely chopped for garnish

In a saucepan, bring broth to a boil. Stir in couscous, remove from heat, cover, and let stand until liquid is absorbed. In a small skillet over medium heat, add olive oil and garlic and sauté until golden brown. Remove skillet from heat, add lemon juice and pepper, and mix ingredients through. Transfer couscous to a large serving bowl. Fluff grains with fingers to separate. Add in garlic mixture, black beans, tomatoes, and onion; stir gently to mix. Garnish with parsley and serve.

Approx. 210 calories per serving
8g protein, 3g total fat, 0.3g saturated fat, 0 trans fat,
37g carbohydrates, 0 cholesterol, 239mg sodium, 5g fiber

ASPARAGUS WITH FRESH GARDEN HERBS

MAKES 4 SERVINGS

1 pound asparagus, tough ends removed
1 tablespoon finely chopped fresh parsley
½ tablespoon finely chopped fresh basil
⅛ teaspoon freshly ground pepper
3 tablespoons trans fat–free canola/olive oil spread, melted
2 Italian plum tomatoes, seeded and chopped
2 tablespoons shredded Parmesan cheese

Steam asparagus for 3–5 minutes until crispy tender. Drain well and place on a serving platter. Combine parsley, basil, pepper, and canola/olive oil spread. Drizzle mixture over asparagus, sprinkle on tomatoes and Parmesan cheese, and serve.

Approx. 85 calories per serving
4g protein, 9g total fat, 1g saturated fat, 0 trans fat,
4g carbohydrates, 2mg cholesterol, 119mg sodium, 2g fiber

BROCCOLI WITH FRESH GARLIC

MAKES 4–6 SERVINGS

10–12 fresh broccoli spears, roughly 6 inches long
3 cups canned low-sodium, fat-free chicken broth
3 tablespoons extra-virgin olive oil
2–3 cloves fresh garlic, crushed
2 tablespoons chopped fresh parsley
Salt to taste
Pinch of freshly ground pepper to taste

Cook spears in a large skillet of chicken broth until slightly undercooked (about 7 minutes). Test with a fork; do not overcook. Drain well and set aside. Heat olive oil in a large skillet over medium-high heat; add garlic and sauté until golden brown. Add broccoli, parsley, and salt and pepper to taste. Turn spears several times, mixing well with seasonings, olive oil, and garlic. Serve immediately.

Approx. 161 calories per serving
11g protein, 9g total fat, 2g saturated fat, 0 trans fat,
16g carbohydrates, 1mg cholesterol, 80mg sodium, 9g fiber

CRISPY TENDER RATATOUILLE
MAKES 8 SERVINGS

2 large eggplants, rinsed and cut into 1½-inch cubes

3 red bell peppers

¾ cup extra-virgin olive oil

2 large onions, chopped

8 cloves fresh garlic, minced

4 small zucchini, cut to 1½-inch cubes

4 large ripe tomatoes, cored and diced

1 cup dry red wine

1 tablespoon of capers, rinsed and drained

1 or 2 pinches of crushed red hot pepper flakes or to taste

Salt and freshly ground pepper to taste

Freshly chopped basil for garnish (optional)

Pitted black olives for garnish (optional)

Place eggplant cubes in a bowl with salt and cover with water. Place heavy plate inside bowl to weight down cubes, submerging them in brine. Set aside for 1½–2 hours. Roast red bell peppers under broiler in oven until skins turn black and are easy to remove. Peel off skins and cut peppers into long strips. Set aside. Heat ¼ cup of olive oil in a large skillet over medium-low heat, add onions and garlic, and cook until soft. Do not brown. Add roasted pepper to mixture. Drain eggplant cubes and pat dry with paper towels. Add another ¼ cup olive oil to skillet, return to medium heat, and sauté eggplant cubes until golden brown (15 minutes). Add zucchini to skillet and cook, adding more olive oil if needed. When zucchini is cooked, add tomatoes, lowering heat slightly; stir in wine and simmer until wine is evaporated and mixture turns to a jam consistency (about 20 minutes). Stir in capers and hot pepper flakes and combine all vegetables with tomato sauce. Use a slotted spoon to stir but don't break up vegetables. Add salt and pepper to taste. Before serving, add basil and olives, if desired.

Approx. 221 calories per serving
2g protein, 21g total fat, 3g saturated fat, 0 trans fat,
9g carbohydrates, 0 cholesterol, 43mg sodium, 2g fiber

GARLICKY SWISS CHARD

MAKES 6 SERVINGS OR 3 CUPS

2 bunches Swiss chard (about 1½ pounds each), cleaned and trimmed

3 tablespoons extra-virgin olive oil

6 cloves fresh garlic, minced

½ cup canned low-sodium, fat-free chicken broth

¼ teaspoon hot cherry peppers, finely minced

½ teaspoon salt or to taste

¼ teaspoon freshly ground pepper

Rinse greens well and cut ribs and stems into 2-inch pieces. Set aside. Break leaves into roughly 2-inch pieces. Heat olive oil in a large heavy-bottomed skillet; add garlic and sauté until golden brown, stirring constantly. Add chard ribs and stems, broth, and hot peppers and cook until almost tender. Add leaves in bunches, stirring to wilt. Stir in salt and pepper. Cook covered, until tender and liquid is evaporated, stirring often.

Approx. 83 calories per serving
2g protein, 7g total fat, 1g saturated fat, 0 trans fat,
4g carbohydrates, 0.1mg cholesterol, 222mg sodium, 1g fiber

GREAT CORN ON THE COB

MAKES 4 SERVINGS

4 teaspoons trans fat–free canola/olive oil spread, melted
Salt and freshly ground pepper to taste
4 ears fresh corn, husks and silk removed
24 large fresh basil leaves

Preheat oven to 450 degrees. Combine canola/olive oil spread and salt and pepper in a small bowl. Brush buttery mixture over corn to coat entire ear. Set each ear in heavy tinfoil. Place 3 basil leaves on the bottom and 3 over the top of each ear. Fold tinfoil over ears and twist ends to seal. Place foil-covered ears on a baking sheet. Bake for 15 minutes or until tender.

Approx. 177 calories per serving
3g protein, 11g total fat, 3g saturated fat, 0 trans fat,
17g carbohydrates, 0 cholesterol, 114mg sodium, 2g fiber

PASS THE PEAS, PLEASE

MAKES 6 SERVINGS

2 tablespoons olive oil
1 white onion, chopped
2 cloves fresh garlic, minced
16 ounces fresh or frozen peas, thawed
½ cup canned low-sodium, fat-free chicken broth
Salt and freshly ground pepper to taste
Pinch of sugar (optional)
Butter spray

Heat olive oil in a skillet over medium heat. Add onion and garlic and sauté until soft, about 4–5 minutes. Add peas, broth, salt and pepper, and sugar, if desired. Cover and cook until peas are tender. Serve hot with a spritz of butter spray.

Approx. 98 calories per serving
4g protein, 5g total fat, 1g saturated fat, 0 trans fat,
10g carbohydrates, 0 cholesterol, 90mg sodium, 3g fiber

BAKED POTATO FINGERS WITH SHALLOTS AND FRESH HERBS

MAKES 4 SERVINGS

4 large Yukon Gold potatoes (about 1½ pounds)
2 tablespoons olive oil
2 large shallots, finely minced
1 tablespoon finely chopped fresh sage leaves
1 tablespoon finely chopped fresh rosemary
Salt and freshly ground pepper to taste
Olive oil cooking spray

Preheat oven to 375 degrees. Scrub skins of potatoes with a vegetable brush and pat dry. Cut potatoes in half lengthwise. Cut each half into 4 lengthwise slices. In a small bowl, combine olive oil, shallots, sage, rosemary, and salt and pepper. Stir to blend. Spray a shallow baking sheet with cooking oil. Arrange potato fingers in a single layer on baking sheet and generously brush them with shallot-herb mixture. Place in oven and roast for 40 minutes, turning once after about 20 minutes. Roast until fingers are browned and tender. Remove from oven and serve.

Approx. 179 calories per serving
3g protein, 7g total fat, 1g saturated fat, 0 trans fat,
27g carbohydrates, 0 cholesterol, 10mg sodium, 4g fiber

KALE WITH ORANGE-MUSTARD DRESSING

MAKES 8 SERVINGS

1 tablespoon olive oil
2 bunches fresh kale, stems removed, leaves cut to bite-sized pieces
2 radishes, sliced thin
1 avocado, deseeded, peeled, and chopped

For Dressing:

2 large oranges, peeled, pith removed, and segments separated
2 tablespoons grainy mustard
¼ cup extra-virgin olive oil
1 teaspoon chopped fresh thyme leaves
Salt and freshly ground pepper to taste

In a large skillet, heat olive oil over medium heat. Add kale, a handful at a time, and sauté, stirring frequently until wilted. Transfer to serving bowl, add radishes, avocado, remaining orange segments from dressing, and dressing. Toss to coat kale mixture, divide into 8 portions, and serve warm.

Dressing:

In a small bowl, squeeze enough orange segment membranes to make 3 tablespoons of juice. Set remaining segments aside. Whisk mustard and olive oil into the juice until combined. Add thyme and salt and pepper to taste. Set dressing aside.

Approx. 157 calories per serving
4g protein, 12g total fat, 1g saturated fat, 0 trans fat,
13g carbohydrates, 0 cholesterol, 51mg sodium, 4g fiber

BROILED AVOCADO HALVES AND CHEDDAR CHEESE

MAKES 4 SERVINGS

2 ripe-but-firm avocados, halved and pitted, with skin on
¼ cup reduced-fat shredded extra-sharp cheddar cheese
1 small jalapeno pepper, finely minced (about 1 teaspoon)
Salt and freshly ground pepper to taste
1 tablespoon fresh lime juice
1 lime, quartered, for garnish

Preheat broiler. Place avocado halves on a lined baking sheet cut side up. In a small mixing bowl, combine cheddar cheese, jalapeno, salt and pepper, and lime juice. Divide the cheese mixture among the tops of avocado halves. Place baking sheet 3–4 inches under heat and broil for about 3–5 minutes or until cheese bubbles and begins to brown. Serve halves warm with lime wedges.

Approx. 185 calories per serving
5g protein, 15g total fat, 2g saturated fat, 0 trans fat,
8g carbohydrates, 3mg cholesterol, 92mg sodium, 6g fiber

BROCCOLI WITH ALMONDS AND OLIVES

MAKES 4 SERVINGS

2 tablespoons extra-virgin olive oil
1 clove fresh garlic, minced
2 teaspoons grated lemon zest
½ tablespoon freshly squeezed lemon juice
12 pitted Kalamata olives, chopped
⅛ teaspoon crushed red hot pepper flakes
¼ cup chopped toasted almonds
1 head fresh broccoli (about 1 pound), florets only, blanched
1½ tablespoons chopped fresh parsley
Salt and freshly ground pepper to taste

Combine olive oil, garlic, lemon zest, lemon juice, olives, hot pepper flakes, and almonds in a large bowl. Add blanched broccoli florets, parsley, and salt and pepper to taste. Toss to coat and serve warm.

Approx. 123 calories per serving
4g protein, 14g total fat, 1g saturated fat, 0 trans fat,
8g carbohydrates, 0 cholesterol, 299mg sodium, 4g fiber

GRILLED POLENTA WITH CHEDDAR CHEESE
AND SUNDRIED TOMATOES

MAKES 6 SERVINGS

6 cups water

Salt to taste

1¾ cups yellow cornmeal

1½ tablespoons chopped fresh oregano

1½ tablespoons chopped fresh basil

3 tablespoons trans fat–free canola/olive oil spread

6 ounces reduced-fat shredded cheddar cheese

6 sundried tomato slices

In a heavy saucepan, bring water to a boil and add salt. Gradually whisk in cornmeal. Reduce heat to low and cook cornmeal mixture until it thickens, stirring often for about 15 minutes. Remove from heat, add oregano, basil, and canola/olive oil spread, and stir until melted into mixture. Transfer to a lightly oiled 7-inch baking dish, spreading out evenly to about ¾-inch thickness. Refrigerate until cold and firm, at least 2–3 hours. When firm, invert polenta onto a clean surface and cut into 2x2-inch pieces. Heat grill to medium heat. Oil both sides of polenta with olive oil and sear each side until golden brown (about 3 minutes). Remove from heat, and while hot sprinkle with cheddar cheese and top with a sundried tomato slice. Serve immediately.

Approx. 208 calories per serving
5g protein, 7g total fat, 2g saturated fat, 0 trans fat,
28g carbohydrates, 5mg cholesterol, 107mg sodium, 3g fiber

COUSCOUS WITH TURNIPS AND GREENS
MAKES 4–6 SERVINGS

2½ cups canned low-sodium, fat free chicken broth

3 tablespoons olive oil, divided

1½ cups pearl couscous

1 bunch baby turnips with greens, peeled and quartered

½ teaspoon cumin seeds

2 cloves fresh garlic, minced

½ medium white onion, finely chopped

Salt and freshly ground pepper to taste

In a medium saucepan, add broth and 1 tablespoon olive oil and bring to boil. Remove from heat, stir in couscous, cover, and let stand.

Cut turnips from greens and wash both heads and greens well, removing any brown or wilted leaves. Tear greens into roughly 1-inch pieces and trim turnips and cut into halves. Set greens and turnips aside.

Add remaining olive oil to a large skillet over medium-high heat. Add cumin and cook for 1 minute until fragrant. Add garlic and continue to cook until soft and fragrant, about 1 more minute. Add onion, then stir and cook until soft. Add turnips, cover pan, and cook until crispy tender, stirring occasionally. Uncover pan, add greens and salt and pepper, and cook until greens wilt.

Fluff couscous with a fork and transfer to a large bowl, add cooked vegetable mixture, fluff all again, and serve immediately.

Approx. 203 calories per serving
14g protein, 19g total fat, 1g saturated fat, 0 trans fat,
18g carbohydrates, 0 cholesterol, 44mg sodium, 1g fiber

OVEN-ROASTED POTATO WEDGES
MAKES 6 SERVINGS

1½ pounds russet potatoes, scrubbed and cut lengthwise into wedges
¼ cup olive oil
½ teaspoon smoky paprika
¼ teaspoon garlic salt or to taste
Cayenne pepper to taste
Freshly ground pepper to taste

Preheat oven to 450 degrees. Combine potato wedges, olive oil, paprika, garlic salt, cayenne, and pepper in a large, resealable plastic baggie. Toss well to coat all sides of potatoes with olive oil and seasonings. Remove from bag, place wedges in a single layer on a foil-lined baking sheet, and bake, turning once after 10–15 minutes, until wedges are golden and crispy (about 25–30 minutes).

Approx. 170 calories per serving
4g protein, 7g total fat, 1g saturated fat, 0 trans fat,
24g carbohydrates, 0 cholesterol, 9mg sodium, 2g fiber

BOILED FRESH RED BEETS
MAKES 4 SERVINGS

8 medium red beets, unpeeled
Water to cover beets
Salt and freshly ground pepper, to taste
Butter-flavored cooking spray (optional)

Wear disposable gloves or kitchen gloves to prevent hands from staining since fresh red beets' skins and juices will stain skin and clothing as well as porous items. Cut stems and root ends from beets. Wash beets, gently rubbing skins to extract as much dirt from beets as possible. Place unpeeled beets in a large pot and cover with water. Boil on medium-high heat until beets are tender. Remove from heat and strain off juice through a strainer; if you like beet root juice, reserve. Hold beets in pot under running cool water and gently peel off skins from beets, again using gloves to avoid beet stains. Season with salt and pepper and a spray of butter, if desired, and serve.

Approx. 44 calories per serving
2g protein, 0 total fat, 0 saturated fat, 0 trans fat,
10g carbohydrates, 0 cholesterol, 76mg sodium, 2g fiber

SAUTÉED KALE AND SPINACH WITH MUSHROOMS AND TOMATO

MAKES 4 SERVINGS

4 tablespoons olive oil, divided

4 tablespoons chopped fresh garlic

3 bunches fresh kale, leaves only

Crushed red hot pepper flakes to taste

1 (9-ounce) bag fresh baby spinach

¼ cup water, if needed

Salt and freshly ground pepper to taste

½ large white onion, chopped

2 (8-ounce) containers fresh white button mushrooms, halved

10–15 grape tomatoes

2 tablespoons fresh garlic paste blend

In a large skillet over medium-high heat, add 2 tablespoons olive oil and garlic and sauté until soft and fragrant. Add kale, a handful at a time, and hot pepper flakes, and cook, stirring often, until kale is wilted. Add baby spinach and continue to cook until wilted. Add water, if needed, to keep moist. Season with salt and pepper to taste. Reduce heat to very low and keep warm.

In a separate skillet over medium heat, add remaining 2 tablespoons olive oil. Add onion, mushrooms, grape tomatoes, and garlic paste. Cook, stirring often, until mushrooms are soft and tomatoes begin to break down. Add salt and pepper to taste. Combine tomato mixture with spinach mixture and return heat to a simmer, stirring to incorporate ingredients and flavors, about 2 minutes, and serve.

Approx. 151 calories per serving

11g protein, 15g total fat, 1g saturated fat, 0 trans fat,

27g carbohydrates, 0 cholesterol, 144mg sodium, 5g fiber

ROASTED BABY ARTICHOKES AND PARMESAN CHEESE

MAKES 4 SERVINGS

4 (9-ounce) boxes frozen baby artichokes hearts

2 cups canned low-sodium, fat-free chicken broth

4 cloves fresh garlic, coarsely chopped

Salt and freshly ground pepper to taste

1 cup panko bread crumbs

½ cup grated Parmesan cheese

Melted trans fat–free canola/olive oil spread, to drizzle

Preheat oven to 350 degrees. In a large pot, add artichoke hearts, broth, garlic, and salt and pepper. Bring to a gentle boil and cook for about 3 minutes until hearts are soft. Drain through a large sifter to retain garlic and artichoke pieces. In a rimmed oven-safe casserole dish, spread out artichokes and garlic evenly, top with a layer of bread crumbs, and then sprinkle on Parmesan cheese. Place in oven and bake until heated through and crumbs are a golden brown. Serve while hot with a drizzle of melted canola/olive oil spread.

Approx. 128 calories per serving (about 12 artichoke hearts per serving)
4g protein, 1g total fat, 1g saturated fat, 0 trans fat,
19g carbohydrates, 0 cholesterol, 155mg sodium, 5g fiber

ITALIAN BROCCOLI
MAKES 4 SERVINGS

2 large stalks of broccoli, stems removed and heads cut in half
1 cup of Italian dressing mix of your choice
⅓ cup dry white wine
Salt and freshly ground pepper to taste
½ cup grated Parmesan cheese (optional)

In a large rimmed baking dish, place broccoli heads cut side down in a single layer. Whisk together Italian dressing and wine and pour over broccoli heads. Lift each head to allow liquid to coat the cut sides of the heads as well. Cover the baking dish with plastic wrap and place in refrigerator to marinate for at least 1 hour. After marinating, place heads in a saucepan, pour marinade over heads, and steam them until tender crispy. Remove heads from remaining liquid and serve hot, seasoned with salt and pepper to taste and a sprinkling of Parmesan cheese.

Approx. 58 calories per serving
1g protein, 1g total fat, 1g saturated fat, 0 trans fat,
3g carbohydrates, 0 cholesterol, 75mg sodium, 0 fiber

CRISPY TENDER BROCCOLINI

MAKES 4 SERVINGS

1 pound (roughly 2 bunches) broccolini
2 tablespoons olive oil
2 teaspoons finely chopped fresh garlic
½ teaspoon crushed red hot pepper flakes
2 tablespoons freshly squeezed lemon juice
Zest from ½ of a lemon
Salt and freshly ground pepper to taste

Rinse broccolini under cold water. If stems are thick, peel back skins to remove tough skin. In a large skillet, heat olive oil over medium-high heat. Add garlic and sauté until fragrant. Add broccolini and sauté for about 3 minutes. Cover with water, add hot pepper flakes, and steam for about 3 minutes or until broccolini is crispy tender. Squeeze lemon juice over broccolini, sprinkle with lemon zest, add salt and pepper to taste, and serve.

Approx. 95 calories per serving
3g protein, 7g total fat, 1g saturated fat, 0 trans fat,
6g carbohydrates, 0 cholesterol, 24mg sodium, 1g fiber

SPICY JULIENNED SWEET POTATO FRIES
MAKES 4 SERVINGS

1 pound sweet potatoes, peeled and julienned
1 tablespoon olive oil
1 tablespoon light brown sugar
1 teaspoon salt or to taste
½ teaspoon chili powder
Pinch of cayenne pepper
¼ teaspoon ground cinnamon

Preheat oven to 450 degrees. Line a large baking sheet with foil. In a large, resealable plastic baggie, combine potatoes, olive oil, brown sugar, salt, chili powder, cayenne, and cinnamon. Toss well to coat and remove from bag. Arrange potatoes in a single layer on baking sheet and bake for roughly 15 minutes. Turn potatoes over and bake for additional 15 minutes or until crispy.

Approx. 55 calories per serving
<0.5g protein, 1g total fat, 0 saturated fat, 0 trans fat,
4g carbohydrates, 0 cholesterol, 14mg sodium, 1g fiber

FRESH STEWED TOMATOES

MAKES 4 SERVINGS

1 tablespoon olive oil

½ cup diced white onion

½ cup chopped celery

⅛ cup finely diced green bell pepper

1 tablespoon freshly minced garlic

¼ teaspoon crushed red hot pepper flakes

1 teaspoon dried basil

2 large tomatoes, peeled and quartered

1½ teaspoons low-calorie baking sweetener

¼ cup chopped fresh parsley

Salt and freshly ground pepper to taste

In a large pot, add olive oil, onion, celery, green bell pepper, garlic, hot pepper flakes, and basil. Cook on medium-low heat, stirring often, until vegetables are soft. Add tomatoes, sweetener, parsley, and salt and pepper to taste. Continue cooking on medium-low heat, stirring often, until tomatoes become very soft and fall apart. Serve as a side with meat, chicken, or fish.

Approx. 54 calories per serving
1g protein, 3g total fat, 0 saturated fat, 0 trans fat,
5g carbohydrates, 0 cholesterol, 14mg sodium, 1g fiber

TWICE-BAKED SWEET POTATOES WITH CHEESE
AND FRESH SAGE

MAKES 2 SERVINGS

1 large sweet potato
Olive oil to drizzle
2 tablespoons freshly grated Parmesan cheese + some to sprinkle
1 tablespoon finely chopped fresh sage
Salt and freshly ground pepper to taste

Preheat oven to 400 degrees. Place sweet potato in a shallow oven-safe platter and lightly drizzle top with olive oil. Bake until soft, roughly 45 minutes. Remove from oven and allow to cool. Reduce oven temperature to 375 degrees. When potato is cool enough to touch, cut in half and gently scoop out the flesh from both halves into a bowl, reserving the skins. Add Parmesan cheese and sage to bowl, mix well, and return mixture to reserved skins. Sprinkle tops with salt and pepper to taste. Return potato halves to oven and bake at 375 degrees for an additional 15–20 minutes until thoroughly heated. Serve with a sprinkling of Parmesan cheese.

Approx. 112 calories per serving
2g protein, 3g total fat, 0 saturated fat, 0 trans fat,
18g carbohydrates, 0 cholesterol, 66mg sodium, 3g fiber

ROASTED ACORN SQUASH

MAKES 2 SERVINGS

1 acorn squash, halved, seeds removed, and quartered into wedges
Pure maple syrup to drizzle
Salt and freshly ground pepper to taste

Preheat oven to 400 degrees. Brush squash wedges with pure maple syrup and season with salt and pepper. Roast in oven until tender, roughly 20–25 minutes.

Approx. 116 calories per serving
1g protein, 3g total fat, 1g saturated fat, 0 trans fat,
23g carbohydrates, 0 cholesterol, 295mg sodium, 4g fiber

SPICY SNOW PEAS

MAKES 2 SERVINGS

½ pound fresh snow peas, trimmed
¼ cup water
1 teaspoon minced fresh garlic
Crushed red hot pepper flakes to taste
Salt and freshly ground pepper to taste
Extra-virgin olive oil to drizzle

In a medium pot, add peas, water, and garlic, and bring to boil. Reduce heat to a simmer, add hot pepper flakes, and cover. Cook until water is evaporated and peas are tender, roughly 2–3 minutes. Season with salt and pepper to taste and drizzle with a scant amount of olive oil just before serving.

Approx. 47 calories per serving
3g protein, 0 total fat, 0 saturated fat, 0 trans fat,
8g carbohydrates, 0 cholesterol, 4mg sodium, 3g fiber

LEMON-ALMOND COUSCOUS

MAKES 4 SERVINGS

¾ cup couscous

¼ cup toasted slivered almonds

1 tablespoon honey

2 teaspoons finely shredded lemon peel

2 tablespoons snipped fresh chives

Salt and freshly ground pepper to taste

Cook couscous as per package directions. Stir in almond slices, honey, lemon peel, chives, and salt and pepper to taste.

Approx. 171 calories per serving
6g protein, 3g total fat, 0 saturated fat, 0 trans fat,
30g carbohydrates, 0 cholesterol, 3mg sodium, 2g fiber

BAKED ACORN SQUASH

MAKES 4 SERVINGS

2 acorn squashes, halved and seeded

¼ cup fat-free half-and-half, divided

8 sprigs fresh thyme

Freshly ground pepper to taste

½ cup freshly grated Parmesan cheese

Preheat oven to 375 degrees. Trim bottoms of halved squash to lie flat, if needed, and place halves cut side up in a rimmed baking sheet. Divide half-and-half into 4 portions and pour into seeded centers of each squash. Place 2 sprigs of thyme on the top of each squash half and season tops with pepper. Bake for roughly 40 minutes or until squash is tender when pierced with fork tines. Sprinkle tops with Parmesan cheese and continue to bake until cheese is melted and golden, about 10–15 minutes more.

Approx. 168 calories per serving
4g protein, 4g total fat, 2g saturated fat, 0 trans fat,
24g carbohydrates, 0 cholesterol, 362mg sodium, 4g fiber

SNAP PEAS WITH BASIL PESTO

MAKES 4 SERVINGS

1 pound fresh snap peas
¼ cup market-fresh pesto sauce
Salt and freshly ground pepper to taste

In a large pot, bring water to a rapid boil. Add snap peas and boil for about 3–4 minutes until crispy tender and bright green. Drain peas and toss with pesto. Season with salt and pepper to taste.

Approx. 108 calories per serving
4g protein, 6g total fat, 1g saturated fat, 0 trans fat,
9g carbohydrates, 1mg cholesterol, 144mg sodium, 3g fiber

SAUTÉED KALE

MAKES 4 SERVINGS

1 teaspoon olive oil
1 medium shallot, finely chopped
1 clove fresh garlic, minced
½ cup canned low-sodium, fat-free chicken broth
1 teaspoon finely shredded lemon peel
1 (12-ounce) package fresh kale
Salt and freshly ground pepper to taste
Lemon wedges for garnish

In a heavy skillet, heat olive oil over medium heat, add shallots and garlic, and sauté until soft. Add chicken broth, lemon peel, and handfuls of kale at a time, stirring constantly until leaves wilt. When kale is wilted, add salt and pepper to taste and serve with lemon wedges.

Approx. 53 calories per serving
3g protein, 1g total fat, 0 saturated fat, 0 trans fat,
8g carbohydrates, 0 cholesterol, 45mg sodium, 2g fiber

CARAMELIZED BRUSSELS SPROUTS WITH GARLIC AND RED CHILI PEPPERS

MAKES 4–6 SERVINGS

2 tablespoons trans fat–free canola/olive oil spread
2 tablespoons olive oil
4 cloves fresh garlic, thinly sliced
½ red chili pepper or to taste, deseeded and cut into ⅛-inch thick slices
2 pounds fresh brussels sprouts, halved from top through stem
Salt and freshly ground pepper to taste

In a 12-inch heavy-bottomed skillet, melt canola/olive oil spread with olive oil over medium-low heat. Add slices of garlic and red chili pepper and sauté until brown and crisp. With a slotted spoon, remove garlic and chili pepper slices, reserving them. Turn heat to low and place brussels sprouts cut side down in skillet, keeping cut side in direct contact with pan. Cook sprouts (do not turn) for 10–15 minutes or until they are well caramelized. If the skillet becomes dry, drizzle with small amounts of olive oil as needed. Remove sprouts and skillet juices and place into warm bowl and toss with the reserved garlic and red chili pepper slices. Sprinkle with salt and pepper to taste.

Approx. 138 calories per serving
5g protein, 9g total fat, 2g saturated fat, 0 trans fat,
13g carbohydrates, 0 cholesterol, 41mg sodium, 6g fiber

CARAMELIZED ONIONS AND ROASTED KALE

MAKES 8 SERVINGS

3 large red onions

4 tablespoons olive oil, divided

Salt and freshly ground pepper to taste

½ cup canned low-sodium, fat-free chicken broth

3 tablespoons balsamic vinegar

1 tablespoon trans fat–free canola/olive oil spread

2 bunches kale, stems removed and leaves coarsely chopped

4 cloves fresh garlic, minced

⅛ teaspoon crushed red hot pepper flakes

Preheat oven to 375 degrees. Cut onions into wedges. In a large skillet, heat 1 tablespoon olive oil, then add onions and salt and pepper to taste. Cook over medium-high heat for about 5 minutes, stirring often, until onions begin to brown. Reduce heat to medium and add broth and vinegar. Cover and cook until onions are soft. Add canola/olive oil spread, increase heat to high, and cook 2–4 minutes longer, stirring onions with a wooden spoon as they caramelize. Scrape bottom of pan with spoon to loosen any bits of onion. Set aside.

Using heavy tinfoil, place kale leaves in center of foil and curl up sides of foil to form a basket. Drizzle remaining olive oil over leaves, add garlic and hot pepper flakes, and season with salt and pepper to taste. Toss mixture and roast uncovered in oven for 15–20 minutes, tossing kale several times during roasting. Remove from oven and toss with onion mixture. Serve while hot.

Approx. 70 calories per serving
0 protein, 8g total fat, 1g saturated fat, 0 trans fat,
6g carbohydrates, 0 cholesterol, 17mg sodium, 1g fiber

ROASTED BROCCOLI

MAKES 4 SERVINGS

1¼ pounds fresh broccoli florets (about 8 cups)
3½ tablespoons olive oil, divided
4 cloves fresh garlic, minced
¼ teaspoon crushed red hot pepper flakes
Salt and freshly ground pepper to taste
Grated Parmesan cheese to sprinkle (optional)

Preheat oven to 450 degrees. Combine broccoli and 3 tablespoons olive oil in a resealable plastic baggie and toss to coat broccoli. Transfer broccoli to a baking sheet and roast for 15 minutes. Remove from oven and set aside.

Combine remaining olive oil, garlic, and hot pepper flakes in a small bowl and drizzle mixture over broccoli, tossing to coat. Return broccoli to oven and roast until florets begin to brown, about 6–8 minutes. Season with salt and pepper and serve immediately with a sprinkling of Parmesan cheese, if desired.

Approx. 154 calories per serving
1g protein, 12g total fat, 1g saturated fat, 0 trans fat,
9g carbohydrates, 0 cholesterol, 46mg sodium, 1g fiber

FRESH SPINACH WITH ROASTED MUSHROOMS

MAKES 4 SERVINGS

8 ounces white button mushrooms, cleaned and quartered
2¼ teaspoons garlic paste blend
2 tablespoons olive oil, divided
Pinch of crushed red hot pepper flakes (optional)
1 (10-ounce) bag fresh spinach leaves
2 teaspoons grated lemon zest
Salt and freshly ground pepper to taste
¼ cup chopped fresh parsley

Preheat oven to 425 degrees. Place mushrooms on a baking sheet and brush tops of mushrooms with garlic paste. Drizzle with 1 tablespoon of olive oil and a pinch of hot peppers flakes, if desired. Roast for about 20 minutes until golden brown.

Toss together spinach, lemon zest, and remaining olive oil. Add spinach mixture to mushrooms and roast for another 2–3 minutes until spinach is wilted. Season with salt and pepper and toss with parsley to serve.

Approx. 88 calories per serving
4g protein, 7g total fat, 1g saturated fat, 0 trans fat,
4g carbohydrates, 0 cholesterol, 59mg sodium, 1g fiber

BAKED PARSNIP FRIES WITH ROSEMARY

MAKES 6 SERVINGS

2½ pounds parsnips, cleaned and trimmed
1 tablespoon finely chopped fresh rosemary sprigs
2 large cloves fresh garlic, finely minced
3 tablespoons olive oil
5–6 sprigs rosemary, leaves only
1 teaspoon ground cumin or to taste
Salt to taste
½ teaspoon freshly ground pepper

Preheat oven to 400 degrees. Peel parsnips, cutting them into roughly 3x1½-inch strips. Try to keep strips about the same size so they roast evenly. Place strips in a resealable plastic baggie and add rosemary sprigs, garlic, and olive oil. Toss to coat parsnips. Remove strips from bag and place on a flat baking sheet in a single layer. Crumble rosemary leaves over parsnips, then sprinkle with cumin, and salt and pepper. Roast for about 30 minutes, turning parsnips once after about 15 minutes or when they start to brown. Remove from oven when they are lightly browned but still have a little crispy texture.

Approx. 145 calories per serving
1g protein, 8g total fat, 1g saturated fat, 0 trans fat,
20g carbohydrates, 0 cholesterol, 12mg sodium, 5g fiber

ROASTED CAESAR PARMESAN ROMAINE

MAKES 4 SERVINGS

2 large heads of romaine

2 cloves fresh garlic, minced

1 teaspoon olive oil

¼ cup panko bread crumbs

¼ cup grated Parmesan cheese

4–6 anchovy fillets in olive oil, chopped

1 lemon, quartered

Preheat oven to 450 degrees. Cut heads of romaine in half. Trim off any spoiled leaves. Rinse halves under cold running water to remove any dirt, then pat dry with paper towels. Place romaine halves on a flat baking sheet, cut side up, and scatter garlic over tops. Drizzle each half with olive oil and sprinkle with bread crumbs and Parmesan cheese. Bake on upper rack of oven until leaves start to brown at edges and bread crumbs and Parmesan cheese are lightly browned. Remove from heat and garnish tops with anchovies and a lemon wedge.

Approx. 98 calories per serving
7g protein, 5g total fat, 2g saturated fat, 0 trans fat,
10g carbohydrates, 7mg cholesterol, 247mg sodium, 4g fiber

LEMON GARLIC ASPARAGUS
MAKES 4–6 SERVINGS

3 tablespoons extra-virgin olive oil

2 pounds fresh asparagus, cleaned, with ends trimmed

1 clove fresh garlic, crushed

Salt and freshly ground pepper to taste

2 tablespoons sweet orange juice

¾ teaspoon grated lemon peel

1 cup shredded fresh Parmesan cheese

In a large non-stick skillet, heat olive oil over medium heat. Add asparagus, garlic, and salt and pepper; turn several times to coat asparagus with olive oil. Cover skillet and cook for 6–7 minutes or until asparagus is tender and lightly browned. Remove from heat. Sprinkle with orange juice and lemon peel. Transfer to serving platter and top with Parmesan cheese.

Approx. 134 calories per serving
8g protein, 11g total fat, 4g saturated fat, 0 trans fat,
3g carbohydrates, 11mg cholesterol, 228mg sodium, 1g fiber

FAVA BEANS WITH PESTO SAUCE

MAKES 6 SERVINGS

Spicy Garlicky Pesto Sauce (page 484)
3 (15-ounce) cans cooked fava beans, rinsed and drained
6 large lettuce leaves
1 small red onion, chopped
½ red bell pepper, diced
½ yellow pepper, diced
Salt and freshly ground pepper to taste
Tomato wedges for garnish

In a small bowl, mix pesto sauce with fava beans. Arrange lettuce on platter or on individual plates. Pile pesto-bean mixture on top of lettuce. Scatter onion and diced peppers over bean mixture. Add salt and pepper to taste and garnish with tomato wedges.

This dish also makes a great quick lunch.

Approx. 240 calories per serving
12g protein, 3g total fat, 0.6g saturated fat, 0 trans fat,
40g carbohydrates, 0 cholesterol, 500mg sodium, 10g fiber

MASHED PARSNIPS AND CARROTS

MAKES 4–6 SERVINGS

2 pounds parsnips, cleaned, peeled, and chopped
1 pound carrots, cleaned, peeled, and chopped
3 cloves fresh garlic, chopped
1 medium onion, chopped
Salt and freshly ground pepper to taste

In a pot, add all vegetables and cover them with water. Bring to a boil, reduce heat to medium-high, and cook until carrots are soft. Drain off liquid and transfer vegetable mixture to a food processor and process until smooth. Remove from processor with a rubber spatula and serve hot or warm, seasoned with salt and pepper to taste.

Approx. 191 calories per serving
4g protein, 0 total fat, 0 saturated fat, 0 trans fat,
13g carbohydrates, 0 cholesterol, 105 mg sodium, 10g fiber

FETA AND MIXED BEANS
MAKES 6–8 SERVINGS

1 (16-ounce) can light red kidney beans

1 (16-ounce) can cannellini beans, rinsed and drained

1 (16-ounce) can chickpeas, rinsed and drained

3 ounces fresh feta cheese, crumbled

1 cup finely chopped red onion

3 tablespoons chopped fresh mint

1½ tablespoons non-caloric sweetener

2 cloves fresh garlic, finely chopped

¼ teaspoon salt or to taste

¼ teaspoon freshly ground pepper

2 tablespoons + 1 teaspoon fresh squeezed lemon juice

1 tablespoon balsamic vinegar

1 teaspoon extra-virgin olive oil

4 cups mixed greens

Combine all beans, feta cheese, onion, mint, and sweetener and mix well. Add garlic, salt and pepper, lemon juice, vinegar, and olive oil to bean mixture. Toss again. Place 1 cup of greens on each plate; divide bean mixture into 4 servings, top each plate of greens with bean mixture, and serve.

This dish also makes a great quick lunch.

Approx. 151 calories per serving
11g protein, 3g total fat, 2g saturated fat, 0 trans fat,
26g carbohydrates, 9mg cholesterol, 449mg sodium, 8g fiber

TUSCAN BRAISED FENNEL

MAKES 4 SERVINGS

2 medium fennel bulbs
4 tablespoons extra-virgin olive oil
2 cloves fresh garlic, peeled and sliced
Salt and freshly ground pepper to taste
2 cups canned low-sodium vegetable broth
Garnish with grated Parmesan cheese

Wash and trim bulbs, then cut off tops and reserve for garnish. Pat bulbs dry and cut into quarters. Place pieces of fennel, flat-side down, in a heavy skillet, together with olive oil, garlic, and salt and pepper to taste. Cook over medium heat, turning, until fennel pieces are browned. Add broth, bring to a boil, cover, and reduce heat to simmer. Cook another 30–40 minutes until fennel is tender and liquid is absorbed. Sprinkle with Parmesan cheese and serve.

Approx. 174 calories per serving
2g protein, 14g total fat, 2g saturated fat, 0 trans fat,
8g carbohydrates, 0 cholesterol, 103mg sodium, 1g fiber

GRILLED JUMBO PORTOBELLO MUSHROOMS

MAKES 4 SERVINGS

4 large (4–6-inch) portobello mushrooms
1 tablespoon balsamic vinegar
1 tablespoon Worcestershire sauce
⅓ cup extra-virgin olive oil
Salt and freshly ground pepper to taste

Wash and clean mushrooms. Mix liquid ingredients together, place mushrooms in a resealable plastic baggie, and pour marinade over mushrooms. Seal bag and gently toss mushrooms and marinade to cover mushrooms. Refrigerate and marinate for 1–2 hours. Heat grill, place mushrooms on grill, and brush tops with remaining marinade. Grill each side for 5–6 minutes or until mushrooms are soft. Turn mushrooms over once, brushing marinade mixture onto other side.

Approx. 98 calories per serving
0.6g protein, 9.8g total fat, 1g saturated fat, 0 trans fat,
2g carbohydrates, 0 cholesterol, 39mg sodium, 0.4g fiber

CHICKPEAS WITH COUSCOUS

MAKES 4 SERVINGS

1½ cups canned low-sodium, fat-free chicken broth

⅓ cup couscous

1 (15-ounce) can chickpeas, rinsed and drained

1 medium tomato, chopped

10 medium pitted black olives, sliced

1 stalk celery, finely chopped

2 scallions, green and white parts, sliced into 1-inch pieces

¼ cup black seedless raisins

½ teaspoon cumin

¼ cup non-fat plain yogurt for garnish

Chopped fresh parsley (optional)

Bring chicken broth to a boil, remove from heat, and add couscous. Cover and let stand until couscous is tender and liquid is absorbed. Fluff with a fork and transfer to a bowl. Add chickpeas, tomato, olives, celery, scallions, raisins, and cumin. Stir to mix well and garnish each serving with 1 tablespoon of yogurt and parsley. This dish also makes a great quick lunch.

Approx. 207 calories per serving
10g protein, 3g total fat, 0.3g saturated fat, 0 trans fat,
38g carbohydrates, 0.25mg cholesterol, 362mg sodium, 6g fiber

SPICY COUSCOUS
MAKES 4–6 SERVINGS

2¼ teaspoons extra-virgin olive oil

4 cloves fresh garlic, minced

1 small onion, coarsely chopped

3 cups canned low-sodium vegetable broth or low-sodium, fat-free chicken broth

6 ounces couscous

2 teaspoons ground cayenne pepper or to taste

1 teaspoon Harissa (page 476)—add more or less according to degree of spiciness desired

Cilantro leaves, finely chopped, to taste

Salt and freshly ground pepper to taste

In a skillet, heat 1 teaspoon olive oil, add garlic and onion, and sauté until golden. In a saucepan, bring broth and remaining olive oil to a boil. Place couscous in oven-safe dish and pour hot broth and garlic mixture over couscous; stir to mix. Let stand for 10 minutes, until broth is absorbed. Add cayenne, Harissa, cilantro, and salt and pepper to taste as you fluff couscous between fingers to separate grains. Cover tightly to keep warm. Sprinkle a small amount of cayenne and cilantro on top just before serving.

Approx. 124 calories per serving
4g protein, 1g total fat, 1g saturated fat, 0 trans fat,
24g carbohydrates, 0 cholesterol, 47mg sodium, 1g fiber

SAUTÉED VEGETABLES WITH FRESH THYME

MAKES 4 SERVINGS

2 medium leeks
1 medium red bell pepper
2 medium celery stalks
2 (6–7-ounce) zucchini
1 medium eggplant
4 tablespoons extra-virgin olive oil
Salt and freshly ground pepper to taste
2 tablespoons minced fresh thyme
5 medium cloves fresh garlic, minced
2 tablespoons minced fresh parsley

Clean sand from leeks. Cut 2-inch pieces of white and green parts of leek, flatten each piece, and cut into ⅓-inch slices. Separate slices. Cut red bell pepper in half, deseed, and cut into 2-inch strips. Peel strings from celery and cut into 2-inch pieces. Cut zucchini in half and then into pieces roughly ¼ inch by ¼ inch. Peel eggplant and cut into pieces roughly 2 inches by ½-inch thick. In a large skillet, heat 2 tablespoons of olive oil; sauté eggplant over medium heat. Sprinkle with salt, tossing constantly until crispy tender. Remove eggplant from skillet and set aside on a paper towel–dressed platter, to absorb excess oil from eggplant; place platter in heated oven to keep eggplant warm. Heat additional tablespoon of olive oil in eggplant skillet, add leeks, and cook about 5 minutes, stirring often. Add red bell pepper, celery, salt and pepper, and thyme; continue cooking, tossing often, until vegetables are crispy tender. With a slotted spoon, transfer mixture to eggplant platter. Add zucchini and remaining tablespoon of olive oil, if needed, to skillet, and cook zucchini until tender. Remove zucchini to eggplant platter. Add garlic to skillet and sauté for about 30 seconds; do not brown. Add parsley and heat an additional 2–3 seconds. Transfer all vegetables from eggplant platter to a clean platter. Pour garlic and parsley mixture over vegetables and toss, mixing well. Serve immediately.

Approx. 177 calories per serving
2g protein, 14g total fat, 2g saturated fat, 0 trans fat,
13g carbohydrates, 0 cholesterol, 22mg sodium, 2g fiber

CINNAMON COUSCOUS
MAKES 6–8 SERVINGS

3 cups warmed water
Pinch of salt
½ tablespoon extra-virgin olive oil
6 ounces couscous
2 tablespoons ground cinnamon
¼ cup black seedless raisins
¼ cup low-calorie baking sweetener
4 tablespoons Mazahar (orange blossom water)
Coarsely chopped walnuts for garnish

Bring water to a boil; add salt and olive oil. Place couscous in an oiled oven-safe dish and pour liquid over couscous. Add 1 tablespoon cinnamon, raisins, sweetener, and Mazahar; let stand for about 10 minutes or until liquid is absorbed. Fluff couscous with fingers to separate grains. When ready to serve, top couscous with remaining cinnamon and walnuts.

Approx. 87 calories per serving
3g protein, 1g total fat, 1g saturated fat, 0 trans fat,
19g carbohydrates, 0 cholesterol, 4mg sodium, 1g fiber

SWISS CHARD AND ARBORIO RICE

MAKES 6 SERVINGS

5 cups canned low-sodium, fat-free chicken broth

2½ tablespoons extra-virgin olive oil

1 medium onion, chopped

1¾ cups Arborio or other short-grain rice

1 bunch Swiss chard (about 10 leaves), spines cut to ¼-inch pieces, leaves coarsely chopped

½ teaspoon dried rosemary, crumbled

½ cup dry white wine

Salt and freshly ground pepper to taste

½ cup freshly grated Parmesan cheese (reserve a small amount for garnish, if desired)

Bring broth to a simmer, cover, set aside, and keep moderately hot. In a heavy-bottomed skillet, heat olive oil and sauté onion until translucent. Add rice, chard, and rosemary; stir until chard wilts. Add wine and simmer until liquid is absorbed. Add 4½ cups of broth and simmer until rice is tender and creamy, stirring often, then add remaining ½ cup of broth slowly as needed if mixture appears too dry, cooking about 20 minutes. Add salt and pepper and Parmesan cheese to taste. Serve immediately, garnished with a small amount of Parmesan cheese, if desired.

Approx. 371 calories per serving
12g protein, 10g total fat, 2g saturated fat, 0 trans fat,
56g carbohydrates, 7mg cholesterol, 306mg sodium, 1g fiber

BASIC RICE PILAF

MAKES 6 SERVINGS

3 cups canned low-sodium, fat-free chicken broth
2½ tablespoons extra-virgin olive oil
¼ cup chopped blanched almonds
¼ cup toasted pine nuts
1 medium onion, finely chopped
1½ cups long-grain rice
2 cups frozen peas
Salt and freshly ground pepper to taste
Chopped fresh cilantro for garnish

Heat chicken broth to a slow simmer. Place 2 tablespoons olive oil in a heavy-bottomed skillet and gently sauté almonds and pine nuts—toast but do not burn. Remove nuts from heat with a slotted spoon and set aside. Add onion to olive oil, sauté, and cook until soft; do not brown. Add rice to olive oil and sauté over medium heat for 10–15 minutes, stirring constantly until rice is crispy. Pour in hot chicken broth, and add peas, remaining olive oil, and salt and pepper to taste. Reduce heat, cover, and simmer until liquid is absorbed, about 20 minutes. Remove from heat, gently fold in both nuts, cover, and set aside for 5 minutes before serving. Garnish with chopped cilantro.

Approx. 327 calories per serving
9g protein, 16g total fat, 2g saturated fat, 0 trans fat,
40g carbohydrates, 1mg cholesterol, 6mg sodium, 1g fiber

BAKED EGGPLANT WITH GARLIC AND BASIL
MAKES 4–6 SERVINGS

2 medium eggplants
Olive oil cooking spray
4 cloves fresh garlic, finely chopped
4 tablespoons extra-virgin olive oil
1½ teaspoons chopped fresh basil
1 tablespoon tomato paste
2 tablespoons freshly grated Parmesan cheese for garnish
Finely chopped fresh rosemary for garnish
Salt and freshly ground pepper to taste

Wash and dry eggplants, then cut each in half lengthwise. With a sharp knife, make a crisscross pattern in the skin of each eggplant. Put eggplants skin side down on a lightly oiled baking sheet and set aside. Mix together garlic, olive oil, basil, and tomato paste. Spread mixture onto tops of eggplants and bake at 350 degrees for 45 minutes or until tender. Remove from oven, garnish with Parmesan cheese and rosemary, and season with salt and pepper to taste.

Approx. 97.6 calories per serving
1g protein, 10g total fat, 2g saturated fat, 0 trans fat,
3g carbohydrates, 1mg cholesterol, 51mg sodium, 1g fiber

POLENTA
MAKES 4–6 SERVINGS

3 cups water
1 cup polenta
Extra-virgin olive oil (optional)
Grated Parmesan cheese for garnish (optional)
Salt and freshly ground pepper to taste

Bring water to boil in a saucepan. Slowly add polenta and bring back to a boil, stirring constantly. Lower heat to a simmer; stir frequently for roughly 20–25 minutes or until polenta thickens. Serve drizzled with olive oil and sprinkled with Parmesan cheese. Add salt and pepper to taste.

Approx. 35 calories per serving
1g protein, 4g total fat, 0 saturated fat, 0 trans fat,
6g carbohydrates, 0 cholesterol, 82mg sodium, 0 fiber

SAUTÉED PORTOBELLOS WITH GARLIC AND PARSLEY
MAKES 4 SERVINGS

2 tablespoons extra-virgin olive oil
12 ounces portobello mushrooms, cut into chunks
Salt and freshly ground pepper to taste
4 cloves fresh garlic, finely minced
1 tablespoon finely chopped fresh parsley

In a skillet, heat olive oil and sauté mushrooms over high heat for about 4 minutes. Add salt and pepper to taste. Sprinkle with garlic and parsley and serve hot.

Approx. 81 calories per serving
2g protein, 7g total fat, 1g saturated fat, 0 trans fat,
4g carbohydrates, 0 cholesterol, 3mg sodium, 1g fiber

GARLICKY CANNELLINI BEANS

MAKES 4–6 SERVINGS

2 (15-ounce) cans cannellini beans
4–5 large cloves fresh garlic, minced
2 tablespoons extra-virgin olive oil
½ cup canned low-sodium, fat-free chicken broth
Salt and freshly ground pepper to taste
Pita wedges (optional)

Rinse and drain beans. Cook garlic and olive oil in a skillet over medium heat until garlic softens, then add chicken broth and beans and simmer until most of the liquid is evaporated. Season with salt and pepper and serve with toasted pita.

Approx. 123 calories per serving
6g protein, 5g total fat, 0.6g saturated fat, 0 trans fat,
18g carbohydrates, 0.2mg cholesterol, 372mg sodium, 7g fiber

POLENTA WITH MUSHROOMS AND GARLIC

MAKES 4–6 SERVINGS

1 tablespoon extra-virgin olive oil
3 large cloves fresh garlic, minced
3 ounces white button mushrooms, cleaned and sliced
2 sprigs fresh thyme, stalks removed
3 cups water
1 cup polenta
Salt and freshly ground pepper to taste

In a skillet, heat olive oil and gently sauté garlic and mushrooms until soft. Add thyme, stir to blend, and set aside. Bring water to a boil, add polenta, and continue boiling for 2–3 minutes before reducing to a simmer. Cook, stirring frequently, for about 20–25 minutes, until polenta thickens and liquid is absorbed. Remove from heat, transfer to a bowl, stir in mushroom mixture, and add salt and pepper to taste.

Approx. 59 calories per serving
1g protein, 3g total fat, 0.3g saturated fat, 0 trans fat,
7g carbohydrates, 0 cholesterol, 83mg sodium, 0.2g fiber

GRILLED EGGPLANT

MAKES 4 SERVINGS

1 tablespoon extra-virgin olive oil

2 tablespoons fresh oregano leaves

2 plum tomatoes, diced

1½ pounds eggplant, cut lengthwise into ½-inch thick slices

Olive oil cooking spray

2 large cloves fresh garlic, finely minced

1 teaspoon chopped dried rosemary

Salt and freshly ground pepper to taste

¼ cup crumbled feta cheese

Lemon wedges

Fresh oregano sprigs for garnish

Heat olive oil in saucepan, add oregano leaves, then remove pan from heat. Add tomatoes to oregano and allow to bathe in hot olive oil until ready to serve. Meanwhile, spray both sides of eggplant slices with cooking oil, sprinkle with garlic, rosemary, and salt and pepper, and place on medium-hot grill. Cover grill and cook eggplant until tender and browned on both sides, turning once. Remove eggplant to platter, drizzle with oregano-tomato oil, and top with feta cheese. Garnish with lemon wedges and oregano sprigs.

Approx. 74 calories per serving
4g protein, 6g total fat, 1g saturated fat, 0 trans fat,
10g carbohydrates, 5mg cholesterol, 86mg sodium, 0.2g fiber

GINGERED GREEN BEANS AND PEA PODS

MAKES 4 SERVINGS

8 ounces fresh green beans, washed and trimmed

2 cups canned low-sodium, fat-free chicken broth

2 teaspoons extra-virgin olive oil

2 cloves fresh garlic, finely chopped

½ teaspoon freshly ground ginger

4 ounces snow peas, washed, with strings removed (do not remove peas from pods)

4 ounces sugar peas, washed, with strings removed (do not remove peas from pods)

1 tablespoon low-sodium soy sauce

Freshly ground pepper to taste

In a large pan, steam green beans in chicken broth for about 3–4 minutes. Drain beans. In a clean skillet, add 1 teaspoon olive oil and green beans; sauté for about 2–3 minutes until green beans start to brown. Add remaining olive oil, garlic, ginger, snow peas, and sugar peas. Continue sautéing for another 2–3 minutes, until pea pods are crispy tender. Stir in soy sauce and pepper and serve while hot.

Approx. 63 calories per serving
4g protein, 2g total fat, 0 saturated fat, 0 trans fat,
5g carbohydrates, 0 cholesterol, 187mg sodium, 3g fiber

STEAMED ARTICHOKES

MAKES 4 SERVINGS

4 medium globe artichokes (about 10–11 ounces each)
4 cups canned low-sodium, fat-free chicken broth
10 cloves fresh garlic
Salt and freshly ground pepper to taste
Extra-virgin olive oil or *melted trans fat–free canola/olive oil spread to drizzle (optional)*

Wash artichokes under running water. Remove the sharp tips of each leaf with poultry scissors, keeping the globe intact. Place artichokes, broth, and garlic in a large pot. Cover pot and bring to a boil. Reduce heat to medium, keep pot covered, and continue to steam artichokes, turning over once while steaming. If necessary, add water to pot to keep artichokes bathed in liquid while steaming. Steam until you can pierce the globe stem area of the artichoke with a fork without much resistance. Remove chokes with a slotted spoon to serving dishes, sprinkle with salt and pepper, and drizzle with olive oil or melted canola/olive oil spread, if desired. Serve while warm.

To eat this delectable vegetable, simply pull off the leaves one by one and run the soft flesh of the leaf over your bottom front teeth, extracting the flesh from the inner part of the leaf. In the center of all the leaves is the best part; the heart of the choke connected to the stem is also very good. The only part not considered edible by most people is the crown of fuzzy little leaves that sits directly on top of the heart. Simply remove these fuzzy little leaves with your fingers before eating the heart and stem.

Approx. 76 calories per serving
5g protein, 0.2g total fat, 0.1g saturated fat, 0 trans fat,
17g carbohydrates, 0 cholesterol, 153mg sodium, 5g fiber

MOM'S BROWN RICE

MAKES 8 SERVINGS

4 cups canned low-sodium, low-fat chicken broth

2 cups brown rice

6 cloves fresh garlic

½ cup pine nuts

6 scallions, white and green parts, trimmed and sliced

8 pitted large black olives, drained and coarsely chopped

½ tablespoon extra-virgin olive oil

Salt and freshly ground pepper to taste

Chopped chives for garnish

In a saucepan, bring broth and rice to a boil; reduce heat to medium, cover, and continue boiling until all liquid is absorbed, stirring occasionally if needed. While rice is boiling, sauté garlic, pine nuts, scallions, and olives in olive oil until garlic is soft and pine nuts are lightly toasted. When rice is ready, fluff with a fork and stir in garlic and pine nut mixture; add salt and pepper to taste. Transfer to serving platter and garnish with chives.

Approx. 249 calories per serving
7g protein, 9g total fat, 1g saturated fat, 0 trans fat,
38g carbohydrates, 1mg cholesterol, 58mg sodium, 1g fiber

BAKED SWEET POTATO FRIES WITH BASIL PESTO

MAKES 2 SERVINGS

2 (6-ounce) sweet potatoes
1 tablespoon fresh Basil Pesto Sauce (page 488) or market-fresh basil pesto
Salt and freshly ground pepper to taste
Low-fat or fat-free sour cream, for garnish (optional)

Clean skins of sweet potatoes under cold running water and pat potatoes dry with paper towels. Cut potatoes in half and then each half into fry strips. Place fries in a single layer on a non-stick baking sheet and brush with pesto sauce. Add salt and pepper to taste. Place baking sheet in oven and bake fries at 400 degrees until tender and lightly browned around edges. Divide fries into 2 servings and garnish with a dollop of sour cream, if desired.

Approx. 211 calories per serving
4g protein, 7g total fat, 1g saturated fat, 0 trans fat,
34g carbohydrates, 5mg cholesterol, 152mg sodium, 4g fiber

GREEN BEANS AND BABY PORTOBELLOS

MAKES 4 SERVINGS

12 ounces fresh green beans, ends snipped
1¼ cups sliced baby portobello mushrooms
1½ tablespoons finely chopped fresh garlic
½ teaspoon onion powder
2 tablespoons trans fat–free canola/olive oil spread
Salt and freshly ground pepper to taste

In a medium saucepan add beans and mushrooms plus enough water to fill ⅓ of pan. Bring to a boil, then reduce heat and cook until beans are tender. Drain well and transfer beans and mushrooms to a large heavy-bottomed skillet. Add chopped garlic, onion powder, and canola/olive oil spread, and heat over low heat to melt spread, stirring often to coat beans and mushrooms. Continue to cook on low heat for at least 15 minutes to marry flavors. Add salt and pepper to taste.

Approx. 74 calories per serving
2g protein, 5g total fat, 1g saturated fat, 0 trans fat,
7g carbohydrates, 0 cholesterol, 52mg sodium, 2g fiber

GARLIC ROASTED CAULIFLOWER

MAKES 4 SERVINGS

1 jumbo fresh garlic clove, finely chopped

1 medium head of cauliflower (about 3 pounds), cut into 1½-inch florets

2 tablespoons extra-virgin olive oil

Garlic salt or *seasoning of choice to taste (optional)*

Place garlic, florets, and olive oil in a large resealable plastic baggie and toss to coat florets. Arrange florets in a single layer in a shallow baking pan and sprinkle with seasoning, if desired. Place pan on middle rack of 425-degree oven and roast cauliflower until tender and golden brown (about 20–30 minutes). Stir and turn florets over occasionally while roasting.

Approx. 91 calories per serving

3g protein, 7g total fat, 0.8g saturated fat, 0 trans fat,

7g carbohydrates, 0 cholesterol, 20mg sodium, 3g fiber

SAUTÉED GARLIC SPINACH

MAKES 4 SERVINGS

1½ cups canned low-sodium, fat-free chicken broth

4–6 cloves fresh garlic, chopped

3 (10-ounce) bags fresh spinach leaves

Freshly ground pepper to taste

Salt to taste

In a heavy-bottomed skillet over medium heat add chicken broth and garlic. Add handfuls of spinach while stirring, moving wilted leaves to one side, until all of the spinach has been added and wilted. Reduce heat to low, add pepper, and stir occasionally to blend garlic and spinach, until broth has evaporated. Add salt to taste. Serve while hot.

Approx. 54 calories per serving

5g protein, 0.2g total fat, 0 saturated fat, 0 trans fat,

7g carbohydrates, 2mg cholesterol, 174mg sodium, 4.5g fiber

ARTICHOKE RISOTTO

MAKES 4–6 SERVINGS

1 (15-ounce) can quartered artichokes
2 tablespoons extra-virgin olive oil
1 small white onion, finely chopped
2 cloves fresh garlic, finely chopped
1½ cups of short-grain rice
3 cups canned low-sodium, fat-free chicken broth, warmed
Salt and freshly ground pepper to taste
2 tablespoons finely chopped fresh parsley
¼ cup freshly grated Parmesan cheese (optional)
Sprig of fresh parsley for garnish

Drain liquid from artichokes and set aside. Heat olive oil over medium heat; add onion and garlic and sauté until soft. Add drained artichokes and cook another 5 minutes. Turn heat up to medium-high, add rice, and sauté another 2 minutes, stirring often to keep rice from burning. Add already-warmed chicken broth 1 cup at a time, stirring often and allowing rice to absorb most of the broth before adding the second and third cup. Cook until rice is tender and broth is absorbed (about 15–20 minutes). Add salt and pepper to taste and stir in parsley and Parmesan cheese. Mix well and serve garnished with a sprig of parsley.

Approx. 229 calories per serving
5g protein, 4g total fat, 0.3g saturated fat, 0 trans fat,
41 carbohydrates, 0 cholesterol, 124mg sodium, 3g fiber

Wraps and Sandwiches

ROASTED RED PEPPER SANDWICH

MAKES 2 SERVINGS

1 whole wheat pita loaf
2 large pieces Roasted Peppers (page 311) or 2 large pieces red bell pepper
1 ounce hard Parmesano-Reggiano cheese, sliced in thin pieces
½ cup alfalfa sprouts
4–6 Romaine lettuce leaves, broken
Salt and freshly ground pepper to taste
Garnish with a few black olives

Split pita loaf in half, open pocket of each side of loaf, and lightly toast. Insert 1 large piece of roasted pepper into each ½ pita pocket; split Parmesan-Reggiano cheese, sprouts, lettuce and add to each pocket. Sprinkle each pocket with salt and pepper to taste. Serve garnished with olives.

Approx. 145 calories per serving
8g protein, 3.6g total fat, 2.3g saturated fat, 0 trans fat,
2g carbohydrates, 11mg cholesterol, 215mg sodium, 3g fiber

LAMB WRAP

MAKES 4 SERVINGS

⅓ cup medium-grain bulgur

½ cup diced tomatoes

½ cup finely chopped fresh parsley

¼ cup finely chopped fresh mint leaves, no stems

2 scallions, thinly sliced

2½ tablespoons extra-virgin olive oil, divided

Juice from ½ lemon

2 cloves fresh garlic, minced

½ pound lean ground lamb

Salt and freshly ground pepper to taste

4 ounces plain non-fat yogurt

¾ cup diced cucumber

1 tablespoon chopped fresh mint

4 (6-inch) whole wheat pita loaves (do not split open)

1 cup chopped fresh spinach leaves

4 ounces crumbled fat-free feta cheese

Cover bulgur in a bowl with fresh cold water to a depth of roughly ½ inch. Let stand until water is absorbed (about 30 minutes). Fluff with a fork to separate grains. Grains should be plump and slightly moist; if too moist, spread grains on towel, fold towel, and squeeze to remove excess water. Combine tomatoes, parsley, mint, scallions, and 2 tablespoons olive oil. Add bulgur and toss gently. Squeeze lemon juice over tabbouleh mixture and refrigerate. Heat remaining olive oil, and sauté garlic, lamb, and salt and pepper over medium-high heat until browned, stirring constantly to crumble. Drain well and set aside. Combine yogurt, cucumber, and mint in small bowl, stir well, and set aside. Stack pita rounds and wrap in waxed paper; microwave on high for 45 seconds. In a bowl, combine lamb mixture, spinach, and feta cheese. Spoon ½ cup tabbouleh mixture and ¼ lamb mixture in the center of each pita round. Top with yogurt mixture and roll up pita. To secure, wrap bottom portion of pita roll-up with waxed paper.

Approx. 462 calories per serving
21g protein, 22g total fat, 6g saturated fat, 0 trans fat,
43g carbohydrates, 43mg cholesterol, 635mg sodium, 5g fiber

VEGGIE WRAP

MAKES 6 SERVINGS

Olive oil cooking spray
2 medium tomatoes, cut into ½-inch thick slices
2 small cucumbers, sliced lengthwise into ½-inch thick slices
2 small onions, cut into ½-inch thick slices
1 green bell pepper, cut into strips
2 medium zucchini, sliced lengthwise into ½-inch thick slices
Extra-virgin olive oil to drizzle
¾ tablespoon crumbled dried oregano
¼ tablespoon crumbled dried rosemary
¾ teaspoon dried thyme
½ (15-ounce) can chickpeas, rinsed and drained
¼ teaspoon cumin (optional)
Salt and freshly ground pepper to taste
6 whole wheat flat breads (8–10-inch), warmed
Alfalfa sprouts (optional)

Spray non-stick pan with cooking spray. Place tomatoes, cucumbers, onions, green bell pepper, and zucchini on pan, and drizzle with olive oil. Sprinkle with oregano, rosemary, and thyme, and roast for 15–20 minutes at 425 degrees. Add chickpeas and cumin, plus salt and pepper to taste, and cook an additional 15–20 minutes until tender. Fill warmed flat bread with bean and veggie mix, top with alfalfa sprouts, if desired, roll up, and serve.

Approx. 170 calories per serving
8g protein, 1g total fat, <0.3g saturated fat, 0 trans fat,
36g carbohydrates, 0 cholesterol, 325mg sodium, 6g fiber

CRAB AND AVOCADO STUFFED PITA POCKETS

MAKES 8 SERVINGS

⅔ cup light mayonnaise

4 tablespoons fresh lemon juice

2 tablespoons chopped Roasted Peppers (page 311)

Pinch cayenne pepper

1 pound (about 2 cups) lump crabmeat, well drained

1 cup chopped pre-cooked shrimp

2 small avocados, chopped

3 tablespoons finely chopped white onion

Salt and freshly ground pepper to taste

4 whole grain pita loaves, cut in half

1 cup alfalfa sprouts

Blend together mayonnaise, lemon juice, roasted pepper, and cayenne, then refrigerate to chill (about 1 hour). Mix together crab, shrimp, avocados, onion, and salt and pepper to taste. Fill each pita loaf half with crab mixture and top with ⅛ of mayonnaise mixture. Add ⅛ cup of alfalfa sprouts to each filled pita and serve.

Approx. 171 calories per serving
11.6g protein, 12.4g total fat, 1.7g saturated fat, 0 trans fat,
4.6g carbohydrates, 61.5mg cholesterol, 216mg sodium, 1g fiber

GRILLED JUMBO PORTOBELLO MUSHROOM SANDWICH
MAKES 4 SERVINGS

4 large (4–6-inch) portobello mushrooms
1 tablespoon balsamic vinegar
1 tablespoon Worcestershire sauce
⅓ cup extra-virgin olive oil
Salt and freshly ground pepper to taste
4 whole grain hamburger buns
Condiments of choice (optional)

Wash and clean mushrooms. Mix together vinegar, Worcestershire sauce, olive oil, and salt and pepper, then place mushrooms in a resealable plastic baggie and pour mixture over mushrooms. Seal bag and gently toss mushrooms and marinade to cover mushrooms. Refrigerate and marinate for 1–2 hours. Heat grill, place mushrooms on grill, and brush tops with remaining marinade. Grill each side for 5–6 minutes or until mushrooms are soft. Turn mushrooms over once, brushing marinade mixture onto other side before grilling. Place on whole grain bun and add condiments of choice, if desired.

Approx. 248 calories per serving
5g protein, 11.8g total fat, 1.5g saturated fat, 0 trans fat,
29g carbohydrates, 0 cholesterol, 39mg sodium, 2.4g fiber

STUFFED WHOLE WHEAT KHUBZ

MAKES 8 SERVINGS

4 (6-inch) pita loaves

2 tablespoons stone-ground mustard

1 teaspoon finely chopped fresh cilantro

2 cloves fresh garlic, finely crushed

⅛ teaspoon freshly ground pepper

Garlic salt to taste

1½ teaspoons extra-virgin olive oil

¼ teaspoon balsamic glaze

½ medium red onion, finely sliced

10 medium pitted black olives

1½ cups shredded lettuce

½ cup chopped carrot

½ cup diced celery

1 large tomato, diced

4 ounces crumbled feta cheese

Split pita loaves crosswise in half, spread open pockets (to keep from sealing shut), and lightly toast. Spread thin layer of mustard inside of toasted pockets. Set aside. Mix cilantro, garlic, pepper, and garlic salt with olive oil and glaze; stir together to blend well and then set aside. Combine onion, olives, lettuce, carrot, celery, and tomato, toss to mix, and fill pockets with vegetable blend. Drizzle each stuffed loaf with glaze mixture and add crumbled feta cheese. Serve.

Approx. 152 calories per serving
6g protein, 4g total fat, 2g saturated fat, 0 trans fat,
18g carbohydrates, 12mg cholesterol, 353mg sodium, 3g fiber

SPICY HUMMUS IN TOASTED PITA LOAVES

MAKES 6 SERVINGS

1 (15-ounce) can chickpeas, well rinsed and drained
Juice from 1 lemon
¼ cup water
1 large clove fresh garlic
2 tablespoons tahini paste
Dash of salt
Pinch of crushed red hot pepper flakes
3 (6-inch) whole wheat pita loaves
8 slices tomato, ¼-inch thick
½ cucumber, peeled and thinly sliced
Alfalfa sprouts

In a food processor add chickpeas, lemon juice, and water, and blend to desired consistency. Add garlic, tahini paste, salt, and hot pepper flakes; blend again. Cut pita loaves in half and toast lightly. Divide mixture into 4 portions and stuff loaves with mixture. Top each half loaf with tomato, cucumber, and alfalfa sprouts.

Approx. 152 calories per serving
3g protein, 3g total fat, 0.3g saturated fat, 0 trans fat,
27g carbohydrates, 0 cholesterol, 235mg sodium, 4g fiber

CHICKPEA PITA POCKETS

MAKES 8 SERVINGS

1 (15-ounce) can chickpeas, rinsed and drained

1 cup shredded fresh spinach

⅔ cup halved seedless red grapes

½ cup finely chopped red bell pepper

⅓ cup thinly sliced celery

½ medium cucumber, diced

¼ cup finely chopped onion

¼ cup light mayonnaise

1 tablespoon balsamic syrup

½ tablespoon poppy seeds

4 (6-inch) whole wheat pita loaves, cut in half

In a large bowl combine chickpeas, spinach, grapes, red bell pepper, celery, cucumber, and onion. Whisk together mayonnaise, balsamic syrup, and poppy seeds. Add poppy seed mixture to chickpea mixture and stir until well blended. Lightly toast pita halves and fill with chickpea filling. Serve.

Approx. 152 calories per serving
7g protein, 3g total fat, 0.3g saturated fat, 0 trans fat,
29g carbohydrates, 3mg cholesterol, 294mg sodium, 5g fiber

SPICY MUSHROOM WRAP

MAKES 2 SERVINGS

Olive oil cooking spray
1 tablespoon extra-virgin olive oil
2 large portobello mushrooms, sliced
2 teaspoons minced fresh garlic
½ small white onion, thinly sliced
2 teaspoons spicy brown mustard
½ pound arugula, trimmed and steamed
10 cherry tomatoes, halved
¼ cup shredded part-skim mozzarella cheese
2 light whole grain trans fat–free wraps
¼ hot cherry pepper, diced (optional)

Spray baking dish with cooking oil. In a large skillet, heat olive oil and sauté mushrooms, garlic, and onion for about 5 minutes, stirring constantly. Put mustard, arugula, tomatoes, mozzarella, and cooked mushroom mixture on each wrap. Sprinkle hot peppers down center, if desired; roll up and place seam side down in oiled baking dish. Bake uncovered for 10 minutes or until mozzarella cheese is melted. Serve.

Approx. 199 calories per serving
15g protein, 13g total fat, 2.5g saturated fat, 0 trans fat,
20g carbohydrates, 8mg cholesterol, 513mg sodium, 10mg fiber

CHICKPEA AND FRESH SPINACH SANDWICH

MAKES 4 SERVINGS

1 (15-ounce) can chickpeas
2 teaspoons extra-virgin olive oil
2 cloves fresh garlic, minced
½ medium white onion, diced
Salt and freshly ground pepper to taste
Crushed red hot pepper flakes, if desired
8 slices whole wheat grain bread
1 clove fresh garlic, cut in half
5–6 ounces fresh spinach leaves

Rinse and drain chickpeas thoroughly. Mash to a paste and set aside. In 1 teaspoon olive oil, sauté garlic and onion until golden brown. Add chickpea paste, salt and pepper to taste, and hot pepper flakes, if desired. Drizzle paste with remaining teaspoon of olive oil and set aside. Toast whole wheat bread slices and rub one side of each piece with fresh garlic halves. Divide paste mixture and spinach leaves into 4 portions and make into 4 sandwiches. Serve.

Approx. 227 calories per serving
15g protein, 5g total fat, 0.3g saturated fat, 0 trans fat,
40g carbohydrates, 0 cholesterol, 600mg sodium, 11g fiber

SMOKED FISH AND ROASTED PEPPER SANDWICH

MAKES 4 SERVINGS

2 tablespoons extra-virgin olive oil

1 clove fresh garlic, mashed into a paste

8 slices whole wheat grain bread

3 ounces smoked white fish

3 ounces smoked sturgeon

4 tablespoons shredded romaine lettuce

4 teaspoons diced Roasted Peppers (page 311)

2 teaspoons light mayonnaise

Combine olive oil and garlic, reserving 1 teaspoon of olive oil. Lightly brush both sides of bread with mixture and toast in oven at 350 degrees for 4 minutes or until golden brown. Set aside. Mix fish, lettuce, and roasted peppers together; set aside. Blend mayonnaise and reserved olive oil and add to fish mixture. Divide mixture into 4 servings and spread onto bread, making 4 sandwiches.

Approx. 228 calories per serving
19g protein, 11g total fat, 1g saturated fat, 0 trans fat,
20g carbohydrates, 8mg cholesterol, 463mg sodium, 4g fiber

PORTOBELLO MUSHROOM BURGER
WITH CARAMELIZED ONIONS

MAKES 4 SERVINGS

3 tablespoons olive oil, divided

1 tablespoon balsamic vinegar

3 cloves fresh garlic, minced

4 large portobello mushrooms, stems removed

3 cups thinly sliced red onion

2 tablespoons water

¼ cup red port wine

Salt and freshly ground pepper to taste

½ cup fresh goat cheese (about 3 ounces)

4 whole grain sandwich buns, thin type, toasted

1 cup mixed field greens

4 thick slices tomato

Dijon mustard

Whisk 2 tablespoons olive oil, vinegar, and garlic together in a bowl. Generously brush mixture all over mushrooms and allow to stand for at least 30 minutes. Meanwhile, heat remaining olive oil in a large skillet over high heat. Add onion and cook, stirring frequently, until it begins to brown. Reduce heat to a simmer, add water, and continue to cook until onions soften, about 15 minutes. Add port and cook, stirring occasionally, until liquid evaporates, about 3 minutes. Add salt and pepper to taste. Remove from heat and cover.

Preheat grill to medium. Add salt and pepper to mushrooms and grill gill-side down, about 5 minutes. Flip over, top inside with goat cheese, and continue to grill until mushrooms are tender. Toast buns and divide onions among the mushrooms and goat cheese. Place on buns with cheese-side up, add greens, tomato, and mustard, and serve.

Approx. 247 calories per serving
11g protein, 14g total fat, 4g saturated fat, 0 trans fat,
22g carbohydrates, 10mg cholesterol, 288mg sodium, 7g fiber

GREAT TUNA SALAD ON WHOLE GRAIN TOAST

MAKES 4 SERVINGS

3 (5-ounce) cans solid white albacore tuna, packed in water

¼ cup minced onion

8 manzanilla-stuffed green olives, sliced

1 celery rib, finely chopped

Salt and freshly ground pepper to taste

Squeeze of fresh lemon juice

¼ cup light mayonnaise

8 slices light whole grain bread, toasted

4 crisp Romaine lettuce leaves

4 thick slices tomato

Drain tuna through a strainer and press dry with paper towels. Transfer to a medium bowl and mash with a fork until finely flaked. Add onion, olive slices, celery, salt and pepper, lemon juice, and mayonnaise. Stir to blend ingredients well. Divide tuna mixture into 4 equal portions. Top each of 4 slices of toasted whole grain bread with tuna mixture, lettuce, tomato, and salt and pepper, if desired. Add top piece of toast and serve.

Approx. 153 calories per serving (50 calories per slice of bread)
13g protein, 0 total fat, 0 saturated fat, 0 trans fat,
20g carbohydrates, 4mg cholesterol, 378mg sodium, 4g fiber

MEATLESS SLOPPY JOE

MAKES 4 SERVINGS

2 tablespoons olive oil

1 large yellow onion, chopped

2 tablespoons minced fresh garlic

1 jalapeño pepper, diced

Salt to taste

¼ teaspoon freshly ground pepper

1 green bell pepper, seeded and diced

½ cup grated carrot

1½ cups black beans, rinsed, drained, and mashed

1 tablespoon chili powder or to taste

1 teaspoon light brown sugar

1 tablespoon Worcestershire sauce

2 cups canned low-sodium diced tomatoes, well drained

4 whole wheat or multigrain sandwich buns, toasted

Shredded low-fat cheddar cheese (optional)

In a large skillet over medium-low heat, add olive oil, onion, garlic, jalapeño pepper, salt and pepper, and green bell pepper, and sauté until soft. Add carrot, beans, chili powder, sugar, Worcestershire sauce, and tomatoes. Bring to a boil, reduce heat, and cook for roughly 10 minutes or until sauce thickens. Serve over buns with cheddar cheese, if desired.

Approx. 247 calories per serving
11g protein, 8g total fat, 2g saturated fat, 0 trans fat,
39g carbohydrates, 0 cholesterol, 595mg sodium*,12g fiber

PEAR, CREAM CHEESE, AND RED ONION SANDWICH

MAKES I SERVING

2 slices light whole grain bread
Olive oil cooking spray
2 tablespoons light cream cheese
1 thin slice of red onion
4 slices Bosc or Anjou pear
1 tablespoon crumbled blue cheese
2 fresh basil leaves, cut into thin strips

Lightly spray bread slices with cooking oil and toast in oven or toaster oven until lightly crispy. Spread 1 tablespoon of cream cheese on each slice of bread. Top one slice with onion, pear slices, blue cheese, and basil. Top with remaining slice of bread.

Approx. 207 calories per serving (50 calories per slice of bread)
12g protein, 9g total fat, 4g saturated fat, 0 trans fat,
22g carbohydrates, 26mg cholesterol, 461mg sodium, 4g fiber

GOAT CHEESE AND PESTO SANDWICH

MAKES I SERVING

2 slices light whole grain bread
Olive oil cooking spray
1 tablespoon soft goat cheese
1 tablespoon market-fresh pesto sauce
2 thin slices tomato
4 thin slices red bell pepper
Salt and freshly ground pepper to taste

Lightly spray bread slices with cooking oil. Toast slices until slightly crusty. Set aside to cool. When cooled, divide goat cheese and pesto into 2 portions. Lightly spread top of each slice with a layer of soft goat cheese, followed by pesto sauce. Add tomato and red bell pepper slices. Add salt and pepper to taste. Serve as an open sandwich.

Approx. 294 calories per serving (50 calories per slice of bread)
19g protein, 16g total fat, 8g saturated fat, 0 trans fat,
25g carbohydrates, 25mg cholesterol, 491mg sodium, 4g fiber

GRILLED CHILI TUNA SANDWICH
MAKES 4 SERVINGS

8 slices light whole grain bread

3 tablespoons olive oil

2 (6–8 ounces) tuna fillets, about 1-inch thick

2 teaspoons chili powder, divided

Salt to taste

½ cup low-fat sour cream

1 tablespoon freshly squeezed lemon juice

2 cups watercress

Heat grill to medium-high. Lightly brush bread slices with olive oil. Brush one side of each tuna fillet with olive oil and sprinkle with ½ teaspoon of chili powder and salt. Place seasoned side down on grill. Turn tuna once during cooking, grilling each side for roughly 4–6 minutes. Before turning tuna fillets, lightly brush the tops with olive oil and season tops with ½ teaspoon of chili powder. Grill bread, turning once, until browned, about 1 minute for each side. Gently whisk together sour cream and lemon juice in a small bowl. Slice tuna into thin slices, cutting with the grain. Spread tops of each grilled bread slice with sour cream mixture and add ½ cup of watercress to 4 slices of bread. Place equal amounts of sliced tuna over watercress and top each with remaining 4 slices of bread.

Approx. 301 calories per serving (50 calories per slice of bread)
28g protein, 12g total fat, 2g saturated fat, 0 trans fat,
21g carbohydrates, 42mg cholesterol, 273mg sodium, 4g fiber

APPLE-WALNUT RAISIN WRAP

MAKES 4 SERVINGS

4 tablespoons trans fat–free canola/olive oil spread, divided

2 large apples (Granny Smith or Gala) to yield about 3½ cups diced

1 (1½-ounce) box black raisins

¼ cup maple syrup

1 teaspoon ground cinnamon

Pinch of salt

½ cup walnut pieces

4 (8-inch) flour tortillas

Low-fat vanilla yogurt or fat-free vanilla ice cream (optional)

In a large skillet, heat 2 tablespoons of canola/olive oil spread over medium heat until melted. Add apples, raisins, maple syrup, cinnamon, and salt. Reduce heat to a simmer and cook, stirring occasionally, until apples are tender, about 8–10 minutes. Stir in walnut pieces and cook for an additional 2–3 minutes, until heated through.

In a separate skillet, melt remaining 2 tablespoons of canola/olive oil spread over low heat. Add tortillas, one at a time, and heat, turning once, until lightly browned. Place tortillas on a work surface and spoon apple mixture down the centers of the tortillas. Fold ends over filling and roll up. Serve warm with an optional dollop of yogurt or ice cream on the side, if desired.

Approx. 383 calories per serving
5g protein, 24g total fat, 5g saturated fat, 0 trans fat,
41g carbohydrates, 0 cholesterol, 431mg sodium, 4g fiber

CHICKEN PESTO WRAP

MAKES 2 SERVINGS

Olive oil cooking spray
4 (4-ounce) skinless, boneless chicken tenderloins
Salt and freshly ground pepper to taste
4 tablespoons market-fresh pesto sauce
2 (8-inch) whole grain wraps
8 slices sundried tomato, packed in olive oil
Fresh arugula

Lightly spray a heavy-bottomed skillet with cooking oil. Heat skillet over medium heat, add chicken, season with salt and pepper to taste, and cook tenders until cooked through. Spread 2 tablespoons of pesto onto each wrap and add 2–3 slices of sundried tomatoes and a handful of arugula to each wrap. Top each wrap with 2 chicken tender pieces and roll up wrap, folding in ends of wrap. Slice each wrap in half on a diagonal and serve.

Approx. 249 calories per serving
27g protein, 9g total fat, 2g saturated fat, 0 trans fat,
17g carbohydrates, 51mg cholesterol, 440mg sodium, 1g fiber

SHRIMP AND AVOCADO WRAP

MAKES 4 SERVINGS

2 (10-inch) whole grain wraps
2 tablespoons prepared basil pesto
½ ripe avocado, pitted, peeled, and sliced into 8 wedges
½ clove fresh garlic, finely minced
2 tablespoons finely chopped red onion
½ teaspoon freshly squeezed lime juice
Salt and freshly ground pepper to taste
1 cup baby spinach leaves, divided
10 large cooked shrimp, deveined and peeled, divided

Place wraps on a clean, flat surface and spread 1 tablespoon of pesto over top of each wrap. Arrange 4 wedges of avocado down the center of each wrap. Sprinkle garlic and onion over avocado. Drizzle on a scant amount of lime juice. Season with salt and pepper. Divide spinach and shrimp into 2 portions, adding a bed of spinach to each wrap, followed by shrimp on top. Fold over the top and bottom of each wrap and, starting at one end, tightly roll up wrap. Secure with large tooth pick if necessary. Cut wrap in half on diagonal and serve.

Approx. 191 calories per serving
8g protein, 11g total fat, 2g saturated fat, 0 trans fat,
7g carbohydrates, 33mg cholesterol, 283mg sodium, 4g fiber

Breads

Wheat flour is the most common variety of flour used for making bread. However, other types such as barley flour, bran, buckwheat flour, cornmeal, rolled oats, oat flour, and soy flour—to mention just a few—are also suitable for bread making. All flours should be stored in airtight containers. All-purpose and white bread flour can be stored at 70 degrees for up to six months. Any flour, wheat or otherwise, that contains the germ from the grain can easily turn rancid. These flours should be stored in the refrigerator or freezer and can be kept for up to three months.

Homemade Breads

FOCACCIA
MAKES 12 SQUARES

A popular Italian bread found all over Italy. Usually round or rectangular in shape and about ½–1-inch thick. A variety of different toppings are used, such as herbs, coarse salt, a sprinkling of rosemary with hot pepper flakes, olives, or even an array of vegetables.

1¼ cups hot water
1 package rapid-rising active dry yeast
3 tablespoons toasted wheat germ
1 tablespoon extra-virgin olive oil
Pinch of salt
2 cups durum whole wheat flour + extra for kneading
Olive oil for brushing surfaces

Pour water into a medium-sized bowl and sprinkle with yeast. Stir with a wire whisk. Add wheat germ, olive oil, and salt, and whisk again. Add flour, then stir with a wooden spoon until dough forms a ball and leaves sides of bowl. Knead briefly, adding extra flour if needed, until dough is no longer sticky but still soft (about 3 minutes). Turn dough out onto a lightly floured surface; roll out into a rectangle, 11 inches by 17 inches. Lightly dust top with flour while rolling to prevent sticking. Ease dough into a lightly oiled 11x17-inch baking pan, stretch to fit, and cover with sheet of lightly oiled waxed paper, oiled side down. Allow to rise in a warm place for 25 minutes. After dough has risen, press dough with index finger to create little dimples over the surface. Add favorite topping and bake in 450-degree oven until lightly browned on the bottom (about 20–25 minutes). Remove and cool on rack. Slice into 12 large squares and serve.

Approx. 111 calories per square
4g protein, 1g total fat, <0.5g saturated fat, 0 trans fat,
23g carbohydrates, 0 cholesterol, 239mg sodium, 1g fiber

EGYPTIAN KHUBZ (PITA BREAD)

MAKES 12 LOAVES

The Arabs eat bread with every meal. They use it to scoop up sauces, dips, yogurt, and liquids. Pita cut in half can be filled with shish kabobs, falafel, or salads. They consider bread to be a divine gift from God.

1 package dried yeast
¼ teaspoon honey
1½ cups warm water
4 cups durum whole wheat flour
Pinch of salt
½ tablespoon extra-virgin olive oil
Cornmeal to dust baking sheet

Dissolve yeast and honey in 1 cup warm water and set aside for 5 minutes. Mix flour, salt, and olive oil in a large bowl, add yeast mixture and remaining water, and mix well. Knead for 10 minutes until dough is elastic; then place dough in a warm, oiled bowl, cover with a dry cloth and set in a warm place to double its volume (about 2–3 hours). Punch dough down and knead again for about 2 more minutes. Form dough into 12 smooth balls the size of oranges. Place balls on a dry cloth in a warm place and cover to rise for another 30 minutes. Preheat oven to 500 degrees and lightly flour a board with cornmeal and roll out balls into ¼-inch thick circles. Bake loaves 5–8 minutes on a preheated baking sheet on center rack of oven. The loaves will puff up while baking but will collapse when cooled.

Approx. 218 calories per loaf
7g protein, 5g total fat, 0.5g saturated fat, 0 trans fat,
41g carbohydrates, 0 cholesterol, 497mg sodium, 10g fiber

LAVOSH

Same recipe as for pita bread, except bread is left in oven until it is golden brown and crisp. Once cooled, break bread into pieces.

Approx. 218 calories per loaf
7g protein, 5g total fat, 0.5g saturated fat, 0 trans fat,
41g carbohydrates, 0 cholesterol, 497mg sodium, 10g fiber

BANANA-WALNUT LOAF

MAKES I LOAF (YIELDS ABOUT 12 SLICES)

Canola oil cooking spray
1¾ cups all-purpose flour
1½ teaspoons baking soda
1½ teaspoons salt
3 large eggs or ¾ cup liquid eggs
¾ cup low-calorie baking sweetener
1 cup mashed very ripe bananas (roughly 2 large bananas)
½ cup chopped walnuts
½ cup canola oil

Preheat oven to 350 degrees. Spray the inside of a 9x5x3-inch baking loaf pan with cooking oil. Combine flour, baking soda, and salt in a bowl. Whisk in eggs, sweetener, bananas, walnuts, and canola oil, and mix until well blended. Scrape batter into oiled loaf pan and bake for about 60 minutes or until a toothpick inserted into the center of the loaf comes out clean. Remove from oven and place pan on a wire rack, allowing to cool for at least 15 minutes before trying to release loaf from the pan.

Approx. 166 calories per slice
3g protein, 7g total fat, 1g saturated fat, 0 trans fat,
19g carbohydrates, 53mg cholesterol, 307mg sodium, 0 fiber

SESAME BREAD (KERSA)

MAKES 2 16-INCH ROUND LOAVES (12 SLICES/LOAF)

Kersa is a round, flat Moroccan bread that is slightly crunchy on the outside and chewy on the inside, great for dipping in soup or with stews.

1 package of active dry yeast

¼ cup + 2 cups warm water

1 teaspoon low-calorie baking sweetener

4 cups durum whole wheat semolina flour

2 teaspoons salt

⅓ cup cornmeal + extra for dusting

½ tablespoon extra-virgin olive oil

2 teaspoons sesame seeds

Using a small bowl, combine yeast with ¼ cup water, add sweetener, and let set until mixture starts to bubble. In a heavy-duty mixer bowl with dough hook mix flour, salt, and cornmeal. Indent center of dough, pour in yeast mixture and olive oil. Knead dough, adding remaining water as needed until dough takes on an elastic quality. Grease 2 baking sheets and dust with cornmeal. Separate dough to form 2 round balls and place each ball on a separate baking sheet. Press them into 8-inch circles. Sprinkle 1 teaspoon of sesame seeds over each loaf, gently pressing them into surface of dough. Cover dough with a clean cloth and set aside in a warm place for about 1 hour until they double their size. Preheat oven to 425 degrees. Prick the top of loaves with a fork and bake for 10 minutes. Lower heat to 375 degrees and bake loaves until top is crusty and golden brown, about 15–20 minutes.

Approx. 84 calories per slice
3g protein, 2g total fat, <0.5g saturated fat, 0 trans fat,
16g carbohydrates, 0 cholesterol, 90mg sodium, 1g fiber

Bread-Machine Breads

HONEY WHOLE WHEAT BREAD
MAKES 20—22 SLICES

⅔ cup + 3 tablespoons water

2 tablespoons canola oil

1½ teaspoons sodium-free salt substitute

1 tablespoon low-calorie brown sugar blend

2 tablespoons natural fat-free dry milk

2 tablespoons pure honey

2¾ cups whole wheat flour

2¼ teaspoons active dry yeast (at room temperature)

Remove baking machine canister. First, add water, then canola oil, salt substitute, sweetener, milk, and honey. Cover these ingredients with flour and finally yeast. Do not allow yeast to touch liquids. Return canister to machine per machine instructions, close lid, and follow setting instructions for making whole wheat bread. When machine is finished, remove loaf and allow to thoroughly cool before slicing. Store any unused bread in freezer.

Approx. 73 calories per slice
2g protein, 1g total fat, 0 saturated fat, 0 trans fat,
13g carbohydrates, 0 cholesterol, 2g sodium, 2g fiber

CRANBERRY NUT WHOLE WHEAT BREAD

MAKES 20–22 SLICES

¾ cup + 7 tablespoons water

2 tablespoons canola oil

1½ teaspoons sodium-free salt substitute

2 tablespoons low-calorie brown sugar blend

2 tablespoons natural fat-free dry milk

2¾ cups whole wheat flour

½ cup chopped dried cranberries

¼ cup sliced raw almonds

2¼ teaspoons active dry yeast (at room temperature)

Remove baking machine canister. First, add water, then canola oil, salt substitute, sweetener, and milk. Cover liquid ingredients with flour, cranberries, nuts, and finally yeast. Do not allow yeast to touch liquids. Return canister to machine per machine instructions, close lid, and follow setting instructions for making whole wheat bread. When machine is finished, remove loaf and allow to thoroughly cool before slicing. Store any unused bread in freezer.

Approx. 93 calories per slice
4g protein, 2g total fat, 0 saturated fat, 0 trans fat,
14g carbohydrates, 0 cholesterol, 1mg sodium, 3g fiber

MIXED FRUIT AND NUT WHOLE WHEAT BREAD

MAKES 20–22 SLICES

1¼ cups of water

2 tablespoons canola oil

1½ teaspoons sodium-free salt substitute

2 tablespoons low-calorie brown sugar blend

2 tablespoons natural fat-free dry milk

2¾ cups whole wheat flour

⅓ cup lightly salted pumpkin seeds

5 dried apricots, finely chopped

¼ cup white raisins

¼ cup sliced raw almonds

2¼ teaspoons active dry yeast (at room temperature)

Remove baking machine canister. First, add water, then canola oil, salt substitute, sweetener, and milk. Cover these ingredients with flour, seeds, apricots, raisins, almonds, and finally yeast. Do not allow yeast to touch liquids. Return canister to machine per machine instructions, close lid, and follow setting instructions for making whole wheat bread. When machine is finished, remove loaf and allow to thoroughly cool before slicing. Store any unused bread in freezer.

Approx. 88 calories per slice
3g protein, 2g total fat, 1g saturated fat, 0 trans fat,
14g carbohydrates, 0 cholesterol, 3mg sodium, 2g fiber

NUTTY POMEGRANATE WHOLE WHEAT BREAD

MAKES 20–22 SLICES

1¼ cups of water

2 tablespoons canola oil

1½ teaspoons sodium-free salt substitute

2 tablespoons low-calorie brown sugar blend

2 tablespoons natural dry milk

2¾ cups whole wheat flour

Seeds from 1 pomegranate fruit

⅓ cup lightly salted pumpkin seeds

¼ cup sliced raw almonds

1½ teaspoons dried orange peel

2¼ teaspoons active dry yeast (at room temperature)

Remove baking machine canister. First, add water, then canola oil, salt substitute, sweetener, and milk. Cover these ingredients with flour, pomegranate and pumpkin seeds, almonds, orange peel, and finally yeast. Do not allow yeast to touch liquids. Return canister to machine per machine instructions, close lid, and follow setting instructions for making whole wheat bread. When machine is finished, remove loaf and allow to thoroughly cool before slicing. Store any unused bread in freezer.

Approx. 73 calories per slice
3g protein, 2g total fat, 0.1g saturated fat, 0 trans fat,
13g carbohydrates, 0 cholesterol, 2mg sodium, 2g fiber

NUTTY WHOLE WHEAT BREAD

MAKES 20–22 SLICES

1¼ cups of water

2 tablespoons canola oil

1½ teaspoons sodium-free salt substitute

2 tablespoons low-calorie brown sugar blend

2 tablespoons natural fat-free dry milk

2¾ cups whole wheat flour

¼ cup finely chopped raw walnuts

1½ teaspoons dried orange peel

⅓ cup lightly salted pumpkin seeds

2¼ teaspoons active dry yeast (at room temperature)

Remove baking machine canister. First, add water, then canola oil, salt substitute, sweetener, and milk. Cover these ingredients with flour, nuts, orange peel, seeds, and finally yeast. Do not allow yeast to touch liquids. Return canister to machine per machine instructions, close lid, and follow setting instructions for making whole wheat bread. When machine is finished, remove loaf and allow to thoroughly cool before slicing. Store any unused bread in freezer.

Approx. 79 calories per slice
3g protein, 2g total fat, 0.2g saturated fat, 0 trans fat,
12g carbohydrates, 0 cholesterol, 2mg sodium, 2g fiber

SUNDRIED TOMATO BASIL WHITE WHEAT BREAD

MAKES 20–22 SLICES

1½ cups water (room temperature)
2 tablespoons olive oil
2 teaspoons sodium-free salt substitute
3 tablespoons low-calorie brown sugar blend
3 tablespoons natural fat-free dry milk
3 tablespoons fresh sundried tomato pesto
8 large pitted black olives, chopped
10 sundried tomatoes, chopped
2 cups white wheat flour
2 cups bread flour
2 teaspoons active dry yeast

Remove baking machine canister. First, add water, then canola oil, salt substitute, sweetener, milk, pesto, olives, and sundried tomatoes. Cover these ingredients with both flours and finally yeast. Do not allow yeast to touch liquids. Return canister to machine per machine instructions, close lid, and follow setting instructions for making white wheat bread. When machine is finished, remove loaf and allow to thoroughly cool before slicing. Store any unused bread in freezer.

Approx. 104 calories per slice
4g protein, 11g total fat, 0.1g saturated fat, 0 trans fat,
14g carbohydrates, 0 cholesterol, 21mg sodium, 2g fiber

Desserts

FRESH FRUIT AND NUT PLATTER

A platter of seasonal fresh fruits and various types of nuts is often served alone or in mixed company at the end of a Mediterranean meal.

Great fruits to try include bananas, kiwi, figs, dates, strawberries, grapes, peaches, plums, pears, melons, apples, pomegranates, currants, and mandarin oranges.

STRAWBERRY AND POACHED PEARS
MAKES 4 SERVINGS

4 large ripe Anjou or Bartlett pears, peeled and cored
2 tablespoons fresh lemon juice
½ cup red wine (not cooking wine)
1½ cups water
2 tablespoons low-calorie baking sweetener
1 cinnamon stick
1 teaspoon freshly grated orange rind
½ teaspoon freshly grated lemon rind
¼ teaspoon cloves, ground
Fresh mint leaves for garnish

For Strawberry Sauce:
  1 pint fresh strawberries, cleaned and sliced
  3 tablespoons non-caloric sweetener
  1 teaspoon Grand Marnier liqueur

Slice off bottom of pears to allow them to sit flat in a pan. Brush body of pears with lemon juice. In a saucepan combine wine, water, sweetener, cinnamon, orange rind, lemon rind, and cloves. Bring to a boil over medium heat, reduce heat, and simmer for 5 minutes. Add pears, cover, and poach for 20 minutes until tender. Let pears stand in liquid until cool. Refrigerate until ready to serve. When serving, place pears on dessert plates and drizzle with a small amount of strawberry sauce. Garnish with mint leaf.

Sauce:

Put strawberries in bowl and sprinkle with sweetener and Grand Marnier. Let stand at room temperature for 1 hour. Blend or process until puréed, then refrigerate sauce to chill.

Approx. 120 calories per serving
1g protein, 1g total fat, 0 saturated fat, 0 trans fat,
3g carbohydrates, 0 cholesterol, 2mg sodium, 4g fiber

FIGS IN PLAIN YOGURT
MAKES 4 SERVINGS

16 small figs
1½ cups red wine
2 tablespoons honey
¼ teaspoon ground cinnamon
2 cups plain low-fat yogurt
Non-caloric sweetener, as desired
Finely chopped fresh mint for garnish

Slice open skins of figs on one side. Combine wine, honey, and cinnamon in a large saucepan and bring mixture to boil. Reduce to simmer, add figs, and simmer for 10–15 minutes. Remove from heat and allow figs to bathe in liquid for 5–10 minutes. Remove skins from figs and mash insides. Combine mashed figs with yogurt and mix well; add sweetener, if desired. Refrigerate until well chilled. Divide yogurt mixture into 4 dessert bowls. Sprinkle with fresh mint.

Approx. 280 calories per serving
0.5g protein, 2g total fat, 1g saturated fat, 0 trans fat,
48g carbohydrates, 8mg cholesterol, 75mg sodium, 4g fiber

HONEY MOUSSE DELIGHT

MAKES 6 SERVINGS

⅓ cup honey

2 teaspoons freshly grated orange rind

12 ounces part-skim ricotta cheese

2½ cups halved fresh strawberries

2½ cups fresh blackberries

¼ cup fresh orange juice

3 tablespoons non-caloric sweetener

2 tablespoons finely chopped walnuts

Mix honey, orange rind, and ricotta cheese in a medium bowl; cover and refrigerate to chill. Combine berries, juice, and sweetener, gently toss, and let stand for 5 minutes before covering and re-chilling. When well chilled, spoon ⅓ berry mixture (divided equally) into 6 serving bowls and top each with about ¼ cup of ricotta mixture. Divide remaining fruit mixture into 6 portions and add on top of cheese. Sprinkle with walnuts and serve.

Approx. 196 calories per serving
7g protein, 6g total fat, 3g saturated fat, 0 trans fat,
29g carbohydrates, 18mg cholesterol, 71mg sodium, 1g fiber

SPICE CAKE
MAKES 9 (1-INCH-WIDE) SERVINGS

½ teaspoon anise seed

¾ cup water

½ cup honey

½ cup low-calorie baking sweetener

½ teaspoon baking soda

3 cups unbleached white flour

⅛ teaspoon cinnamon

¼ teaspoon fresh grated nutmeg

Pinch of salt

⅛ cup mixed chopped orange and lemon peels

Olive oil cooking spray

In a medium saucepan bring anise seed covered with water to a boil; add honey and sweetener and stir until both are dissolved. Remove mixture from heat and add baking soda. Sift flour, spices, and salt into a large bowl. Add orange and lemon peels. Strain liquid from anise seeds and mix seeds into dry ingredients, stirring constantly. Beat until mixture is smooth, then pour into 9x5x3-inch sprayed and floured baking pan. Bake for 1 hour in a 350-degree oven or until cake just begins to shrink from sides of pan. Remove from oven and let cool slightly. Serve warm or cool.

Approx. 360 calories per serving
8g protein, 0.7g total fat, 0.1g saturated fat, 0 trans fat,
83g carbohydrates, 0 cholesterol, 83mg sodium, 2g fiber

PEACH MARSALA COMPOTE

MAKES 6 SERVINGS

Canola oil cooking spray
12 fresh peaches
6 cups water
¾ cup low-calorie baking sweetener
½ cup Marsala wine
½ teaspoon ground cinnamon
½ teaspoon vanilla extract
½ teaspoon freshly grated nutmeg

Lightly spray a 2-quart baking dish with cooking oil. Blanch the peaches in boiling water for 20 seconds, then remove skin while holding under cold running water. Pit and slice peaches. Add peaches, sweetener, wine, cinnamon, vanilla extract, and nutmeg to a baking dish and bake for 45 minutes to 1 hour in a 350-degree oven. Serve warm or at room temperature.

Approx. 80 calories per serving
1g protein, 0.2g total fat, 0 saturated fat, 0 trans fat,
21g carbohydrates, 0 cholesterol, 126mg sodium, 3g fiber

SAUTÉED PEACHES OR NECTARINES WITH MAPLE SYRUP

MAKES 2 SERVINGS

2 teaspoons canola oil
2 ripe peaches or nectarines, pitted, skinned, and sliced
2 tablespoons pure maple syrup
Dash of ground cinnamon
Dollop of plain yogurt per serving

Heat canola oil in a skillet over medium-high heat and sauté peaches or nectarines until golden, roughly 1–2 minutes. When golden, stir in maple syrup and allow syrup to thicken slightly. Serve warm with a sprinkling of ground cinnamon and a dollop of yogurt.

Approx. 130 calories per serving
1g protein, 0 total fat, 0 saturated fat, 0 trans fat,
31g carbohydrates, 0 cholesterol, 2mg sodium, 3g fiber

SWEET MANGO MOUSSE

MAKES 6 SERVINGS

1¼ cups water

1 cup couscous

4 tablespoons non-caloric sweetener

¾ cup fresh orange juice

2 tablespoons orange-flavored liqueur

1 large ripe mango

1 cup light whipping cream, well chilled

1¼ teaspoons vanilla extract

1 (8-ounce) container low-fat vanilla yogurt

Orange zest, finely minced, for garnish

Bring water to a boil over medium-high heat. Add couscous slowly, stirring once, and remove from heat. Cover and set aside for 12–15 minutes, until couscous is tender. Add 2 tablespoons of sweetener and mix well into couscous. Cover and set aside. In a small saucepan over medium heat, heat juice, stirring constantly until reduced to the consistency of honey (about 4–5 minutes). Stir in liqueur. Set aside. Peel the mango; cut half of flesh into thin wedges; coarsely dice the other half and set aside. Pour cream into a chilled bowl and whip until it peaks. Fold in vanilla extract and remaining sweetener. Divide in half and set half aside. In a clean bowl combine remaining half of whipped cream, yogurt, and diced mango and refrigerate until well chilled. Before serving, combine mango mixture with couscous. Divide into 6 equal portions, and top each portion with a good dollop of the remaining whipped cream and mango wedges. Drizzle with liqueur sauce, sprinkle with orange zest, and serve.

Approx. 316 calories per serving
7g protein, 19g total fat, 7.8g saturated fat, 0 trans fat,
40g carbohydrates, 46mg cholesterol, 44mg sodium, <1g fiber

FRESH FRUIT IN YOGURT WITH RUM

MAKES 2 SERVINGS

¼ cup each of 2 of the following: blueberries, sliced strawberries, grapes, kiwi, or
   raspberries
2 cups low-fat plain yogurt
Dark rum (or other favorite liqueur) to taste
Non-caloric sweetener to taste (optional)

Cut up enough desired fresh fruit for 2 servings; add 2 cups plain yogurt and mix well. Divide mixture into 2 individual glass dessert cups and generously splash each serving with dark rum. Add sweetener, if desired; chill before serving.

Approx. 140 calories per serving
1g protein, 3.5g total fat, 2g saturated fat, 0 trans fat,
16g carbohydrates, 15mg cholesterol, 150mg sodium, 0 fiber

NOTE: Values shown are for yogurt dip only (values for fruit cannot be calculated since they depend on the specific fruits chosen).

FRESH FRUIT KABOBS AND CINNAMON HONEY DIP

MAKES 2 SERVINGS

Assorted bite-sized chunks of your favorite fresh fruits (enough for 2 [8-inch]wooden
   skewers)
1 cup low-fat plain yogurt
2 tablespoons of honey or non-caloric sweetener
Pinch of ground white pepper
6 teaspoons of ground cinnamon or to taste

Prepare fruits on skewers and set aside. Combine yogurt, honey, and white pepper, and mix well. Divide mixture into 2 individual serving bowls; sprinkle cinnamon on top of each serving and gently swirl in. Cover and refrigerate to chill before serving.

Approx. 70 calories per serving
0.5g protein, 2g total fat, 1g saturated fat, 0 trans fat,
8g carbohydrates, 7mg cholesterol, 75mg sodium, 0 fiber

NOTE: Values shown are for yogurt dip only (values for fruit cannot be calculated since they depend on the specific fruits chosen).

STUFFED DATES
MAKES 16 DATES

16 pitted dates
16 whole almonds
6 tablespoons almond paste

Slice dates open on one side. Pull back skin from the meat of the date and stuff each date with 1 almond and 1 teaspoon almond paste. Serve.

Approx. 152 calories per date
9g protein, 14g total fat, 1.2g saturated fat, 0 trans fat,
9g carbohydrates, 0 cholesterol, 0.8mg sodium, 3g fiber

SWEET ITALIAN RICE PUDDING
MAKES 6 SERVINGS

24 ounces evaporated skim milk
¼ cup long-grain rice
3 tablespoons low-calorie baking sweetener
1 teaspoon vanilla extract
Ground cinnamon

Combine 12 ounces milk and rice in a double boiler over water. Simmer, stirring frequently, for about 20 minutes. Add remaining milk and sweetener and mix well. Return to a simmer, stirring often, until the mixture gains a pudding consistency (about 45 minutes). Add vanilla extract and blend into pudding while simmering for an additional few minutes. Remove from heat and sprinkle generously with cinnamon. Cool to room temperature, cover, and refrigerate before serving.

Approx. 117 calories per serving
9g protein, 0.5g total fat, 0.4g saturated fat, 0 trans fat,
19g carbohydrates, 4mg cholesterol, 133mg sodium, <0.5g fiber

CRÈME DE BANANA BAKED APPLES

MAKES 4–6 SERVINGS

4 medium sweet apples, peeled, cored, and halved

6 ounces unsweetened apple juice

2 teaspoons ground cinnamon

3 tablespoons pure honey

1 teaspoon vanilla extract

4 tablespoons Crème de Banana liqueur

1 cup plain fat-free yogurt

Non-caloric sweetener to taste

Place apples cored side up in a snugly fitting shallow baking dish. Add apple juice to just barely cover bottom halves of apples. Sprinkle with 1 teaspoon cinnamon, cover, and bake for 30–40 minutes in a 350-degree oven or until apples are almost tender. Remove from oven and pour off any additional liquid, leaving just enough to cover bottom of dish. Mix together honey, vanilla extract, and liqueur and drizzle over tops of apples. Sprinkle remaining teaspoon of cinnamon over top. Bake for an additional 10 minutes. Remove from oven and divide equally onto 4 dessert plates. Blend yogurt and sweetener together and serve on the side.

Approx. 130 calories per serving
<.05g protein, <0.5g total fat, <.05g saturated fat, 0 trans fat,
27g carbohydrates, <1mg cholesterol, 28mg sodium, 2g fiber

CANTALOUPE SORBET

MAKES 4–6 SERVINGS

1½ cups of water
½ cup low-calorie baking sweetener
2 ripe cantaloupes, peeled, halved, seeded, and chunked
¼ cup fresh lemon juice
¼ cup egg whites
Fresh mint sprigs for garnish

Combine water and sweetener and bring to a boil over medium heat. Reduce heat and simmer for 5 minutes, then allow to cool. In a food processor or blender, add cantaloupe and its juices, lemon juice, and cooled syrup. Puree until smooth. Pour mixture into bowl and freeze until almost frozen. Remove from freezer and beat with an electric beater until mixture is again smooth. Beat egg whites until stiff and fold into frozen fruit mixture. Cover container and freeze again until firm (about 2–3 hours). When ready to serve, scoop into dessert cups and garnish with mint sprigs.

Approx. 67 calories per serving
2g protein, <0.5 total fat, 0 saturated fat, 0 trans fat,
15g carbohydrates, 0 cholesterol, 28mg sodium, 1g fiber

HONEYDEW SORBET
MAKES 4–6 SERVINGS

1½ cups water

½ cup low-calorie baking sweetener

2 ripe honeydews (about 5 inches in diameter each), peeled, seeded, and chunked

¼ cup fresh lemon juice

¼ cup egg whites

Fresh mint sprigs for garnish

Combine water and sweetener, and bring to a boil over medium heat. Reduce heat and simmer for 5 minutes, then allow to cool. In a food processor or blender add honeydew and its juices, lemon juice, and cooled syrup. Puree until smooth. Pour mixture into bowl and freeze until almost frozen. Remove from freezer and beat with an electric beater until mixture is again smooth. Beat egg whites until stiff and fold into frozen fruit mixture. Cover container and freeze again until firm (about 2–3 hours). When ready to serve, scoop into dessert cups and garnish with mint sprigs.

Approx. 117 calories per serving
2g protein, <0.5g total fat, 0 saturated fat, 0 trans fat,
31g carbohydrates, 0 cholesterol, 33mg sodium, 2g fiber

STRAWBERRIES AND BALSAMIC SYRUP
MAKES 4 SERVINGS

2½ cups fresh strawberries, hulled and halved

4 tablespoons Crème de Banana liqueur

Non caloric sweetener to taste

Balsamic syrup

Combine strawberries and liqueur in a large bowl, toss well, cover, and refrigerate 20–30 minutes. When ready to serve, remove strawberries with a slotted spoon and place in a single layer on a dessert platter. Dust generously with sweetener, drizzle with balsamic syrup, and serve.

Approx. 49 calories per serving
<1g protein, 0.4g total fat, <0.1g saturated fat, 0 trans fat,
7g carbohydrates, 0 cholesterol, 1mg sodium, 2g fiber

DRUNKEN PEACHES

MAKES 4 SERVINGS

4 peaches

1½ cups red wine

1⅓ cups water

3 strips lemon peel (yellow part only)

3 tablespoons honey

1 cinnamon stick

Non-caloric sweetener to taste (optional)

Fat-free whipped cream (optional)

Peel skin from peaches. In a saucepan add wine, water, lemon peel, honey, and cinnamon stick, and bring to boil. Add peaches to sauce, submerging under liquid as much as possible, and gently poach for 5–10 minutes, until just tender. Remove peaches from saucepan and place in a bowl; set aside. Boil liquid in the saucepan, stirring constantly, until it becomes thick and syrupy. Remove cinnamon stick and lemon peel before liquid becomes dark. Pour syrup, when cool, over peaches, and serve. Garnish with sweetener and whipped cream, if desired.

Approx. 115 calories per serving
1g protein, <.08g total fat, 0 saturated fat, 0 trans fat,
22g carbohydrates, 0 cholesterol, 0.5mg sodium, 1g fiber

DRUNKEN APRICOTS

MAKES 4 SERVINGS

8 medium apricots
1½ cups red wine
1⅓ cups water
3 strips lemon peel (yellow part only)
3 tablespoons honey
1 cinnamon stick
Non-caloric sweetener to taste (optional)
Fat-free whipped cream (optional)

Peel skin from apricots. In a saucepan add wine, water, lemon peel, honey, and cinnamon stick, and bring to boil. Add apricots to sauce, submerging under liquid as much as possible, and gently poach for 5–10 minutes, until just tender. Remove apricots from saucepan and place in a bowl; set aside. Boil liquid in the saucepan, stirring constantly, until it becomes thick and syrupy. Remove cinnamon stick and lemon peel before liquid becomes dark. Pour syrup, when cool, over apricots, and serve. Garnish with sweetener and whipped cream, if desired.

Approx. 112 calories per serving
1g protein, 0.3g total fat, 0 saturated fat, 0 trans fat,
20g carbohydrates, 0 cholesterol, 1mg sodium, 1g fiber

PHYLLO TARTLETS WITH HONEY-SWEETENED CHERRIES

MAKES 8 TARTLETS

3 tablespoons instant tapioca

5 cups pitted frozen sweet cherries, thawed and drained

¾ cup honey, warmed

1 tablespoon freshly squeezed lemon juice

¾ tablespoon ground cloves

Pinch of salt

Butter-flavored cooking spray

20 sheets (9x14-inch) phyllo dough, thawed and cut in half

Process tapioca in a spice grinder or mini food processor until finely ground. Transfer to a large bowl and add cherries, honey, lemon juice, cloves, and salt. Set aside.

Preheat oven to 325 degrees. Lightly spray the inside of 8 (3-inch wide) tartlet pans with cooking oil. Unroll phyllo sheets on a clean, dry surface, keeping them in a stack. Cut the stack crosswise (so you now have 40 sheets). Cover sheets with waxed paper and a damp kitchen towel to prevent them from drying out while you work. Place 1 half sheet of phyllo in each pan, pressing it into the edges, then lightly spray with cooking oil. Continue adding sheets and lightly spraying with cooking oil until you have 5 layers in each pan. Trim the phyllo, leaving ½–1-inch overhang. Place the tartlets on a baking sheet. Divide the cherry mixture among the pans. Fold the dough over the filling (it won't cover completely). Lightly spray the edges of dough with cooking oil. Bake the tartlets until the filling begins to bubble and the dough is golden brown. Serve warm.

Approx. 247 calories per tartlet

0 protein, 0 total fat, 0 saturated fat, 0 trans fat,

58g carbohydrates, 0 cholesterol, 60mg sodium, 2g fiber

MOROCCAN SWEET ORANGES

MAKES 4 SERVINGS

4 large sweet oranges
Honey, to drizzle
Cinnamon, to sprinkle

Peel oranges and slice crosswise into rounds. Arrange orange slices on a dessert platter, drizzle tops with honey and a sprinkle of cinnamon, and serve.

Approx. 71 calories per serving
1g protein, 0 total fat, 0 saturated fat, 0 trans fat,
18g carbohydrates, 0 cholesterol, 0 sodium, 1g fiber

PUMPKIN PUDDING

MAKES 4 SERVINGS

1¾ cups skim milk
1 (1-ounce) package sugar-free instant vanilla pudding mix
½ cup canned pumpkin
½ teaspoon pumpkin spice

Combine cold milk and pudding mix in a chilled bowl and stir until smooth. Blend in pumpkin and spice and refrigerate to chill before serving.

Approx. 55 calories per serving
5g protein, 0 total fat, 0 saturated fat, 0 trans fat,
9g carbohydrates, 2mg cholesterol, 137mg sodium, 1g fiber

HONEY NESTS

MAKES 4 SERVINGS

½ pound angel hair pasta

8 tablespoons trans fat–free canola/olive oil spread, melted

1½ cups shelled pistachio nuts, chopped, divided

¼ cup low-calorie baking sweetener

⅓ cup honey

⅝ cup water

2 teaspoons freshly squeezed lemon juice

Low-fat plain Greek yogurt for garnish

Preheat oven to 350 degrees. Cook pasta as per package directions and drain thoroughly. Transfer pasta to a bowl and add melted canola/olive oil spread. Toss to coat pasta and allow to cool. Divide pasta into 8 equal portions. Using 4 small oven-safe bowls, press 1 portion of pasta down lightly into each of the 4 bowls and top with half of the nuts. Cover each with a remaining portion of pasta and place bowls on a baking sheet. Bake for 45 minutes or until pasta is golden brown and crispy on the top.

While pasta is baking, combine sweetener, honey, and water in a small saucepan and bring to a boil over low heat, stirring constantly until sweetener is dissolved. Let simmer for another 10 minutes, add lemon juice, and let simmer for 5 more minutes. When pasta is well browned (not burned), remove from oven and carefully transfer angel hair nests to serving dishes. Drizzle honey-lemon mixture over tops of nests and sprinkle with remaining nuts. Allow to cool before serving with a dollop of yogurt.

Approx. 453 calories per serving
11g protein, 16g total fat, 2g saturated fat, 0 trans fat,
73g carbohydrates, 0 cholesterol, 233mg sodium, 5g fiber

STRAWBERRY-RHUBARB QUINOA PUDDING

MAKES 6 SERVINGS

3 cups water, divided

1½ cups chopped rhubarb, fresh or frozen

1 cup chopped strawberries, fresh or frozen, + more for garnish

½ cup quinoa

½ teaspoon ground cinnamon

Dash of salt

¼ cup + 1½ teaspoons low-calorie baking sweetener

½ teaspoon freshly grated lemon zest

1 tablespoon cornstarch

1 cup plain non-fat yogurt

1 teaspoon pure vanilla extract

In a saucepan, combine 2¾ cups water, rhubarb, strawberries, quinoa, cinnamon, and salt. Bring to a boil and reduce heat to a simmer. Cover and cook for about 25 minutes or until quinoa is tender. Stir in ¼ cup sweetener and lemon zest. In a small bowl, combine remaining ¼ cup water with cornstarch and whisk until smooth, then add to quinoa mixture and continue to let simmer, stirring constantly for 1 minute. Remove from heat, divide among 6 serving bowls, and refrigerate to cool for 1 hour. Meanwhile, combine yogurt, vanilla extract, and remaining 1½ teaspoons sweetener in a small bowl. Top each serving with a generous dollop of yogurt mixture and sliced fresh strawberries.

Approx. 106 calories per serving
4g protein, 1g total fat, 0 saturated fat, 0 trans fat,
17g carbohydrates, 1mg cholesterol, 125mg sodium, 2g fiber

DRUNKEN STRAWBERRIES
MAKES 4 SERVINGS

1 pound hulled fresh strawberries, sliced
1½ packets of a non-caloric sweetener
1 tablespoon Grand Marnier liqueur
1 teaspoon freshly squeezed lemon juice
1 cup low-fat plain Greek yogurt

Combine strawberries, sweetener, liqueur, and lemon juice in a bowl. Allow to stand and marinate until strawberries release their juices, roughly 10–15 minutes. Divide mixture into four dessert bowls, add ¼ cup yogurt to each bowl, and serve.

Approx. 22 calories per serving
3g protein, 1g total fat, 0 saturated fat, 0 trans fat,
7g carbohydrates, 3mg cholesterol, 43mg sodium, 1g fiber

DELICIOUSLY SWEETENED YOGURT
MAKES 2 SERVINGS

2 ripe apricots, halved, pitted, and cut to ½-inch wedges
1 cup sweet cherries, halved and pitted
3 teaspoons fresh mint, finely chopped
6 packets non-caloric sweetener, divided
2 cups low-fat plain Greek yogurt
2 teaspoons pure vanilla extract
2 tablespoons shelled, chopped, and toasted pistachios

Toss together apricots, sweet cherries, mint, and 1½ packets of sweetener. Allow to stand for 10–15 minutes until fruits release some of their juices. Meanwhile, combine yogurt, vanilla extract, and remaining sweetener. Stir until well mixed and smooth. Divide yogurt mixture into 2 bowls and top with fruit mixture and a sprinkling of nuts. Serve immediately.

Approx. 228 calories per serving
14g protein, 6g total fat, 2g saturated fat, 0 trans fat,
33g carbohydrates, 16mg cholesterol, 202mg sodium, 1g fiber

EASY PEACH COBBLER

MAKES 15 SERVINGS

½ cup + 1½ teaspoons low-calorie baking sweetener

2 tablespoons cornstarch

1 (29-ounce) can sliced peaches, drained, liquid reserved

½ tablespoon ground cinnamon

2 tablespoons trans fat–free canola/olive oil spread

1 cup self-rising flour

1 tablespoon trans fat–free shortening

½ cup almond milk

Preheat oven to 400 degrees. In a saucepan, combine ½ cup sweetener and cornstarch, gradually stirring in reserved peach juice and bringing to a boil for 1 minute, stirring constantly. Add peaches, pour mixture into a 9x13-inch baking dish, sprinkle with cinnamon, dot with canola/olive oil spread, and set aside. Mix flour and remaining sweetener, cut with shortening, then add milk and stir until ingredients are well blended. Spoon dough onto fruit and bake for 25–30 minutes. Serve warm.

Approx. 76 calories per serving
1g protein, 1g total fat, 0 saturated fat, 0 trans fat,
12g carbohydrates, 0 cholesterol, 20mg sodium, 0 fiber

LEMON CAKES

MAKES 8 SERVINGS

2 tablespoons trans fat–free canola/olive oil spread + more, softened, to coat ramekins
⅓ cup all-purpose flour, spooned and leveled
½ teaspoon baking powder
¼ teaspoon salt
3 large eggs, separated
¼ cup + ⅛ cup low-calorie baking sweetener
1 teaspoon finely grated lemon zest
⅓ cup freshly squeezed lemon juice
1¼ cups almond milk
Confectioners' sugar for dusting, scant amount

Preheat oven to 325 degrees. Brush the sides and bottoms of 8 (6-ounce) ramekins with softened canola/olive oil spread. Place ramekins in a shallow baking casserole. In a bowl, combine flour, baking powder, and salt. In a separate larger bowl, whisk together egg yolks with ¼ cup of sweetener until mixture is pale and smooth. Whisk in 2 tablespoons canola/olive oil spread, lemon zest, lemon juice, milk, and flour mixture. Cover and refrigerate mixture for 3 hours. In another large bowl, using an electric mixer beat egg whites with ⅛ cup sweetener until mixture peaks, about 5 minutes, and fold into chilled batter. With a ladle, divide batter among ramekins, wiping any dripped excess from edges. Add enough water to the casserole to come halfway up sides of the ramekins. Place casserole with ramekins in oven and bake until cakes puff and are slightly golden on top, about 30 minutes. Dust with confectioners' sugar and serve while hot.

Approx. 78 calories per serving
2g protein, 2g total fat, 1g saturated fat, 0 trans fat,
4g carbohydrates, 79mg cholesterol, 219mg sodium, 0 fiber

VANILLA-RHUBARB COMPOTE

MAKES 4 SERVINGS

4 cups diced rhubarb
¼ cup low-calorie baking sweetener
¼ teaspoon ground cinnamon
½ teaspoon pure vanilla extract
4 (store-bought) crêpes
Vanilla yogurt or fat-free ice cream for serving

In a saucepan, combine rhubarb, sweetener, and cinnamon. Bring to a simmer over medium-high heat, then reduce heat to gentle simmer and cook until rhubarb begins to break down, about 5 minutes. Remove from heat and add vanilla extract. Stir and allow to sit for 2–3 minutes to incorporate flavors. On a work surface, lay out crêpes and fill centers with rhubarb mixture. Fold in ends and roll crêpes. Serve warm with vanilla yogurt or fat-free ice cream.

Approx. 137 calories per serving
5g protein, 5g total fat, 1g saturated fat, 0 trans fat,
17g carbohydrates, 78mg cholesterol, 142mg sodium, 2g fiber

COOL REFRESHING ORANGE POPS

MAKES 10 SERVINGS

1 cup concentrated orange juice, thawed
¼ cup low-calorie baking sweetener
2 cups low-fat vanilla yogurt
2 teaspoons pure vanilla extract

In a saucepan, combine orange juice and sweetener over medium-low heat. Cook, stirring constantly, until sweetener dissolves, roughly 3 minutes. Add in yogurt and vanilla extract, stirring to blend. Transfer to a large spouted container and fill 10 (3-ounce) ice-pop molds. Insert popsicle sticks and freeze until pops are solid, about 6 hours—or as long as 1 week. To remove from molds, briefly run molds under hot water to release pops.

Approx. 45 calories per serving
3g protein, 0 total fat, 0 saturated fat, 0 trans fat,
8g carbohydrates, 1mg cholesterol, 0 sodium, 0 fiber

STRAWBERRY-WALNUT TRIFLE

MAKES 15 SERVINGS

1 small, no-sugar-added angel food cake

3 ounces sugar-free strawberry gelatin

10 ounces frozen, unsweetened strawberries, thawed and halved (reserve 1 cup for garnish)

2 bananas, sliced

1 (1½-ounce) package sugar-free instant vanilla pudding mix

3 cups almond milk

Fat-free whipped cream

Chopped walnut pieces, to sprinkle

Tear cake into bite-sized pieces and place in bottom of a glass trifle bowl. Dissolve gelatin in 1 cup boiling hot water and add to strawberries. Spoon strawberry mixture evenly over cake pieces. Add banana slices to top of strawberries and refrigerate while preparing pudding.

Combine pudding mix with almond milk and whisk for roughly 2 minutes until it begins to set. Refrigerate pudding for an additional 5 minutes to set more firmly before adding it to the trifle bowl, spooning evenly over bananas and strawberries. Refrigerate trifle bowl mixture for at least 2 hours before serving. Top each serving with reserved strawberries, a dollop of whipped cream, and a sprinkle of chopped walnuts.

Approx. 72 calories per serving

1g protein, 0 total fat, 0 saturated fat, 0 trans fat,

17g carbohydrates, 0 cholesterol, 150mg sodium, 0 fiber

CHUNKY APPLE SAUCE

MAKES 6 SERVINGS

4 pounds apples (use different varieties for a chunkier texture, such as McIntosh, Gala,
  Fuji, Granny Smith, etc.)
¼ cup freshly squeezed lemon juice
1½ cups water
3 tablespoons light brown sugar
2 (1½-ounce) boxes black raisins

Peel, core, and slice apples. In a large pot, combine apples, lemon juice, water, sugar, and raisins. Bring to a boil over high heat. Reduce heat to a simmer and cook apple mixture until apples are soft and falling apart. With a large fork, mash about half of the apples, leaving the remainder in small- to medium-size chunks. Allow to cool before refrigerating in an airtight container.

Approx. 104 calories per serving
0 protein, 0 total fat, 0 saturated fat, 0 trans fat,
27g carbohydrates, 0 cholesterol, 2mg sodium, 3g fiber

APRICOT SORBET

MAKES 6 SERVINGS

1 cup low-calorie baking sweetener
1 pound very ripe apricots, pitted and sliced + 3 extra, ripe-but-firm apricots, pitted and
  thinly sliced
¾ cup sparkling champagne
2 cups water + extra as needed

Bring sweetener, 1 pound apricots, champagne, and 2 cups water to a boil in a medium saucepan. Reduce heat to a simmer and cook, stirring often, until apricots are very tender. Allow to cool. Transfer mixture to a blender and puree until smooth. Add extra water to mixture as needed to make 4 cups. Transfer mixture to a large, shallow baking dish, gently mix in thin slices of apricots, and freeze mixture until solid (at least 4–5 hours). Scoop into individual bowls when ready and serve.

Approx. 62 calories per serving
0 protein, 0 total fat, 0 saturated fat, 0 trans fat,
13g carbohydrates, 0 cholesterol, 3mg sodium, 3g fiber

CARAMELIZED PINEAPPLE AND PISTACHIOS

MAKES 4 SERVINGS

¼ cup dark brown, low-calorie baking sweetener (firmly packed)

½ cup no-pulp orange juice

3 tablespoons honey

1 medium ripe pineapple, peeled, cored, and cut lengthwise into 8 wedges

⅓ cup unsalted pistachios, coarsely chopped

¼ cup plain low-fat yogurt

Preheat oven to 450 degrees. Line a rimmed baking sheet with parchment paper. In a large bowl, combine sweetener, orange juice, and honey. Stir until sweetener dissolves. Add pineapple wedges and toss to coat. Allow to marinate for 20–25 minutes, tossing occasionally. Place pineapple wedges flat side down on baking sheet and reserve marinade. Roast pineapple for about 15 minutes, turn and brush on marinade, and continue roasting until tender and caramelized. Remove from oven, drizzle remaining marinade over pineapple, and allow to cool to room temperature. Divide among 4 plates, sprinkle each with pistachios, and add a spoonful of yogurt to the side of each plate.

Approx. 184 calories per serving
4g protein, 4g total fat, 0 saturated fat, 0 trans fat,
19g carbohydrates, 0 cholesterol, 12mg sodium, 3g fiber

SPICED APPLES

MAKES 4–6 SERVINGS

⅛ cup low-calorie baking sweetener
⅛ teaspoon ground cinnamon
6 small red apples (about 2½ inches diameter)
1½ teaspoons light amber maple syrup
1½ cups dry white wine
¾ cup (6 ounces) apple cider
Dash nutmeg
½ teaspoon finely minced fresh orange peel

In a small bowl, combine sweetener and cinnamon. Roll apples in syrup then in cinnamon-sweetener mixture. Place apples in a baking dish and bake at 400 degrees for 15 minutes. In a saucepan combine wine, cider, nutmeg, and orange peel; heat on low heat. Pour over baked apples and serve.

Approx. 114 calories per serving
<0.5g protein, <0.5g total fat, 0 saturated fat, 0 trans fat,
20g carbohydrates, 0 cholesterol, 5mg sodium, 3g fiber

STRAWBERRIES AMARETTO

MAKES 8 SERVINGS

3 pints fresh strawberries
2 cups plain low-fat yogurt
1 teaspoon vanilla extract
¼ cup Amaretto liqueur
Fat-free whipped cream (optional)

Set aside 8 strawberries for garnish. Hull remaining strawberries and cut into halves. Place strawberry halves in dessert cups. In a bowl combine yogurt, vanilla extract, and liqueur; blend well. Pour over strawberries and garnish each cup with a reserved berry. Add whipped cream, if desired.

Approx. 96 calories per serving
4g protein, 0.6g total fat, <0.5 saturated fat, 0 trans fat,
9g carbohydrates, <0.5mg cholesterol, 42mg sodium, 3g fiber

LEMON SHERBET
MAKES 4–6 SERVINGS

3 large lemons
½ cup honey
2½ cups water
¼ cup liquid egg whites

Remove zest from lemons and set aside. Squeeze all 3 lemons to get ⅔ cup of fresh lemon juice and set juice aside. In a saucepan add zest, honey, and water. Bring to a rapid boil for 5 minutes, then allow to cool to room temperature. Strain lemon juice through a sieve. When honey mixture has cooled, add strained lemon juice, pour into freezer container, and freeze until mushy. When mushy, stir ice crystals from edges of container. Do this every hour for 4 hours, then remove from freezer and whisk until smooth. Beat egg whites to stiffen and fold into whisked lemon mixture. Cover and return to freezer for another 2–3 hours, until mixture has the consistency of packed snow. Serve immediately.

This recipe can also be used to make orange sherbet, substituting oranges for lemons.

Approx. 91 calories per serving
1g protein, 0 total fat, 0 saturated fat, 0 trans fat,
22g carbohydrates, 0 cholesterol, 16mg sodium, 0 fiber

SOUR CREAM AND WALNUT COOKIES

MAKES 20–25 COOKIES

Canola oil cooking spray
½ cup trans fat–free canola/olive oil spread
⅔ cup low-calorie baking sweetener
⅔ cup low-fat sour cream
1½ cups all-purpose unbleached flour
1 teaspoon baking soda
½ cup chopped walnuts

Lightly coat 2 cookie sheets with cooking spray. In a bowl combine canola/olive oil spread and sweetener. Use an electric beater on very low to whip mixture into a soft consistency. Add sour cream and whip again for a few seconds to blend. Sift flour and baking soda into sour cream mixture. With a wooden spatula, fold flour and baking soda into mixture until well blended. Add walnuts to dough mixture. Drop 1 tablespoon of dough on the cookie sheet for each cookie. Allow room between cookies. Press cookies flat with a wooden spatula and bake at 350 degrees, until golden brown (about 10–15 minutes). Remove from the oven and allow cookies to cool before serving.

Approx. 82 calories per cookie
3g protein, 3g total fat, 1g saturated fat, 0 trans fat,
5g carbohydrates, 2mg cholesterol, 38mg sodium, <1g fiber

MERINGUE KEY LIME DESSERT CUPS
MAKES 6–8 SERVINGS

1½ cups low-calorie baking sweetener
¼ cup cornstarch
¼ teaspoon sodium-free salt substitute
¼ cup + 2 tablespoons fresh Key lime juice
½ cup cold water
¾ cup whole egg substitute
2 tablespoons trans fat–free canola/olive oil spread
½ cup boiling water
2 teaspoons grated fresh lime zest

For Meringue:

¾ cup egg whites
¼ teaspoon cream of tartar
½ cup low-calorie baking sweetener
8 thin slices fresh lime for garnish

Combine sweetener, cornstarch, and salt substitute in a large saucepan. Add lime juice, water, and egg substitute; blend well. Add canola/olive oil spread and slowly blend in boiling water. Heat mixture to boiling over medium heat and cook for 2–3 minutes, stirring constantly. Add in lime zest, remove mixture from heat, and set aside to cool.

Meringue:

Place egg whites in a bowl and whip on low speed until they start to bubble. Turn speed to medium-high; add cream of tartar and whip until mixture holds a peak. Continue whipping on high while gradually adding sweetener. Meringue will stiffen and peak. Fill oven-safe dessert cups with Key lime mixture and top with a healthy dollop of meringue. Place in a 350-degree oven until meringue lightly browns. Serve warm or cold, garnished with fresh lime slices.

Approx. 58 calories per serving
5g protein, 2g total fat, 0.4g saturated fat, 0 trans fat,
16g carbohydrates, 0 cholesterol, 109mg sodium, 0 fiber

HOMESTYLE APPLE PIE

MAKES 8 SERVINGS

For Crust:

> 1 cup pastry flour
> 6 tablespoons canola oil
> 3 tablespoons water
> All-purpose flour

For Filling:

> 6 sweet apples, cored, peeled, and sliced (Red or Yellow Delicious, Gala, or Macintosh)
> ⅔ cup low-calorie baking sweetener
> ⅛ teaspoon salt
> ¾ teaspoon cinnamon
> ¾ teaspoon nutmeg
> 1½ tablespoons trans fat–free canola oil/olive oil spread
> Fat-free whipped cream (optional)

Crust:

Prepare dough by combining pastry flour with canola oil and water. Mix well and form into a ball. Use a small amount of all-purpose flour to coat work surface, place dough on surface, and sprinkle a small amount of all-purpose flour on dough to keep it from sticking to the rolling pin. Roll out dough into a flat circle large enough to cover the inside and sides of a 9-inch pie pan.

Filling:

Place sliced apples in a bowl, add sweetener, salt, cinnamon, and nutmeg, and stir to coat apple slices with dried ingredients. Transfer apple mixture to dough-lined pie pan. Spread apples out evenly. Place dots of canola/olive oil spread onto the top of apples and put pie into oven. Bake at 450 degrees for 15 minutes. Reduce oven temperature to 350 degrees and bake for another 45 minutes. Remove from oven and cool slightly before cutting. Serve warm with fat-free whipped cream, if desired.

Approx. 111 calories per serving
1g protein, 2g total fat, 0 saturated fat, 0 trans fat,
23g carbohydrates, 0 cholesterol, 88mg sodium, 3g fiber

TOASTED CRÊPE CUPS WITH FRESH BERRIES IN A LEMON YOGURT SAUCE

MAKES 4 SERVINGS

4 (prepared) flat crêpes (use only trans fat-free brands)

Canola oil cooking spray

½ cup + 4 tablespoons low-fat plain yogurt

½ cup fat-free cream cheese

4 teaspoons fresh lemon juice

2 teaspoons non-caloric sweetener

10 pecan halves, chopped

1 cup blueberries, fresh or frozen (thawed)

8 fresh strawberries, hulled and sliced

4 whole fresh strawberries for garnish (optional)

4 fresh mint leaves for garnish (optional)

Invert 4 oven-safe dessert cups on a baking sheet and lightly spray the outside of each cup with cooking oil. Form 1 flat crêpe around each dessert cup, folding crêpes down the center to fit cup size better if necessary (crêpes will not adhere completely to cups but will take on enough of its form to give them a cup shape when baked). Spray tops of crêpes very lightly with cooking oil and place baking sheet in oven. Bake crêpes until golden brown and crispy (about 6–7 minutes). Remove from oven and allow to cool before removing crêpes from cups. Meanwhile, combine yogurt and cream cheese in a bowl. Stir until well blended. Add in lemon juice and sweetener. Stir until all ingredients are well blended. Add pecans to mixture and gently fold in blueberries and strawberries. Divide mixture into 4 portions and spoon into formed crêpe cups. Garnish with a fresh whole strawberry and a fresh mint leaf, if desired.

Approx. 133 calories per serving
5g protein, 3g total fat, 0 saturated fat, 0 trans fat,
16g carbohydrates, 23mg cholesterol, 180mg sodium, 2g fiber

TOASTED SAUTÉED BANANA AND STRAWBERRY CRÊPES

MAKES 4 SERVINGS

Canola oil cooking spray
2 small bananas, sliced lengthwise
Cinnamon and non-caloric sweetener for sprinkling
4 teaspoons fat-free cream cheese
4 (prepared) flat crêpes (use only trans fat–free brands)
½ cup fresh strawberries, sliced
⅛ cup raw sliced almonds
Fat-free sour cream for garnish (optional)

Lightly spray a heavy-bottomed skillet with cooking oil and sauté the bananas (sprinkled with cinnamon and sweetener) until lightly browned. Remove from heat and set aside. Spread 1 teaspoon of cream cheese down the center of each crêpe. Place a sautéed banana half on top of the cheese and add strawberries. Fold crêpes over to form a pocket while folding in the ends. Place folded crêpes on a baking sheet lightly sprayed with canola oil cooking spray; also spray tops of crêpes. Sprinkle tops of crêpes with almond slices and sweetener. Place in oven and bake until crêpes are golden brown and crispy (about 7–9 minutes). Serve warm with a dollop of sour cream, if desired.

Approx. 119 calories per serving
4g protein, 1g total fat, 0 saturated fat, 0 trans fat,
21g carbohydrates, 5mg cholesterol, 67mg sodium, 4g fiber

FRUITED NUTTY PASTRY ROLLS

MAKES 20 PIECES

Canola oil cooking spray
4 tablespoons trans fat–free canola/olive oil spread
¼ cup low-calorie baking sweetener
1 egg
1 teaspoon almond extract
⅔ cup all-purpose unbleached flour, sifted
4 tablespoons natural chunky peanut butter
4 tablespoons low-sugar fruit jam
⅛ cup finely chopped walnuts

Lightly coat a baking sheet with cooking spray. In a bowl beat together canola/olive oil spread and sweetener until soft and fluffy. Crack the egg and separate the yolk from the white; reserve white. Beat the egg yolk and almond extract into the spread and sweetener mixture. Add in flour. Stir to mix all ingredients and form firm dough ball. Add in a small amount of extra flour if dough is too soft. Divide the dough in half and roll each half into a log about 10 inches long. Place both logs on the baking sheet. Lightly spray the handle of a dinner knife with cooking spray. Starting about ⅛ inch from the beginning of each log, use the knife handle to make a channel down the center, stopping about ⅛ inch before the end of the log. Whisk the egg white gently and brush it over each log. Fill the channel with peanut butter and top with jam. Sprinkle with walnut pieces. Chill logs for about 30–45 minutes. Heat oven to 350 degrees and bake chilled logs until they are a light golden brown (about 10–12 minutes). Remove from oven and allow logs to cool until jam sets. Slice each roll diagonally into 10 slices before serving.

Approx. 78 calories per piece
4g protein, 6g total fat, 1g saturated fat, 0 trans fat,
5g carbohydrates, 11mg cholesterol, 50mg sodium, <0.5g fiber

MERINGUE COOKIES
MAKES 20–24 COOKIES

1 cup liquid egg whites
Pinch of cream of tartar
¼ cup low-calorie baking sweetener
1 teaspoon white wine vinegar
1 teaspoon vanilla extract

Preheat oven to 275 degrees. Line 2 cookie trays with parchment paper. Place egg whites in a mixing bowl and slowly whisk on low speed with an electric beater until they begin to bubble. Add cream of tartar and increase speed slightly; whisk until the mixture begins to peak. Increase speed to medium and slowly add sweetener, vinegar, and vanilla extract. Continue whisking until mixture is satiny and firmly holds peak. Ladle a soup spoon–sized portion of mixture onto parchment-lined trays to make 20–24 cookies. Put trays of meringues in oven and bake for about 1 hour. Turn off oven and allow cookies to stand in closed oven for an additional hour to dry. When meringues are pierced with a toothpick that comes back dry, they are ready. Transfer cookies to cooling racks to continue to cool.

Approx. 5 calories per cookie
1g protein, 0 total fat, 0 saturated fat, 0 trans fat,
<0.1g carbohydrates, 0 cholesterol, 15mg sodium, 0 fiber

RASPBERRY MERINGUES

MAKES 30–40 COOKIES

¾ cup liquid egg whites

½ cup sliced raw almonds

2 tablespoons low-calorie baking sweetener

¼ teaspoon almond extract

⅛ teaspoon sodium-free salt substitute

⅓ cup non-caloric sweetener

⅓ cup low-calorie raspberry jam

Egg whites need to be at room temperature for 30 minutes before use. Preheat oven to 275 degrees. Line cookie sheets with parchment paper. Combine sliced almonds and 2 tablespoons of sweetener in a food processor or blender, and process until finely ground. In a large bowl add egg whites, almond extract, and salt substitute, and whip on medium speed until mixture begins to bubble. Gradually add ⅓ cup of sweetener a little at a time, increasing speed to high, and whip until mixture forms stiff peaks. Gently fold in almond mixture. Ladle soup spoon–sized portions of mixture onto parchment paper, making about 30–40 cookies. Bake for 20–25 minutes. Turn oven off and allow cookies to stand in closed oven for an additional hour to dry. Transfer cookies to cooling racks to continue to cool. When completely cooled, spoon a small amount of raspberry jam into center of each cookie.

Approx. 11 calories per cookie
6g protein, 0.7g total fat, 0 saturated fat, 0 trans fat,
8g carbohydrates, 0 cholesterol, 6mg sodium, .03g fiber

BROWNIES
MAKES 24 BROWNIES

1¼ cups cake flour (or substitute a combination of all-purpose flour and cornstarch as
    follows: 2½ tablespoons of cornstarch plus enough flour to fill 1¼ cups)
½ teaspoon sodium-free salt substitute
¾ teaspoon baking powder
3 tablespoons unsweetened dark baking cocoa
2¼ cups low-calorie baking sweetener
1 cup liquid egg substitute
4 tablespoons canola oil
1 tablespoon vanilla extract

Combine all dry ingredients in a large bowl and whisk to incorporate. In a separate bowl combine egg, canola oil, and vanilla extract. Pour egg mixture into dry ingredients and mix until batter is smooth and blended. Pour batter into a non-stick 9x13-inch baking pan and spread batter out evenly over bottom. Place pan on middle shelf in a 350-degree oven. Bake brownies for roughly 30 minutes; the center should spring back when touched with a finger, or you can insert a toothpick into the center. Brownies are done when the toothpick comes out with just a few moist crumbs on it. Do not overbake brownies or they will be dry. Immediately remove pan from oven and allow brownies to cool on cooling rack before cutting.

Approx. 54 calories per brownie
2g protein, 3g total fat, <0.4g saturated fat, 0 trans fat,
5g carbohydrates, 0 cholesterol, 33mg sodium, <0.5g fiber

SWEET PLUM COMPOTE

MAKES 6 SERVINGS

Canola oil cooking spray
3 pounds ripe plums, halved and pitted
¼ cup low-calorie baking sweetener
1 cup water
1 tablespoon Crème de Cassis liqueur

Lightly spray a baking dish with cooking oil. Add plums to baking dish. Combine sweetener and water in a saucepan and bring to a boil; cook for about 5 minutes, stirring constantly, or until liquid becomes syrupy. Pour syrup over plums and drizzle with Crème de Cassis. Bake mixture for 45 minutes to 1 hour in a 350-degree oven. Serve warm or cool.

Approx. 130 calories per serving
2g protein, 1g total fat, 0.1g saturated fat, 0 trans fat,
28g carbohydrates, 0 cholesterol, 1mg sodium, 1g fiber

ORANGE MACAROONS

MAKES 15 COOKIES

Canola oil cooking spray
½ cup liquid egg whites
2 tablespoons low-calorie baking sweetener
1 teaspoon finely grated fresh orange zest
¼ teaspoon vanilla or orange extract
Dash of salt (optional)
1½ cups sweetened dried flaked coconut

Line a cookie sheet with parchment paper and spray lightly with cooking spray. In a bowl add egg whites, sweetener, zest, extract, salt, and coconut. Stir to incorporate ingredients. Drop tablespoons of mixture onto parchment paper to make about 15 cookies. Allow about 1½ inches between each cookie. Bake in an oven preheated to 325 degrees on the middle oven rack for roughly 15–20 minutes or until the tops are a pale golden brown. Remove from oven and allow to cool.

Approx. 37 calories per cookie
1g protein, 3g total fat, 2g saturated fat, 0 trans fat,
2g carbohydrates, 0 cholesterol, 11mg sodium, <0.2g fiber

FRESH PINEAPPLE IN SPICY RUM SYRUP

MAKES 6 SERVINGS

1 fresh pineapple (roughly 3 pounds)
2½ cups water
½ cup low-calorie baking sweetener
8 slices fresh ginger
3 tablespoons dark rum
12 fresh mint leaves
Fat-free whipped cream

Trim top off pineapple and peel. Cut in half, core, and cut each half into ¼-inch slices. Set slices aside. In a large heavy-bottomed skillet, bring water, sweetener, and ginger to a boil. Stir mixture constantly until sweetener dissolves and continue boiling uncovered for an additional 3–4 minutes. Remove from heat and let stand uncovered for another 10–12 minutes to allow the liquid to be infused with the ginger's flavor. With a slotted spoon remove ginger and discard. Add pineapple slices, cover, and simmer, stirring often, until pineapple looks translucent (about 6–8 minutes). With a slotted spoon remove pineapple to a heat-proof bowl. Boil liquid to a reduction of 1 cup of syrup, stirring constantly (about 8–10 minutes). Add rum to syrup and return to a gentle boil for another 1 minute. Pour syrup over pineapple, allow all to come to room temperature, and then chill for 1 hour. Serve garnished with fresh mint leaves and a dollop of fat-free whipped cream.

Approx. 75 calories per serving
0.5g protein, 0.5g total fat, .05g saturated fat, 0 trans fat,
15g carbohydrates, 0 cholesterol, 1mg sodium, 1g fiber

HEALTHY CHOCOLATE CUPCAKES

MAKES 12 CUPCAKES

1¼ cups pastry flour

3 tablespoons ground flaxseed

1 cup low-calorie baking sweetener

½ cup unsweetened dark cocoa

½ teaspoon baking soda

½ teaspoon baking powder

½ teaspoon sodium-free salt substitute

½ cup concentrated pomegranate juice or other clear concentrated juice

¾ cup vanilla soy milk

3 tablespoons canola oil

⅓ cup chopped walnuts

Mix together flour, flaxseed, sweetener, cocoa, baking soda, baking powder, and salt substitute. Blend all ingredients well with a whisk. Make a well in the center of the mixture. In a separate bowl add juice, soy milk, canola oil, and ⅔ of the walnuts (reserve ⅓ for garnish). Stir ingredients well and pour mixture into the well of the flour mixture. With a spatula, blend all ingredients until well mixed. Line a 12-cup cupcake pan with paper cupcake liners and fill each liner until almost full. Sprinkle a small amount of the reserved chopped walnuts on top of each cupcake. Place pan in a 350-degree oven on center rack and bake for 18–20 minutes or until a toothpick inserted in the center of a cupcake comes out clean. Do not overbake. Allow to cool for 10–15 minutes before serving.

Approx. 135 calories per cupcake
7g protein, 7g total fat, 1g saturated fat, 0 trans fat,
17g carbohydrates, 0 cholesterol, 79mg sodium, 1g fiber

HEALTHY BANANA-NUT MUFFINS

MAKES 12 MUFFINS

1 cup (8 ounces) of soy flour

2 teaspoons baking powder

2 tablespoons low-calorie baking sweetener

¼ cup finely chopped walnuts

2 medium-sized ripe bananas, mashed

1 teaspoon vanilla extract

1¼ cups vanilla soy milk

¼ cup egg substitute

2 tablespoons canola oil

2 tablespoons dry oatmeal

Line a 12-cup muffin pan with paper muffin cups. Sift soy flour and baking powder together into a mixing bowl. Add sweetener and walnuts and stir to mix ingredients. Make a well in the center of the mix and add bananas, vanilla extract, soy milk, egg substitute, and canola oil. Pour batter into muffin cups, sprinkle tops with oatmeal, and bake in a 350-degree oven for 20–25 minutes or until muffins are firm and a toothpick inserted into the center of a muffin comes back dry. Remove from oven and allow to cool.

Approx. 100 calories per muffin
5g protein, 6g total fat, 0.6g saturated fat, 0 trans fat,
9g carbohydrates, 0 cholesterol, 22mg sodium, 2g fiber

CARAMELIZED PEARS

MAKES 6 SERVINGS

3 ripe Bartlett pears, peeled, cut in half, and cored

3 tablespoons fresh lemon juice

1 tablespoon vanilla extract

3 tablespoons trans fat–free canola/olive oil spread

½ cup low-calorie baking sweetener

6 tablespoons low-fat plain yogurt

6 lemon slices for garnish (optional)

Preheat oven to 400 degrees. Place pears in a large bowl; add lemon juice and vanilla extract. Gently toss ingredients to coat pears. Melt spread in an oven-safe skillet over medium-high heat. Add sweetener and stir to distribute sweetener evenly in pan. Place pears cut side down in skillet and drizzle remaining lemon juice mixture from bowl over pears. Cook until sweetener begins to dissolve and mixture bubbles, shaking pan often to move mixture around and under pears while cooking. Cook for about 5 minutes. Transfer skillet to oven and bake until pears are soft and juices are golden colored (about 15–20 minutes). Serve pears warm, drizzled with mixture from pan; add a tablespoon of yogurt on the side and garnish with a lemon slice.

Approx. 102 calories per serving
2g protein, 5g total fat, 1.5g saturated fat, 0 trans fat,
14g carbohydrates, 1mg cholesterol, 61mg sodium, 2g fiber

PLUM SORBET

MAKES 10–12 SERVINGS

1 pound (about 14) red plums, halved and pitted
6 ounces sweet red sherry
¾ cup water
1½ cups non-caloric sweetener
1 cinnamon stick
1 teaspoon vanilla extract
Zest from half a lemon

Place the freezer canister of an ice cream maker in the freezer. Combine plums, sherry, water, sweetener, cinnamon stick, vanilla extract, and zest in a heavy sauce-pan and cook, covered, over medium heat, stirring occasionally, until plums fall apart (about 20–30 minutes). Remove cinnamon stick. Place plum mixture in a blender or food processor and process until smooth. Strain pureed mixture through a mesh strainer to separate any remaining large pieces. Allow to cool, then trans-fer mixture to cold ice cream canister and return to freezer uncovered for about 2 hours. When sorbet is cold, transfer to an airtight freezer container for at least 1 more hour before serving.

Approx. 56 calories per serving
0.6g protein, 0.23 total fat, 0 saturated fat, 0 trans fat,
11g carbohydrates, 0 cholesterol, 1mg sodium, 1g fiber

DARK DOUBLE CHOCOLATE PUDDING
MAKES 6–8 SERVINGS

¼ cup egg substitute

3 cups skim milk

⅔ cup low-calorie baking sweetener

¼ cup cornstarch

3 tablespoons unsweetened dark cocoa powder

⅛ teaspoon low-sodium salt

½ teaspoon pure vanilla extract

2 ounces dark chocolate chips

Fat-free whipped cream for garnish (optional)

Beat egg substitute lightly and set aside. Gradually heat milk over low heat until it begins to bubble. Remove from heat and add sweetener, cornstarch, cocoa, and salt. Bring mixture to a boil over medium heat while whisking constantly. When mixture thickens slightly, remove from heat. Slowly add egg substitute to 1 cup of milk mixture (do this so that egg subsitute does not immediately cook) and whisk. Pour egg mixture into remaining milk mixture and return to a boil, whisking constantly. When mixture thickens to pudding consistency, remove from heat and add vanilla extract and chocolate chips. Stir to incorporate, then pour into bowl and cover with plastic wrap. Push wrap down into bowl so it touches top of pudding; this keeps pudding from developing a skin on the top. Refrigerate until ready to serve and garnish with whipped cream, if desired.

Approx. 92 calories per serving
4g protein, 1.7g total fat, 0.39g saturated fat, 0 trans fat,
13g carbohydrates, 2mg cholesterol, 97mg sodium, 0.4g fiber

ORANGE ANGEL FOOD CUPCAKES
MAKES 6 LARGE CUPCAKES

1½ cups egg whites

1 teaspoon cream of tartar

¼ teaspoon low-sodium salt

1 teaspoon orange extract

Zest and juice from a small orange

¾ cup low-calorie baking sweetener

½ cup + 1 tablespoon cake flour

Fat-free whipped cream and maraschino cherries for garnish (optional)

In a mixing bowl beat egg whites with electric beater on high until foamy. Add cream of tartar, salt, orange extract, and orange zest and juice. Beat again until mixture is stiff and peaks. Add sweetener, ¼ cup at a time, while continuing to beat. With a wooden spoon, fold in flour and gently stir to mix. Line a cupcake tin with 6 paper liners and spoon mixture into liners. Bake on the bottom rack of a 350-degree oven for 15–20 minutes or until the center of cupcakes springs back when touched. Remove from oven and allow to cool before serving. Garnish with whipped cream and a maraschino cherry, if desired.

Approx. 58 calories per cupcake
6g protein, 0 total fat, 0 saturated fat, 0 trans fat,
8g carbohydrates, 0 cholesterol, 140mg sodium, 0 fiber

CHOCOLATE SWEET TREATS

MAKES ABOUT 40 PIECES

¾ cup ground flaxseed

3 tablespoons chocolate-flavored whey protein

1½ teaspoons ground cinnamon

½ cup fat-free, sugar-free chocolate syrup

2 tablespoons natural chunky peanut butter

1 tablespoon unsweetened dark cocoa powder

Mix flaxseed, whey protein, cinnamon, syrup, and peanut butter together in a bowl; stir to blend well. Spoon 35–40 teaspoon-sized portions onto a cookie sheet covered with parchment paper. Lightly sprinkle each treat with a small amount of cocoa powder and refrigerate to chill; let harden for about 2 hours.

Approx. 20 calories per piece
1g protein, 1g total fat, 0.1g saturated fat, 0 trans fat,
1g carbohydrates, <0.1mg cholesterol, 8mg sodium, 1g fiber

Smoothies and Coolers

NOTE: The delicious smoothies listed below can also be prepared without whey protein.

BLUEBERRY BURST WHEY SMOOTHIE

MAKES 1 16-OUNCE SERVING

½ cup cold water
¼ cup fresh or unsweetened frozen blueberries
2 packets non-caloric sweetener
¼ cup plain non-fat yogurt
1 scoop natural-flavored whey protein powder
8 ice cubes
Fat-free whipped cream
Sprinkle of crushed almonds for garnish

In an ice-crushing blender, add water, berries, and sweetener and blend until smooth. Add yogurt and whey and blend until smooth again. Add ice cubes and chop until crushed. Pour into glass and top with whipped cream and almonds.

Approx. 124 calories per serving
22g protein, 1g total fat, 0 saturated fat, 0 trans fat,
10g carbohydrates, 2mg cholesterol, 88mg sodium, 1g fiber

SUMMER RHUBARB COOLER

MAKES 3 CUPS

¼ cup low-calorie baking sweetener
1 cup water
½ pound fresh rhubarb, trimmed and cut into 1-inch pieces
1 cup sliced fresh strawberries + extra for garnish
3 tablespoons freshly squeezed lemon juice
3 drinking glasses chilled in freezer

Bring sweetener and water to a boil in a large saucepan over high heat. Cook, stirring often, to dissolve sugar, about 2 minutes. Reduce heat to medium and add rhubarb, then cook until tender. Add strawberries and lemon juice and cook for 2 additional minutes. Strain mixture through a sieve to remove solids. Pour strained mixture into a 9x13-inch baking dish, cover with plastic wrap, and place in freezer. Every 30 minutes stir mixture with tips of fork to break up any forming ice chunks. Freeze mixture until slushy and frozen, about 3 hours. When frozen, scoop into 3 chilled glasses and garnish with remaining sliced strawberries.

Approx. 35 calories per cup
0 protein, 0 total fat, 0 saturated fat, 0 trans fat,
7g carbohydrates, 0 cholesterol, 3mg sodium, 2g fiber

STRAWBERRY SUNDAE WHEY SMOOTHIE
MAKES 1 16-OUNCE SERVING

½ cup cold water
½ cup fresh or unsweetened frozen strawberries
¼ teaspoon vanilla extract
2 packets non-caloric sweetener
¼ cup plain non-fat yogurt
1 scoop natural-flavored whey protein powder
8 ice cubes
Fat-free whipped cream
Fat-free, sugar-free chocolate syrup to drizzle

In an ice-crushing blender, add water, strawberries, vanilla extract, and sweetener, and blend until smooth. Add yogurt and whey, and blend until smooth again. Add ice and chop until crushed. Pour into glass and top with whipped cream and chocolate syrup.

Approx. 134 calories per serving
21g protein, 1g total fat, 0 saturated fat, 0 trans fat,
11g carbohydrates, 2mg cholesterol, 94mg sodium, 2g fiber

CHOCOLATE MOUSSE WHEY SMOOTHIE

MAKES 1 16-OUNCE SERVING

½ cup cold water

½ cup plain fat-free yogurt

1 scoop natural-flavored whey protein powder

2 packets non-caloric sweetener

1 tablespoon fat-free, sugar-free chocolate syrup

1 teaspoon almond extract

8 ice cubes

Fat-free whipped cream

Fat-free, sugar-free chocolate syrup to drizzle

Sprinkle of crushed almonds for garnish (optional)

In an ice-crushing blender, add water, yogurt, whey, sweetener, chocolate syrup, and almond extract, and blend until smooth. Add ice and chop until crushed. Pour into a glass and top with whipped cream, chocolate syrup, and almonds, if desired.

Approx. 145 calories per serving
24g protein, 1g total fat, 0 saturated fat, 0 trans fat,
11g carbohydrates, 3mg cholesterol, 148mg sodium, 0 fiber

PINEAPPLE DELIGHT WHEY SMOOTHIE

MAKES 1 16-OUNCE SERVING

½ cup cold water
½ cup fresh pineapple, diced
1 teaspoon pineapple extract
2 packets non-caloric sweetener
¼ cup plain non-fat yogurt
1 scoop natural-flavored whey protein powder
8 ice cubes
Fat-free whipped cream
Crushed walnuts for garnish

In an ice-crushing blender, add water, pineapple, pineapple extract, and sweetener, and blend until smooth. Add yogurt and whey and blend until smooth again. Add ice and chop until crushed. Pour into a glass and top with whipped cream and walnuts.

Approx. 149 calories per serving
20g protein, 1g total fat, 0 saturated fat, 0 trans fat,
16g carbohydrates, 1mg cholesterol, 88mg sodium, 1g fiber

BANANA PEACH VANILLA SOY MILK SMOOTHIE

MAKES 1 SMOOTHIE

1 cup light vanilla soy milk
1 medium banana
1 medium peach, pitted and sliced
1 cup ice
1 teaspoon vanilla extract
Non-caloric sweetener

In a blender combine soy milk, banana, peach, and ice. Process to desired consistency; with machine running, add vanilla extract and sweetener. Serve immediately.

Approx. 204 calories per smoothie
5g protein, 3g total fat, 0 saturated fat, 0 trans fat,
19g carbohydrates, 0 cholesterol, 2mg sodium, 3g fiber

CHOCOLATE RASPBERRY SOY MILK SMOOTHIE

MAKES 1 SMOOTHIE

1 cup light chocolate soy milk
1 medium banana
1 cup frozen unsweetened raspberries
1 cup ice
1 teaspoon vanilla extract
Non-caloric sweetener to taste

In a blender combine soy milk, banana, raspberries, and ice. Process to desired consistency; with machine running, add vanilla extract and sweetener. Serve immediately.

Approx. 317 calories per smoothie
8g protein, 4g total fat, 0.5g saturated fat, 0 trans fat,
66g carbohydrates, 0 cholesterol, 136mg sodium, 9g fiber

MELON MADNESS WHEY SMOOTHIE

MAKES 1 16-OUNCE SERVING

½ cup cold water
½ (5–6-inch) fresh cantaloupe
2 packets non-caloric sweetener
¼ cup plain non-fat yogurt
1 scoop natural-flavored whey protein powder
8 ice cubes
Fat-free whipped cream
Crushed almonds for garnish

In an ice-crushing blender, add water, cantaloupe, sweetener, yogurt, and whey, and blend until smooth. Add ice and chop until crushed. Pour into glass and top with whipped cream and almonds.

Approx. 204 calories per serving
22g protein, 1g total fat, 0 saturated fat, 0 trans fat,
27g carbohydrates, 1mg cholesterol, 111mg sodium, 2g fiber

Appetizers, Dips, and Snack Foods

Appetizers

ROASTED GARLIC
MAKES 4–5 SERVINGS

1 jumbo fresh elephant garlic head
Extra-virgin olive oil to drizzle
Dry seasonings of choice (optional)

Holding entire head of garlic, cut off the top leaf points of each clove to expose a small portion of the clove. Keep the remainder of leaves intact around the body of the garlic head. Place trimmed garlic head in a tight-fitting oven-safe bowl, trimmed side up. Drizzle a small amount of olive oil over the top of the head and down around the sides. Sprinkle with your favorite seasoning (optional). Place garlic on middle rack of oven and bake at 400 degrees for 20–30 minutes or until cloves are soft and a light golden brown. Remove from oven and spread garlic on crusty bread or add to vegetables, omelets, or pasta.

Approx. 59 calories per serving
3g protein, 0.2g total fat, <1g saturated fat, 0 trans fat,
13g carbohydrates, 0 cholesterol, 7mg sodium, 1g fiber

STUFFED GRAPE LEAVES (DOLMAS)

MAKES 20 SERVINGS

3 tablespoons extra-virgin olive oil, divided
1 cup chopped red onion
½ cup chopped scallions
1 cup basmati rice
4 cloves fresh garlic, minced
1 teaspoon ground cumin
½ teaspoon freshly ground pepper
2 cups canned low-sodium vegetable broth
¼ cup chopped fennel
¼ cup chopped fresh dill
¼ cup finely chopped fresh parsley
2 tablespoons dried mint
1 (16-ounce) jar grape leaves
1–2 lemons, thinly sliced to make about 20 slices
2 cups water

For Yogurt Sauce:

2 cups plain non-fat yogurt
4 scallions, minced
1 clove fresh garlic, minced
1 teaspoon salt

In a skillet over medium heat, add 1 tablespoon olive oil, onions, and scallions; cook until soft and transparent. Add rice and cook until grains are slightly browned, stirring constantly. Add garlic, cumin, pepper, and vegetable broth. Reduce heat to simmer, cover, and cook until rice is tender and all liquid is absorbed. Allow rice to cool, then stir in fennel, dill, parsley, and mint. Set aside. Drain grape leaves and cover with water; bring to a rolling boil. Blanch leaves for 1–2 minutes, drain, and allow to cool. With leaf shiny side down, fill with rice mixture and roll starting at the stem and folding in sides. Repeat until all 20 leaves are filled. Line a heavy-bottomed pan with 10 of the unfilled grape leaves. Pack the rolled leaves in tightly side by side, seam side down. Top rolled leaves with lemon slices and cover lemon slices with remaining unfilled grape leaves. Mix together water and remaining olive oil and pour over grape leaf rolls. Place an object like a heavy plate on top of rolls to help hold them below the water level during cooking, and simmer for about 1 hour, checking to make sure they haven't boiled dry. Remove pan from stove and allow to cool. Remove rolls from pan and chill. Serve chilled or at room temperature. Serve with yogurt sauce on the side as a dip.

Yogurt Sauce:

Mix together plain yogurt, scallions, garlic, and salt to taste. Chill until ready to serve.

Approx. 59 calories per serving
1g protein, 2g total fat, 0.2g saturated fat, 0 trans fat,
9g carbohydrates, 0 cholesterol, 123mg sodium, 1g fiber

TOMATO AND GARLIC BRUSCHETTA
MAKES ENOUGH FOR 8 SERVINGS

8 slices (½-inch thick) of a French baguette or a crusty whole grain bread
1 teaspoon extra-virgin olive oil
1¼ cups chopped plum tomatoes
1½ teaspoons minced fresh garlic
1 teaspoon balsamic vinegar
½ teaspoon dried basil
¼ teaspoon of non-caloric sweetener
¼ teaspoon freshly ground pepper

Place slices of bread on ungreased baking sheet. Brush each slice with olive oil and bake at 500 degrees for 3–4 minutes until golden brown. Combine tomatoes, garlic, vinegar, basil, sweetener, and pepper in a small bowl. Mix well and spoon mixture over bread slices.

Approx. 57 calories per serving
2.5g protein, 0.7g total fat, 0.4g saturated fat, 0 trans fat,
11g carbohydrates, 0 cholesterol, 106mg sodium, 1g fiber

TOMATO AND FRESH PARMESAN CHEESE BRUSCHETTA
MAKES 8 SLICES

8 slices (½-inch thick) of a French baguette or crusty whole grain bread

2 cloves fresh garlic, finely minced

1 teaspoon extra-virgin olive oil + more for brushing

1 small onion, diced

1 medium tomato, diced

Pinch dried oregano, crumbled

Pinch freshly ground pepper

2 tablespoons freshly grated Parmesan cheese

Scantly brush slices of bread on both sides with olive oil, then toast. Remove from oven and evenly distribute garlic on one side of bread. Rub garlic into bread with handle of knife and set aside; keep warm. Heat teaspoon of olive oil in skillet, add onion, and lightly sauté until golden brown. Remove from heat. Preheat broiler. Combine onion, tomato, oregano, and pepper; spread evenly over garlic bread and sprinkle with Parmesan cheese. Place bread with Parmesan cheese under broiler for 1 minute until lightly browned. Serve immediately.

Approx. 70 calories per serving
3g protein, 1.7g total fat, 0.3g saturated fat, 0 trans fat,
13g carbohydrates, 1mg cholesterol, 127mg sodium, 1g fiber

ITALIAN CROSTINI

MAKES APPROXIMATELY 25–27 SERVINGS

1 French baguette roughly 10–12 inches long, cut into ½-inch thick slices
Extra-virgin olive oil cooking spray
2½ teaspoons fresh garlic paste
Minced dry or fresh basil, parsley, or chives
Salt and freshly ground pepper to taste

Lightly spray both sides of each slice of bread with a scant amount of cooking oil. Rub a scant amount of garlic paste onto one side of each slice, then slightly sprinkle herb of choice over garlic. Add salt and pepper to taste. Place slices on a non-stick cookie sheet and place in a 375-degree oven on middle rack to bake until slices are a light golden brown (about 3–5 minutes). Serve as is or add your favorite topping (smoked mozzarella, chopped fresh tomatoes, chopped black olives, roasted garlic, etc.), if desired.

Approx. 41 calories per serving
1g protein, 0.2g total fat, 0.03g saturated fat, 0 trans fat,
10g carbohydrates, 0 cholesterol, 101mg sodium, 1g fiber

MUSHROOM CROSTINI

MAKES 4 SERVINGS

1 (10–12-inch) loaf of crusty whole grain bread

Olive oil cooking spray

1½ tablespoons trans fat–free canola/olive oil spread

1 tablespoon extra-virgin olive oil

3 tablespoons minced shallots

2 tablespoons freshly minced garlic

4 cups assorted mushrooms (such as crimini, shiitake, button, or portobello), sliced

½ cup sherry

1 tablespoon freshly chopped parsley

1 teaspoon freshly chopped thyme

Salt and freshly ground pepper to taste

Freshly grated Parmesan cheese for garnish (optional)

Slice bread loaf into 8 thick slices. Lightly spray slices on both sides with cooking oil and place on a non-stick baking sheet. Bake until slices are crispy and golden brown. Allow canola/olive oil spread to come to room temperature. In a large skillet heat olive oil, add shallots and garlic, and cook until soft. Add mushrooms and sherry to garlic mixture and cook until mushrooms are tender and most of the liquid has evaporated (gently stir during cooking to blend flavors). When mushrooms are soft, blend in canola/olive oil spread, parsley, thyme, and salt and pepper to taste. Spoon mushroom mixture onto the toasted bread slices and sprinkle with scant amounts of Parmesan cheese, if desired.

Approx. 115 calories per serving
2g protein, 7g total fat, 1g saturated fat, 0 trans fat,
15g carbohydrates, 0 cholesterol, 38mg sodium, 2g fiber

ANTIPASTI

MAKES 10–15 SERVINGS

Antipasti means "before the pasta" (traditionally, pasta is the first main course in Italian cuisine). Antipasti tend to include a number of different appetizers laid out on one large platter.

Fruits (choose whatever is in season), cut into manageable pieces

Cheese (use soft and hard, and spicy and mild, cheeses, leaving some in whole wedges and slicing or chunking others)

Seafood (try large to jumbo cooked shrimp, tails on but otherwise shelled; cooked calamari; steamed clams; mussels; smoked oysters; smoked fish)

Other items (try adding marinated artichokes, black and green olives of various flavors, oil-soaked and seasoned sundried tomatoes, roasted peppers, pickled pearl onions, and bread sticks with thin slices of prosciutto wrapped around the tips; use any red fatty meats sparingly)

Use a large platter for presentation (about 15x15 inches) and place items in some semblance of order: fruits by cheese, cheese by meats, pickled items near each other, and so on. Make sure all items are drained of liquid before adding to platter. Serve your antipasti with a tray of crunchy whole grain bread or bread sticks.

AVOCADO SPREAD WITH CRUSTY GARLIC TOAST

MAKES 2 SERVINGS

1 large ripe avocado, pitted and peeled

½ cup fresh cilantro leaves

1 clove fresh garlic, chopped

2 tablespoons minced scallions

1 tablespoon freshly squeezed lemon juice

1 tablespoon extra-virgin olive oil

Salt and freshly ground pepper to taste

4 slices (½-inch thick) whole grain baguette

Olive oil cooking spray

½ teaspoon garlic powder

1 tablespoon shredded Parmesan cheese

4 thin slices jalapeño pepper (optional)

Preheat broiler. Combine avocado, cilantro, garlic, scallions, lemon juice, olive oil, and salt and pepper in a food processor and process until buttery smooth. Set aside. Spray both sides of each baguette slice with cooking oil and place on a foil-covered baking sheet. Sprinkle baguette tops with garlic powder and Parmesan cheese. Place baking sheet about 6 inches under broiler and broil slices until lightly toasted. Remove from heat, allow to cool, and cover with avocado spread. Top with very thin slices of jalapeño and serve.

Approx. 270 calories per serving
4g protein, 21g total fat, 3g saturated fat, 0 trans fat,
15g carbohydrates, 2mg cholesterol, 130mg sodium, 7g fiber

BABY SHRIMP ON TOASTED RYE

MAKES 12–16 SERVINGS

½ cup reduced-fat mayonnaise
2 tablespoons finely minced shallot
1 tablespoon finely chopped fresh parsley
1 teaspoon Dijon mustard
½ teaspoon chopped capers
16 slices cocktail-sized, thin rye bread
Garlic/olive oil cooking spray
1 bag cooked salad shrimp, thawed
Scant splash of freshly squeezed lemon juice
16 paper-thin slices lemon

In a small bowl, whisk together mayonnaise, shallot, parsley, mustard, and capers. Cover and refrigerate for no less than 1 hour to blend flavors. Meanwhile, spray rye slices lightly with garlic/olive oil spray and toast in a toaster oven or oven at 300 degrees until slightly crispy. Remove from oven and spread 1 teaspoon of mayonnaise mixture on each slice of rye toast. Top with 4–5 shrimp and a scant splash of lemon juice. Add a slice of lemon for garnish and serve.

Approx. 47 calories per serving
2g protein, 2g total fat, 0 saturated fat, 0 trans fat,
4g carbohydrates, 5mg cholesterol, 157mg sodium, 1g fiber

HUMMUS AND ALFALFA SPROUTS

MAKES 12 SERVINGS

12 large whole grain crackers
1½ cups hummus
12 slices low-fat cheddar cheese
12 tablespoons alfalfa sprouts
Freshly ground pepper
Lemon wedges for garnish

Arrange crackers on a platter. Spread hummus equally on top of crackers. Top each cracker with a slice of cheddar cheese, sprouts, and a sprinkling of pepper. Garnish platter with lemon wedges to squeeze over crackers before enjoying.

Approx. 121 calories per serving
8g protein, 4g total fat, 1g saturated fat, 0 trans fat,
9g carbohydrates, 6mg cholesterol, 274mg sodium, 1g fiber

APPLE, GORGONZOLA, AND WALNUT CROSTINI

MAKES 24 SERVINGS

24 thin slices French bread
Olive oil cooking spray
2 Granny Smith apples, cored and thinly sliced
8 ounces crumbled gorgonzola cheese
1 cup chopped walnuts

Preheat broiler. Lightly spray both sides of bread slices with a scant amount of cooking oil. Place slices on a baking sheet and toast under broiler on both sides, turning once, until lightly browned. Remove from broiler and place 2 slices of apple on each piece of toast. Top each slice with a mound of gorgonzola cheese. Press walnut pieces into cheese and return to broiler. Broil until cheese melts and both cheese and walnuts are lightly browned. Serve while warm.

Approx. 234 calories per serving
8g protein, 5g total fat, 1g saturated fat, 0 trans fat,
35g carbohydrates, 4mg cholesterol, 468mg sodium, 2g fiber

AVOCADO AND MANGO SALSA

MAKES 4 SERVINGS

½ red onion, finely chopped
1 ripe avocado, peeled and cut into ½-inch cubes
2 ripe mangoes, peeled and cut into ½-inch cubes
½ jalapeño pepper, seeds removed and finely diced
2 tablespoons fresh cilantro, finely chopped
Juice from 1 lime
Salt and freshly ground pepper to taste

Combine onion, avocado, mango, jalapeño, cilantro, and lime juice in a bowl. Blend well to incorporate ingredients. Season with salt and pepper to taste. Cover and refrigerate to chill. Use as topping for fish or as a dip with chips.

Approx. 147 calories per serving
1g protein, 7g total fat, 1g saturated fat, 0 trans fat,
21g carbohydrates, 0 cholesterol, 5mg sodium, 5g fiber

BAY SCALLOPS WITH SMOKED PAPRIKA

MAKES 10 SERVINGS

1½ tablespoons olive oil
1½ tablespoons trans fat–free canola/olive oil spread
1 pound fresh bay scallops (about 100 scallops)
Smoked paprika to coat
1 lemon, halved, one half to squeeze and the other thinly sliced for garnish
10 small wood skewers

In a large heavy-bottomed skillet, heat olive oil and canola/olive oil spread over medium-high heat. Add scallops and coat tops of scallops generously with smoked paprika. Stir frequently as scallops begin to brown. Drizzle with freshly squeezed juice from half of a lemon and cook for about 3 minutes or until cooked through. Do not overcook. Skewer 10 scallops on each skewer and serve with thin slices of lemon to squeeze over skewers.

Approx. 73 calories per serving
8g protein, 4g total fat, 0 saturated fat, 0 trans fat,
1g carbohydrates, 14mg cholesterol, 111mg sodium, 0 fiber

CROSTINI WITH PESTO, PROSCIUTTO, MOZZARELLA, AND SUNDRIED TOMATOES

MAKES 8 SERVINGS

8 (½-inch thick) slices rustic whole grain bread
Scant amount of olive oil
Salt and freshly ground pepper to taste
1 tablespoon market-fresh pesto sauce
16 slices sundried tomatoes, packed in olive oil
8 thin slices provolone-mozzarella cheese
8 pieces thinly sliced prosciutto (about 4–6 ounces)
1 cup baby arugula

Preheat oven to 425 degrees. On a rimmed baking sheet, arrange bread slices in a single layer and lightly brush tops with olive oil. Season with salt and pepper to taste. Bake until golden brown, about 10–15 minutes. Remove from oven and top each crostini with a thin layer of pesto sauce. Add 2 slices of sundried tomatoes to each crostini, followed by a slice of provolone-mozzarella cheese and a slice of prosciutto. Top with a few sprigs of arugula and serve.

Approx. 180 calories per serving
13g protein, 6g total fat, 3g saturated fat, 0 trans fat,
18g carbohydrates, 29mg cholesterol, 669mg sodium, 1g fiber

ROASTED TOMATO BOATS

MAKES 4 SERVINGS

2 tablespoons olive oil
2 cloves fresh garlic, minced
Salt and freshly ground pepper to taste
6 plum tomatoes, halved and deseeded
⅔ cup panko bread crumbs
½ cup crumbled feta cheese
Chopped fresh parsley for garnish

Whisk together olive oil, garlic, and salt and pepper to taste. Place tomato halves in a resealable plastic baggie and add olive oil mixture to the bag. Toss to coat tomatoes and marinate for 20 minutes. Preheat oven to 350 degrees. Mix bread crumbs and feta cheese together in a small bowl. Place tomato halves on a baking sheet and fill cavities with cheese mixture. Bake tomatoes for 30 minutes, until soft and cheese is melted. Serve with a sprinkle of chopped fresh parsley.

Approx. 156 calories per serving
5g protein, 10g total fat, 4g saturated fat, 0 trans fat,
10g carbohydrates, 17mg cholesterol, 235mg sodium, 1g fiber

CHEESY CRAB BITES

MAKES 15 SERVINGS

4 ounces low-fat cream cheese, softened

¼ cup low-fat shredded cheddar cheese

2 tablespoons light mayonnaise

1 teaspoon freshly squeezed lemon juice

½ teaspoon seafood seasoning mix (such as Old Bay)

½ teaspoon garlic powder

1 scallion, thinly sliced

1 (13-ounce) can crabmeat, picked through and flaked apart

1 (2-ounce) box mini phyllo shells

Dash of paprika

Preheat oven to 350 degrees. In a bowl, gently blend together cream cheese, cheddar cheese, mayonnaise, and lemon juice. Fold seafood seasoning, garlic powder, scallions, and crabmeat into mixture. Fill phyllo shells with mixture, add a dash of paprika on top of each shell, and place shells on a flat baking sheet. Bake for roughly 15 minutes, or until shells are golden brown and mixture is heated through. Serve warm.

Approx. 62 calories per serving

5g protein, 1g total fat, 0 saturated fat, 0 trans fat,

2g carbohydrates, 29mg cholesterol, 168mg sodium, 0 fiber

CRISPY CHICKEN PARMESAN TENDERS

MAKES 12 TENDERS

½ cup liquid eggs
½ teaspoon garlic powder
Salt and freshly ground pepper to taste
1 cup panko bread crumbs
½ cup grated Parmesan cheese
1 teaspoon paprika
1 teaspoon dry Italian seasoning mix
1 pound chicken tenders
Olive oil cooking spray

Preheat oven to 425 degrees. In a shallow dish, combine eggs, garlic powder, and salt and pepper to taste. In a separate shallow dish, combine bread crumbs, Paremsan cheese, paprika, and Italian seasoning. Dip each tender into egg mixture, coating all sides with mixture, then dip into bread crumb mixture, again coating all sides of chicken. Place coated tenders on a baking sheet, spray the tenders with cooking oil, and place in oven to bake. Cook for 20 minutes until outsides are lightly browned and crispy and chicken juices run clear when pierced. Cut each tender into bite-sized pieces, if desired, and spear with a toothpick for easy serving.

Approx. 75 calories per tender
8g protein, 1g total fat, 1g saturated fat, 0 trans fat,
4g carbohydrates, 20mg cholesterol, 107mg sodium, 0 fiber

PIZZA ZUCCHINI BOATS

MAKES 8 LARGE BOATS

4 large zucchini
¾ pound ground turkey sausage
1 teaspoon dry Italian seasoning mix
1 (15-ounce) can diced, low-sodium tomatoes, well drained
½ cup shredded, part-skim mozzarella cheese, divided
Salt and freshly ground pepper to taste

Preheat oven to 350 degrees. Wash and trim zucchini, then halve lengthwise. With a small spoon, scoop out the flesh, being careful not to break through the shell of the zucchini. In a small bowl, mix together zucchini flesh, sausage, and Italian seasoning. Transfer mixture to a skillet and cook on medium heat for roughly 5 minutes or until browned. Drain mixture and add drained tomatoes, ¼ cup of mozzarella cheese, and salt and pepper to taste. Place zucchini halves on a rimmed baking sheet. Fill zucchini shells with sausage mixture and bake for 20 minutes or until zucchini is tender crispy. Sprinkle tops of zucchini with remaining mozzarella cheese and bake for an additional 3–5 minutes or until cheese is melted. Remove from oven and allow to cool slightly before slicing each zucchini into pieces. Each boat can be cut into roughly 35–40 bite-sized pieces.

Approx. 102 calories per large boat
9g protein, 3g total fat, 1g saturated fat, 0 trans fat,
7g carbohydrates, 25mg cholesterol, 276mg sodium, 4g fiber

AVOCADO TOASTS

MAKES 4 SERVINGS

Olive oil cooking spray
4 (½-inch thick) slices crusty country bread
¼ teaspoon fresh garlic paste blend
1 avocado, peeled, pitted, and sliced into 4 portions
¼ cup sliced black olives
¼ cup radish sprouts
Salt and freshly ground pepper to taste
1 lemon, cut into wedges (optional)

Preheat oven to 350 degrees. Lightly spray a baking sheet with cooking oil. Place bread slices on the sheet and lightly spread tops with garlic paste and a light spray of olive oil. Bake until tops are golden brown. Remove from oven and transfer to a plate. Top each toast with avocado slices, black olives, radish sprouts, and salt and pepper to taste. Use the lemon wedges to squeeze lemon juice on toasts, if desired, and serve.

Approx. 169 calories per serving
4g protein, 8g total fat, 1g saturated fat, 0 trans fat,
21g carbohydrates, 0 cholesterol, 226mg sodium, 4g fiber

CRISPY POLENTA TOPPED WITH A SPICY MARINARA

MAKES 9 (2½-INCH SLICE) SERVINGS

Canola oil cooking spray
1 (18-ounce) tube of mushroom and onion polenta
Garlic salt to taste (optional)
Freshly ground pepper to taste
9 tablespoons spicy diced tomatoes, well drained
9 tablespoons simple marinara sauce
Grated Parmesan cheese, to sprinkle

Preheat oven to 400 degrees. Cover a baking sheet with aluminum foil. Lightly spray foil with cooking oil. Slice polenta into 2½-inch wide round pieces. Place rounds on baking sheet in a single layer. Lightly spray each round with cooking oil and sprinkle each piece with a scant amount of garlic salt, if desired, and pepper. Place baking sheet in hot oven on top rack and cook until rounds are crispy and golden brown. While the polenta is browning, combine tomatoes and marinara sauce in a saucepan and warm. When the polenta is generously browned and crispy, remove from oven and place rounds on warmed serving tray. Top each round piece with 1 tablespoon of the marinara mixture and sprinkle with Parmesan cheese. Serve immediately.

Approx. 88 calories per serving
2g protein, 0 total fat, 0 saturated fat, 0 trans fat,
17g carbohydrates, 0 cholesterol, 356mg sodium, 1g fiber

Dips

CHILLED AVOCADO DIP

MAKES I CUP

2 tablespoons lemon juice

2 tablespoons tahini paste

1 large ripe avocado, halved, pitted, and peeled

¼ cup freshly chopped parsley

1 tablespoon extra-virgin olive oil

⅛ cup chopped onion

3 cloves fresh garlic, peeled and chopped

3 tablespoons low-calorie mayonnaise

⅛ teaspoon cayenne pepper

Salt and freshly ground pepper to taste

Dash of paprika

Blend lemon juice and tahini paste, then add avocado, parsley, olive oil, onion, garlic, mayonnaise, cayenne, and salt and pepper to taste. Blend until smooth, transfer to serving bowl, and chill. When ready to serve, sprinkle with paprika.

Approx. 90 calories per 2 tablespoons
1g protein, 9g total fat, 1.3g saturated fat, 0 trans fat,
3g carbohydrates, 2g cholesterol, 52mg sodium, 1g fiber

SMOKED TROUT DIP

MAKES 2 CUPS—ROUGHLY 64 SERVINGS

1 (8-ounce) package reduced-fat cream cheese, softened
½ cup chopped scallions, white and green parts
¼ cup reduced-fat sour cream + more to thin
1 tablespoon chopped fresh dill
½ teaspoon hot pepper sauce
½ teaspoon low-sodium Cajun seasoning
8 ounces smoked trout fillets, broken into rough pieces
Salt and freshly ground pepper to taste
⅛ cup chopped red onion
2 ounces capers, drained
Toasted slices of baguette or assorted crackers

Put cream cheese in a medium bowl and beat with electric beater until smooth. Add in scallions, sour cream, dill, hot sauce, and Cajun seasoning. Continue to beat until well blended. Reduce beater speed to low, fold in trout, and beat until smooth. If mixture is too thick, add additional sour cream to thin until desired consistency. Season with salt and pepper to taste, then cover and refrigerate until well chilled. Serve chilled and topped with red onion, capers, and toasted bread slices or crackers.

Approx. 1,246 calories for 2 cups of dip (bread slices or crackers not included)
110g protein, 77g total fat, 37g saturated fat, 0 trans fat,
17g carbohydrates, 386mg cholesterol, 1,694mg sodium, 0 fiber

MEDITERRANEAN SALSA

MAKES 2 CUPS

2 cups finely chopped Italian (plum) tomatoes
4 tablespoons extra-virgin olive oil
2 tablespoons cider vinegar
2 tablespoons chopped fresh basil leaves
1 tablespoon chopped fresh oregano
½ teaspoon onion salt
Pita wedges

In a medium bowl, combine all ingredients and toss to mix. Allow to stand at room temperature for 30 minutes to blend flavors. Serve with toasted pita wedges or other chips.

Approx. 545 calories per 2 cups salsa
3g protein, 57g total fat, 7g saturated fat, 0 trans fat,
14g carbohydrates, 0 cholesterol, 18mg sodium, 4g fiber

CUCUMBER SALSA

MAKES ABOUT 3 CUPS

2 cups finely diced cucumber, peeled and deseeded
½ cup finely diced red onion
½ cup chopped fresh cilantro
1 clove fresh garlic, minced
1 finely diced jalapeño pepper
3 tablespoons fresh lime juice
1 tablespoon extra-virgin olive oil
Salt and freshly ground pepper to taste

In a medium bowl, combine cucumber, onion, cilantro, garlic, and jalapeño. Toss to mix, then add in lime juice, olive oil, and salt and pepper to taste. Toss again and refrigerate for 15 minutes to allow flavors to blend. Let cool to room temperature before serving. Serve as a great addition over grilled fish, like tuna or swordfish.

Approx. 152 calories per 3 cups salsa
1g protein, 15g total fat, 1g saturated fat, 0 trans fat,
6g carbohydrates, 0 cholesterol, 6mg sodium, 2g fiber

MANGO CHUTNEY

MAKES 6 SERVINGS

1 ripe mango, peeled, pitted, and diced into small cubes
1 bunch cilantro, finely chopped
½ teaspoon crushed red hot pepper flakes
¼ cup extra-virgin olive oil
2 tablespoons freshly squeezed lime juice
Salt and freshly ground pepper to taste

In a bowl, combine mango, cilantro, hot pepper flakes, olive oil, and lime juice. Stir to blend, then add salt and pepper to taste. Serve with fish or chicken.

Approx. 82 calories per serving
0 protein, 7g total fat, 1g saturated fat, 0 trans fat,
6g carbohydrates, 0 cholesterol, 53mg sodium, 1g fiber

REMOULADE DIPPING SAUCE

MAKES 1 CUP

⅔ cup light mayonnaise
2 scallions, white and green parts, chopped
1 tablespoon finely minced fresh parsley
1½ tablespoons minced fresh dill
2 teaspoons freshly squeezed lemon juice
2 tablespoons prepared horseradish, well drained
4 tablespoons spicy mustard
1 tablespoon ketchup
1 teaspoon Worcestershire sauce
1 tablespoon paprika
Salt and freshly ground pepper to taste
Tabasco sauce to taste

Combine all ingredients in a small bowl and refrigerate for up to 1 hour to blend flavors. Serve as a dip for crab cakes or cooked shrimp.

Approx. 404 calories per cup
0 protein, 38g total fat, 5g saturated fat, 0 trans fat,
19g carbohydrates, 55mg cholesterol, 1,375mg sodium, 1g fiber

HUMMUS DIP

MAKES 1½ CUPS

1 (19-ounce) can chickpeas, drained, ¼ cup liquid reserved
¼ cup tahini paste
2 cloves fresh garlic, peeled and chopped
6 tablespoons lemon juice
Salt and freshly ground pepper to taste
Extra-virgin olive oil to drizzle
1 tablespoon finely chopped fresh mint for garnish

In food processor, process chickpeas, ⅛ of reserved liquid, tahini paste, garlic, lemon juice, and salt and pepper until smooth; it should be the consistency of butter. Use remaining reserved liquid to achieve desired consistency, if necessary. Place on serving plate, drizzle with olive oil, and garnish with mint.

Approx. 79 calories per 2 tablespoons
2g protein, 6g total fat, 0.3g saturated fat, 0 trans fat,
5g carbohydrates, 0 cholesterol, 46mg sodium, 1g fiber

GREEK FETA AND WALNUT DIP

MAKES 2 CUPS

½ pound feta cheese
2 tablespoons extra-virgin olive oil
⅔ cup low-fat milk
1 cup finely ground walnuts
Pinch of cayenne pepper
2 tablespoons minced fresh parsley

Drain feta cheese, then combine all ingredients in a food processor and process until smooth. Let mixture stand for 1 hour before serving.

Approx. 88 calories per tablespoon
4g protein, 7.7g total fat, 2.5g saturated fat, 0 trans fat,
2g carbohydrates, 13mg cholesterol, 164mg sodium, <0.5g fiber

GREEK BEAN DIP

MAKES 3¾ CUPS

2 (15-ounce) cans Great Northern beans, rinsed and drained
4-ounce package light cream cheese
4 ounces feta cheese
3 cloves minced fresh garlic
2 tablespoons lemon juice
1 tablespoon chopped fresh oregano
½ teaspoon freshly ground pepper
¼ teaspoon salt
½ cup deseeded and finely chopped tomato
¼ cup sliced ripe olives

In a food processor or blender, process beans, cream cheese, feta cheese, garlic, lemon juice, oregano, pepper, and salt until smooth. Transfer mixture to a 1½-quart baking dish, cover, and bake at 350 degrees for 25 minutes or until heated through. Remove from heat, sprinkle tomato and olives over dip, and serve.

Approx. 23 calories per 1 tablespoon
2g protein, 0.7g total fat, <0.5g saturated fat, 0 trans fat,
2g carbohydrates, 1mg cholesterol, 51mg sodium, <0.5g fiber

HERB CUCUMBER YOGURT DIP

MAKES 2 CUPS

1 English cucumber
Salt to taste
2 cloves fresh garlic, chopped
2 teaspoons white wine vinegar
2 tablespoons extra-virgin olive oil
2 cups plain low-fat yogurt
2 teaspoons fresh dill
2 teaspoons dried mint
Freshly ground pepper to taste
2 tablespoons chopped fresh mint for garnish

Peel and slice cucumber (if very seedy, remove seeds). Place in bowl and sprinkle with a little salt; let sit for about 15 minutes to draw out water. In a separate bowl, mash garlic into a paste; add pinch of salt, vinegar, and olive oil, and stir. Add yogurt, dill, and dried mint, and mix well. Rinse salt from cucumber slices and pat dry, removing any excess water. Combine cucumber with yogurt mixture; add salt and freshly ground pepper to taste. Garnish with fresh chopped mint and serve.

Approx. 16 calories per ⅛ cup
<0.5g protein, 1g total fat, <0.5g saturated fat, 0 trans fat,
1g carbohydrates, 2mg cholesterol, 7mg sodium, 0 fiber

ROASTED PEPPER DIP

MAKES 1½ CUPS

4 large red bell peppers
1 tablespoon red wine vinegar
3 tablespoons extra-virgin olive oil
2 cloves fresh garlic, peeled and minced
Salt and freshly ground pepper to taste

Wash red bell peppers and pat dry. Place on moderately hot grill, turning often until skin is charred and blistered (about 15–20 minutes). Remove from grill and let peppers cool. Rub off blackened skins. Cut each bell pepper in half, remove stalks and seeds, and cut into ½-inch strips. In a food processor add vinegar and bell peppers and pulse, adding olive oil slowly until bell peppers are smooth. Transfer pepper mixture from processor to a bowl. Mash garlic and stir into pepper mixture; add salt and pepper to taste.

Approx. 22 calories per 1 tablespoon
<0.2g protein, 2g total fat, <0.2g saturated fat, 0 trans fat,
2g carbohydrates, 0 cholesterol, 0.5mg sodium, 0.5g fiber

HUMMUS WITH TAHINI DIP

MAKES ABOUT 2 CUPS

4 cups canned chickpeas, rinsed and drained
3 tablespoons tahini paste
3 tablespoons freshly squeezed lemon juice
4 cloves fresh garlic, crushed into a paste
Salt to taste
1 tablespoon chopped fresh cilantro for garnish
4 tablespoons extra-virgin olive oil

Puree chickpeas in a food processor or blender. Blend together the tahini, lemon juice, garlic, and salt. Combine this with the chickpeas and blend until it becomes a smooth paste. Serve garnished with cilantro and drizzled with olive oil.

Approx. 84 calories per tablespoon
3g protein, 4.5g total fat, 1g saturated fat, 0 trans fat,
8g carbohydrates, 0 cholesterol, 150mg sodium, 3g fiber

Snack Foods

CHOCOLATE BITES

MAKES 24 BITES

½ cup unsweetened cocoa powder

Pinch of salt

¼ cup low-calorie baking sweetener, divided

3 large eggs, whites only

¼ teaspoon cream of tartar

1 teaspoon pure vanilla extract

1 tablespoon confectioner's sugar (optional)

Preheat oven to 400 degrees. Line a baking sheet with foil. In a small bowl, sift together cocoa powder, salt, and ⅛ cup sweetener. Set aside. In a large bowl, combine egg whites and cream of tartar. Beat with an electric beater until peaks form. Slowly add in remaining sweetener and beat until meringue forms stiff peaks. Fold in cocoa mixture and vanilla extract. Drop rounded teaspoons of mixture 1 inch apart onto baking sheet. Bake for 25 minutes then remove from oven. Lightly dust with confectioner's sugar, if desired, and serve.

Approx. 14 calories per bite

1g protein, 0 total fat, 0 saturated fat, 0 trans fat,

1g carbohydrates, 26mg cholesterol, 36mg sodium, <0.5g fiber

CINNAMON AND FLAXSEED WAFERS
MAKES 12–16 WAFERS

3 cups ground flaxseed
2 tablespoons ground cinnamon
6 packets non-caloric sweetener
1½ cups water
Canola oil cooking spray

Preheat oven to 350 degrees. In a large bowl, mix together flaxseed, cinnamon, and sweetener. Stir to blend ingredients. Add water and keep stirring until well blended. Set aside. Lay parchment paper or waxed paper down on a flat surface. Form mixture into palm-sized balls and roll out to ⅛-inch thickness with a rolling pin lightly sprayed with cooking oil. Cut rolled-out mixture into desired size for wafer pieces and place on a baking sheet lined with foil and lightly sprayed with cooking oil. Bake for about 30–35 minutes until crispy. Remove from heat and allow to cool before serving.

Approx. 90 calories per wafer
4g protein, 7g total fat, 0 saturated fat, 0 trans fat,
6g carbohydrates, 0 cholesterol, 0 sodium, 6g fiber

Quick and Easy Snacks

- Any type of fresh fruit or raw vegetable

  Nutritional values depend on type of fruit or vegetable choices.

- 10–20 raw almonds or walnuts with 8-ounce glass of water

  Approx. 140 calories
  5g protein, 12g total fat, 0.8g saturated fat, 0 trans fat,
  4g carbohydrates, 0 cholesterol, 0 sodium, 4g fiber

- Whey protein smoothies
  - Blueberry Burst (page 439)
  - Stawberry Sundae (page 441)
  - Chocolate Mousse (page 442)
  - Pineapple Delight (page 443)
  - Melon Madness (page 444)

For nutritional values see page numbers listed above.

- A fresh raw cucumber with skin intact, quartered and sprinkled with herbs such as garlic powder, salt, onion powder, freshly ground pepper, fresh or dried dill, fresh or dried chives, or a combination

  Approx. 39 calories
  2g protein, 0.4g total fat, <0.1g saturated fat, 0 trans fat,
  9g carbohydrates, 0 cholesterol, 6mg sodium, 3g fiber

- A fresh ripe tomato, sliced and seasoned with fresh or dried basil, dried cilantro, garlic powder, salt, freshly ground pepper, dried thyme, marjoram, or a combination

  Approx. 38 calories
  2g protein, 0.6g total fat, < 0.1g saturated fat, 0 trans fat,
  8g carbohydrates, 0 cholesterol, 16mg sodium, 2g fiber

- Popcorn rice cake (trans fat–free) with 1 tablespoon fresh hummus

  Approx. 61 calories
  2g protein, 1g total fat, 0.2g saturated fat, 0 trans fat,
  11g carbohydrates, 0 cholesterol, 82mg sodium, 0.2g fiber

- A raw apple with skin intact, sliced, and 2 teaspoons fresh peanut butter thinly spread onto slices

  Approx. 139 calories
  2g protein, 6g total fat, 0.8g saturated fat, 0 trans fat,
  23g carbohydrates, 0 cholesterol, 37mg sodium, 5g fiber

- 2 Bavarian (no salt added) pretzels (trans fat–free)

  Approx. 100 calories
  2g protein, 0 total fat, 0 saturated fat, 0 trans fat,
  20g carbohydrates, 0 cholesterol, 20mg sodium, 3 fiber

- 1 (3–4 ounce) cup sugar-free, fat-free Jello with 2 tablespoons fat-free whipped cream

  Approx. 15 calories
  2g protein, 0 total fat, 0 saturated fat, 0 trans fat,
  1g carbohydrates, 0 cholesterol, 45mg sodium, 0 fiber

- 1 fat-free, no-sugar-added Fudgsicle

  Approx. 40 calories
  1g protein, 1g total fat, 0.5g saturated fat, 0 trans fat,
  9g carbohydrates, 0 cholesterol, 45mg sodium, 2g fiber

Spices, Sauces, Marinades, and Dressings

Spices

MIXED SPICES
MAKES ABOUT 2 TABLESPOONS

2 teaspoons ground allspice
1 teaspoon ground cinnamon
1 teaspoon ground cloves
1 teaspoon ground coriander
1 teaspoon ground cumin
¼ teaspoon freshly ground pepper

Combine ingredients and store in a small jar with a tight lid in a cool dry place away from light.

HARISSA (RED PEPPER SPICE)

MAKES ABOUT ⅔ CUP

Tunisian kitchens are noted for the spiciness of their food, which comes from a hot pepper sauce called "harissa." The sauce adds piquancy to all types of stews as well as couscous. If you are brave enough, you can even eat it on its own as a spread on bread. Commercial harissa is imported from North Africa and is available in tubes in most gourmet stores where couscous is sold.

½ cup ground fresh cayenne
2 tablespoons finely ground caraway seeds
¼ cup cumin
1 teaspoon coriander seed
2 tablespoons salt
5 cloves fresh garlic, peeled and crushed
1 tablespoon water
½ cup extra-virgin olive oil

Mix all spices together in a mortar. Add crushed garlic and salt to spice mixture and mash together to form a paste. Put paste into a jar and add water and ¼ cup of olive oil; mix well. Spoon remaining olive oil over the top, cover tightly, and refrigerate. It keeps for months.

SPICE RUB

MAKES ENOUGH FOR 1 POUND OF FISH

2 tablespoons curry powder
1 tablespoon cumin powder
1 teaspoon sugar
½ teaspoon salt
½ teaspoon paprika
¼ teaspoon cardamom

Combine ingredients and sprinkle fish before cooking.

CHICKEN RUB
MAKES ENOUGH FOR A 3–4 POUND ROASTER

1 tablespoon Dijon mustard
1 tablespoon dark spicy mustard
2 cloves fresh garlic, finely minced
1 tablespoon extra-virgin olive oil
1 teaspoon dried thyme
Salt and freshly ground pepper to taste

Combine all ingredients, stir well to incorporate flavors, and rub mixture inside chicken cavity as well as over outside of chicken. Place chicken in refrigerator and marinate for 2–3 hours before roasting.

BLACKENING SEASONING MIX
MAKES ¼ CUP

2 teaspoons dried basil
2 teaspoons crushed black peppercorns
1 teaspoon ground white pepper
1 teaspoon ground cumin
1 teaspoon caraway seeds, crushed
1 teaspoon fennel seeds, crushed
1 teaspoon dried thyme
1 teaspoon dried oregano
½ teaspoon salt
½ teaspoon crushed red hot pepper flakes
2 teaspoons paprika

In a skillet over medium-high heat, combine all ingredients, except for paprika, and cook until seeds are lightly browned. Remove from heat and stir in paprika. Store in an airtight container and shake well before using to season fish of your choice.

SPICY CHICKEN RUB
MAKES 5–6 TABLESPOONS

2 teaspoons smoked paprika
1 teaspoon cayenne pepper
2 teaspoons onion powder
1 teaspoon ground cumin
1 teaspoon chili powder
1 teaspoon garlic powder
2 teaspoons dried oregano
2 teaspoons dried thyme
2 teaspoons dry mustard
½ teaspoon salt

Combine all ingredients and rub into chicken before cooking.

Sauces

ORANGE GINGER SAUCE
MAKES 4 SERVINGS

Juice from 3 fresh oranges
¼ cup light mayonnaise
2 tablespoons prepared fresh horseradish
¼ teaspoon honey
¼ teaspoon ground ginger
1 tablespoon extra-virgin olive oil
Salt and freshly ground pepper to taste
Generous pinch of all-purpose flour

Combine orange juice, mayonnaise, horseradish, honey, ginger, olive oil, and salt and pepper in a small saucepan. Whisk to blend on low heat. When sauce begins to simmer, whisk in flour. Cook for 1–2 minutes, whisking constantly, until sauce is smooth.

Approx. 60 calories per serving
0 protein, 5g total fat, 0 saturated fat, 0 trans fat,
5g carbohydrates, 0 cholesterol, 155mg sodium, 0 fiber

SWEET AND SPICY GLAZE

MAKES ENOUGH FOR 1 (1–1½-POUND) WHOLE CHICKEN

2 tablespoons spicy chili sauce
⅓ cup honey

Blend together well and brush over shrimp or chicken. The sauce will caramel-ize when food is grilled.

Approx. 101 calories
0 protein, 0 total fat, 0 saturated fat, 0 trans fat,
25g carbohydrates, 0 cholesterol, 32mg sodium, 0 fiber

RED PESTO SAUCE

MAKES 4 SERVINGS

2 ounces sundried tomatoes in oil, drained and oil reserved
2 cloves fresh garlic, minced
1 cup loosely packed fresh basil leaves
3 tablespoons pine nuts, lightly toasted
4 tablespoons extra-virgin olive oil
4 tablespoons freshly grated Parmesan cheese
Salt and freshly ground pepper to taste
Balsamic vinegar to taste

Combine sundried tomatoes, garlic, basil, and pine nuts in a food processor. Combine olive oil with 2 tablespoons oil reserved from sundried tomatoes (making 6 tablespoons oil in total) and slowly add oil to food processor. Process ingredients to a smooth consistency. Transfer mixture to a closable container. Stir in Parmesan, salt to taste, and a generous amount of pepper. Add vinegar to taste, seal container, and refrigerate. Can be used for up to 1 week.

Approx. 235 calories per serving
5g protein, 21g total fat, 2g saturated fat, 0 trans fat,
9g carbohydrates, 4mg cholesterol, 373mg sodium, 2g fiber

BLACK OLIVE PASTE

MAKES 1½ CUPS (½ TEASPOON GOES A LONG WAY—THERE ARE 144 [½-TEASPOON] SERVINGS IN 1½ CUPS)

1 cup pitted Kalamata olives
5 anchovy fillets
5 cloves fresh garlic, chopped
½ cup extra-virgin olive oil
1 teaspoon dried rosemary
½ teaspoon freshly ground pepper

Combine olives, anchovies, garlic, olive oil, rosemary, and pepper in a food processor and process to a smooth paste. Serve in ½-teaspoon portions or in desired amount as a spread on crostini. Can be added to cooked pasta or used as a garnish to grilled meat (use sparingly; a small amount goes a long way).

Approx. 1,151 calories per 1½ cups
7g protein, 124g total fat, 17g saturated fat, 0 trans fat,
9g carbohydrates, 0 cholesterol, 2,028mg sodium, 4g fiber

LIME SAUCE WITH TOASTED ALMONDS

MAKES 4 SERVINGS

1 tablespoon extra-virgin olive oil
¼ cup sliced almonds
1 tablespoon freshly squeezed lime juice
Salt to taste
¼ cup + 1 tablespoon low-fat plain yogurt
½ shallot, thinly sliced
1 cup torn fresh parsley

In a small saucepan, heat olive oil over medium heat and add almonds. Toast until fragrant and lightly browned. Remove from heat and transfer to a bowl. Allow almonds to cool. Stir in lime juice and add salt to taste. Blend in yogurt until fully combined and chill. To serve with meat or fish entree, put a dollop of sauce on top of each fillet. Add slices of shallot and parsley leaves and serve.

Approx. 78 calories per serving
2g protein, 6g total fat, 1g saturated fat, 0 trans fat,
3g carbohydrates, 1mg cholesterol, 17mg sodium, 2g fiber

HARDY EGGPLANT SAUCE

MAKES 6 SERVINGS

2 tablespoons olive oil
1 medium white onion, coarsely chopped
3–4 large cloves fresh garlic, finely chopped
½ large green bell pepper, coarsely chopped
1 large eggplant (about 1 pound), peeled and cubed
1 (28-ounce) can peeled Italian tomatoes, drained and broken in pieces by hand
½ cup dry red wine
1 teaspoon dried basil
1 teaspoon dried oregano
Salt and freshly ground pepper to taste

In a large heavy-bottomed skillet, heat olive oil over medium heat. Add onion and garlic and sauté until soft and fragrant. Add green bell pepper, eggplant, tomatoes, wine, basil, oregano, and salt and pepper. Cover and let simmer for about 30 minutes or until eggplant and peppers are almost a mushy soft consistency and ingredients are well blended. Serve hot over your favorite pasta.

Approx. 268 calories per serving
2g protein, 4g total fat, 1g saturated fat, 0 trans fat,
12g carbohydrates, 0 cholesterol, 222mg sodium, 5g fiber

EASY BASIL PESTO

MAKES 1 CUP

2 cups packed fresh basil leaves
3 cloves fresh garlic
⅓ cup walnuts
⅔ cup extra-virgin olive oil, divided
½ cup freshly grated Pecorino cheese
Salt and freshly ground pepper to taste

Combine basil, garlic, and walnuts in a food processor and pulse until coarsely chopped. Add ½ cup of oil and process until smooth. Add in Pecorino cheese, salt and pepper, and remaining olive oil and pulse again until blended.

Approx. 1,464 calories per cup
24g protein, 176g total fat, 48g saturated fat, 0 trans fat,
6g carbohydrates, 44mg cholesterol, 767mg sodium, 0 fiber

WHITE WINE SAUCE

MAKES 6 (1½-TABLESPOON) SERVINGS

Olive oil cooking spray
⅓ cup finely chopped white onion
½ cup canned low-sodium, fat-free chicken broth
¼ cup dry white wine (such as Sauvignon Blanc or Pinot Grigio)
2 tablespoons aged white wine vinegar
2 tablespoons trans fat–free canola/olive oil spread, melted
2 teaspoons finely chopped fresh chives

Heat a skillet over medium-high heat and spray skillet with cooking oil. Add onion and sauté for roughly 2 minutes. Stir in chicken broth, wine, and vinegar and bring to a boil. Continue to cook until reduced to ¼ cup, roughly 5 minutes. Remove from heat, add melted canola/olive oil spread and chives, and serve with chicken, pasta, or white fish (such as tilapia).

Approx. 91 calories per serving
0 protein, 6g total fat, 1g saturated fat, 0 trans fat,
6g carbohydrates, 0 cholesterol, 33mg sodium, 0 fiber

MUSHROOM-SHALLOT SAUCE

MAKES 4–6 SERVINGS

2 tablespoons olive oil
1 pound assorted mushrooms, such as button, cremini, or portobello, cleaned and sliced
2 cloves fresh garlic, minced
2 shallots, finely chopped
⅓ cup dry white wine
1 tablespoon Dijon mustard
2 teaspoons fresh snipped thyme

Heat olive oil in a non-stick skillet over medium heat. Combine mushrooms, garlic, and shallots in skillet and cook for about 5 minutes until tender, stirring occasionally. Reduce heat and add wine, mustard, and thyme. Cook for 2–3 minutes more or until well combined and heated through. Serve with chicken or fish.

Approx. 67 calories per serving
2g protein, 4g total fat, 1g saturated fat, 0 trans fat,
2g carbohydrates, 0 cholesterol, 4mg sodium, 1g fiber

SIMPLE QUICK TOMATO SAUCE

MAKES 3 CUPS

3 tablespoons extra-virgin olive oil
4 cloves fresh garlic, peeled and chopped
1 (28-ounce) can peeled whole Roma tomatoes, undrained
Salt and freshly ground pepper to taste
3–4 fresh basil leaves, minced

In a heavy-bottomed pot over medium heat, add olive oil and garlic and sauté, stirring often, until golden brown, about 3 minutes. Add tomatoes with juice and salt and pepper to taste. Increase heat to high, bring sauce to a boil, and cook uncovered for about 5 minutes, reducing liquid slightly. Reduce heat to medium-low and let simmer, stirring occasionally, for about 30 minutes. Add basil and cook for another 15 minutes. Makes enough sauce for 1 pound of pasta.

Approx. 570 calories per 3 cups
7g protein, 42g total fat, 5g saturated fat, 0 trans fat,
35g carbohydrates, 0 cholesterol, 1,330mg sodium, 14g fiber

CORNSTARCH PASTE

Cornstarch
Cold water

Used for thickening sauces, soups, and gravies. For every cup of liquid you want to thicken, combine 1 tablespoon corn starch with 1½ tablespoons cold liquid (for example, water) and stir until smooth and a paste forms. Then, add this cornstarch paste to hot sauces, soups, or gravies to thicken.

THICK POMEGRANATE MOLASSES
MAKES 1 CUP

3 cups fresh pomegranate juice

In a 1½ quart saucepan bring 3 cups of juice to a boil over medium heat. Reduce heat and simmer, uncovered, stirring occasionally and skimming the froth, until juice is reduced to 1 cup. Cool, bottle, and store in refrigerator.

Approx. 255 calories per 1 cup
3g protein, 0 fat, 0 saturated fat, 0 trans fat,
63g carbohydrates, 0 cholesterol, 0 sodium, 0 fiber

SPICY GARLICKY PESTO SAUCE
MAKES 4 SERVINGS

¼ cup extra-virgin olive oil
4 cloves fresh garlic, chopped
¼ teaspoon crushed red hot pepper flakes
Salt and freshly ground pepper to taste
Grated Parmesan cheese (optional)

In a medium-sized skillet over medium heat, warm olive oil. Add garlic and sauté until translucent. Add hot pepper flakes and simmer on very low heat for 3–5 minutes. Serve with your favorite pasta. Garnish with grated Parmesan cheese, if desired.

This sauce is also great on pizza.

Approx. 110 calories per serving
0 protein, 14g total fat, 1.5g saturated fat, 0 trans fat,
1g carbohydrates, 0 cholesterol, 1mg sodium, 0 fiber

SUNDRIED TOMATO PESTO

MAKES 2 CUPS

2 cups boiling water
1 cup sundried tomatoes
¼ cup + ½ tablespoon extra-virgin olive oil
5 cloves fresh garlic
¼ cup pine nuts
½ cup fresh basil
½ cup fresh Italian parsley

Combine boiling water and sundried tomatoes, and let stand until tomatoes soften (about 10–15 minutes). Drain and reserve 1 cup of liquid. In a medium skillet heat ½ tablespoon olive oil over medium-high heat. Add garlic and sauté, stirring often for about 1 minute. Remove from heat. In a food processor, process the garlic, tomatoes, reserved liquid, pine nuts, basil, parsley, and remaining ¼ cup olive oil. Serve over pasta.

This sauce is also great on pizza.

Approx. 50 calories per tablespoon
1g protein, 3.5g total fat, 0.6g saturated fat, 0 trans fat,
2g carbohydrates, 0 cholesterol, 23mg sodium, 1g fiber

TOMATO-BASIL SAUCE

MAKES 4 SERVINGS

1 tablespoon olive oil
4 cloves fresh garlic, minced
1 shallot, finely chopped
1 (14.5-ounce) can diced tomatoes with chilies, well drained
Salt and freshly ground pepper to taste
4 sprigs basil, chopped

In a skillet over medium-high heat, combine olive oil, garlic, and shallot. Sauté garlic and shallot until soft and fragrant. Reduce heat to low. Add tomatoes, salt and pepper, and basil, and cook uncovered until heated through and liquid absorbed. Serve as a chunky sauce over fish or chicken.

Approx. 66 calories per serving
2g protein, 3g total fat, 0 saturated fat, 0 trans fat,
6g carbohydrates, 0 cholesterol, 93mg sodium, 1g fiber

HONEY MUSTARD SAUCE

MAKES 1 CUP

4 tablespoons Dijon mustard
4 tablespoons light mayonnaise
2 tablespoons honey
2 tablespoons red wine vinegar

Combine all ingredients in a covered container and chill in refrigerator to blend flavors for 30 minutes. Serve room temperature with chicken, crab, or shrimp.

Approx. 372 calories per cup
3g protein, 22g total fat, 4g saturated fat, 0 trans fat,
46g carbohydrates, 20mg cholesterol, 402mg sodium, 0 fiber

SPICY PISTACHIO PESTO

MAKES 4 SERVINGS

½ small hot cherry pepper, seeded
3 cloves fresh garlic, peeled
2 medium sweet red peppers, roasted
¼ cup dry-roasted pistachios
Salt and freshly ground pepper to taste
⅓ cup extra-virgin olive oil
¼ cup fresh grated Parmesan cheese

In a food processor combine hot pepper, garlic, red peppers, and pistachios. Season with salt and pepper and pulse while adding olive oil a little at a time until it forms a smooth consistency. Transfer to a bowl and blend in Parmesan cheese.
This sauce is a great topping for fish.

Approx. 233 calories per serving
4g protein, 23g total fat, 3g saturated fat, 0 trans fat,
5g carbohydrates, 5mg cholesterol, 113mg sodium, 1g fiber

SARDINE PASTA SAUCE

MAKES 4 SERVINGS

8–10 small black olives, coarsely chopped

1 (3.75-ounce) tin of sardines in olive oil

2 cloves fresh garlic, pressed

Crushed red hot pepper flakes to taste

¼ cup extra-virgin olive oil

¼ cup finely chopped fresh cilantro

Salt and freshly ground pepper to taste

Combine all the ingredients and mix until sardines are broken into small pieces. Toss with cooked pasta of choice. Add salt and pepper to taste and serve.

Approx. 186 calories per serving
5g protein, 19g total fat, 2.4g saturated fat, 0 trans fat,
<1g carbohydrates, 13mg cholesterol, 121mg sodium, <0.5g fiber

BASIL PESTO SAUCE

MAKES I CUP OF SAUCE

⅓ cup pine nuts, toasted
2½ cups fresh basil leaves
1 teaspoon lemon juice
Dash of salt
4 cloves fresh garlic
½ cup extra-virgin olive oil, divided
¼ cup grated Parmesan cheese
¼ cup grated Pecorino Romano cheese
Freshly ground pepper to taste

In a small skillet toast pine nuts over medium heat for 1–2 minutes. Remove from heat and set aside. Cut basil leaves into strips. Combine lemon juice, salt, and garlic in a mortar and mash into a paste. Add pine nuts and continue to mash until nuts are ground. Add basil strips a few at a time, gradually grounding them into nut mixture. Add a splash of olive oil and mix until paste becomes loose. Add both grated cheeses, pepper to taste, and remaining olive oil as needed to form into desirable consistency.

Sauce can be kept refrigerated for a few days if stored in a jar with a tight-fitting lid. If doing this, add a small amount of olive oil on top of sauce. However, pesto is best if used immediately.

This sauce goes a long way: one spoonful of pesto is all that is needed to flavor minestrone, vegetables, grilled chicken, fish, or pasta.

Approx. 75 calories per tablespoon
2g protein, 7g total fat, 1.2g saturated fat, 0 trans fat,
2g carbohydrates, 5mg cholesterol, 135mg sodium, <1g fiber

RED CLAM SAUCE

MAKES 4 SERVINGS

½ cup white wine

3 cloves fresh garlic, crushed

48 small hard shell clams

2 tablespoons extra-virgin olive oil

1 onion, chopped

2 cups diced plum tomatoes

3 tablespoons chopped fresh basil

1 tablespoon chopped fresh oregano

¼ teaspoon crushed red hot pepper flakes

Salt and freshly ground pepper to taste

1 teaspoon chopped fresh parsley for garnish

In a large pot, cook wine, garlic, and clams in small amount of water until shells open. Remove clams from shells. In a skillet add olive oil and onion and sauté. Add tomatoes, season with basil, oregano, and hot pepper flakes, and cook for 8 minutes. Add clams in their juices and salt and pepper to taste and cook for another 2–3 minutes. Serve over pasta and garnish with parsley.

Approx. 99 calories per serving
15g protein, 8.5g total fat, <1g saturated fat, 0 trans fat,
8g carbohydrates, 26mg cholesterol, 68mg sodium, 1g fiber

ANCHOVY AND GARLIC SAUCE

MAKES 4 SERVINGS

6 tablespoons extra-virgin olive oil

Oil from anchovies

6 cloves fresh garlic, pressed

2-ounce tin of anchovy fillets packed in oil, drained and chopped

Crushed red hot pepper flakes to taste

2 tablespoons fresh cilantro or parsley, finely chopped

6 tablespoons freshly grated Romano cheese

Salt and freshly ground pepper to taste

Combine oils and garlic in a skillet over medium heat and cook about 1–2 minutes. Add anchovies, cook about 30 seconds, and remove from heat. Add in hot pepper flakes and cilantro or parsley. Add to pasta of choice, sprinkle with grated Romano cheese, and serve. Add salt and pepper to taste.

This sauce is also great as a pizza sauce.

Approx. 189 calories per serving
3g protein, 18g total fat, 2g saturated fat, 0 trans fat,
1g carbohydrates, 13mg cholesterol, 387mg sodium, 0 fiber

SIMPLY GREAT MARINARA SAUCE

MAKES 9 CUPS

½ cup yellow onion, finely chopped

6 cloves fresh garlic, finely minced

3 tablespoons extra-virgin olive oil

2 (28-ounce) cans tomato puree with no salt added

1 (28-ounce) can crushed tomatoes

1 tablespoon tomato paste

½ teaspoon dried basil

2½ cups water

1 cup canned low-sodium, fat-free chicken broth

1 teaspoon low-calorie baking sweetener

¼ teaspoon crushed red hot pepper flakes

Salt and freshly ground pepper to taste

Sauté onion and garlic in olive oil over medium heat until soft; do not brown. Add tomato puree, crushed tomatoes, tomato paste, and basil. Stir to blend flavors. Add water, broth, sweetener, hot pepper flakes, and salt and pepper, then bring mixture to a boil, cover, reduce heat to low, and simmer for 1 hour. Store unused sauce (in a sealed container) in the freezer for up to 3–4 months.

Approx. 74 calories per ½ cup sauce
17g protein, 3g total fat, <0.4g saturated fat, 0 trans fat,
12.4g carbohydrates, <0.1mg cholesterol, 131mg sodium, 2g fiber

SIMPLE TOMATO PASTA SAUCE
MAKES 6–8 SERVINGS

1½ pounds fresh tomatoes or 1 (28-ounce) can peeled tomatoes
6 cloves fresh garlic, finely chopped
6 tablespoons extra-virgin olive oil
10 fresh basil leaves, chopped
Salt and freshly ground pepper to taste
1 large carrot, finely chopped
1 large onion, finely chopped
1 stalk celery, finely chopped
1 teaspoon finely chopped fresh parsley
½ teaspoon crushed red hot pepper flakes

If using fresh tomatoes, place them in a large pot of water and bring to a boil. Remove from heat, rinse tomatoes under cold water, and immediately peel off skins. This method allows you to easily remove the skins from the tomatoes. Cut peeled tomatoes in chunks and set aside. If using canned tomatoes, drain off liquid and reserve (to be used later if sauce is too thick). In a large skillet over medium-high heat, lightly sauté garlic in olive oil, then add basil, tomatoes, salt and pepper to taste, carrot, onion, celery, parsley, and hot pepper flakes; cook at medium-high heat for 2–3 minutes. Reduce heat to low and simmer for about 20–25 minutes, stirring often to blend ingredients.

Approx. 119 calories per serving
1g protein, 11g total fat, 1g saturated fat, 0 trans fat,
7g carbohydrates, 0 cholesterol, 15mg sodium, 2g fiber

Marinades

GINGER GARLIC MARINADE

MAKES ENOUGH FOR 1½ POUNDS OF FISH, POULTRY, OR MEAT

3 tablespoons extra-virgin olive oil
2 tablespoons low-sodium soy sauce
2 tablespoons fresh lime juice
1 tablespoon ground ginger
1 tablespoon finely chopped fresh garlic
½ teaspoon dry mustard

Combine all ingredients and stir to blend. Place fish, poultry, or meat in a container and cover with marinade. Cover with a tight-fitting lid and turn container upside down several times to coat all pieces with marinade. Place in refrigerator for a minimum of 30 minutes, up to several hours. Remove fish or meat from marinade when ready to cook and discard marinade.

GREAT FISH MARINADE

MAKES ENOUGH FOR 1½ POUNDS OF FISH

Juice from 2 fresh large limes
1 tablespoon extra-virgin olive oil
2 tablespoons low-sodium soy sauce
2 cloves fresh garlic, finely chopped
½ cup dry vermouth
2 tablespoons fresh mint leaves, minced

Combine all of the ingredients in a small bowl and whisk to blend. Set aside. Score skin of fish and place in a tightly sealable container in a single layer. Pour marinade over fish and turn to coat both sides. Cover and refrigerate for 2–3 hours, turning container upside down several times while marinating to coat fish. Remove fish when ready to cook and discard marinade.

YUMMY MARINADE FOR CHICKEN

MAKES ROUGHLY ½ CUP

½ cup of your favorite Italian dressing
1 teaspoon freshly squeezed lime juice
1½ teaspoons sourwood honey
2 tablespoons minced fresh garlic
1 pound skinless, boneless chicken pieces

Mix Italian dressing, lime juice, honey, and garlic together in a bowl and blend well. Add chicken pieces, making sure to coat all pieces with sauce. Place in refrigerator to marinate for at least 1 hour before cooking.

A GREAT MARINADE

MAKES 6 SERVINGS

⅓ cup olive oil
4 cloves fresh garlic, minced
1 teaspoon crushed red hot pepper flakes
3 tablespoons freshly squeezed lime juice
¼ cup orange juice

In a small pot, combine olive oil, garlic, and hot pepper flakes. Heat over medium heat until garlic is soft. Remove from heat and stir in both juices. Allow to cool before adding to protein. Use to marinate pork, chicken, shrimp, or scallops.

Dressings

YOGURT DRESSING
MAKES 1 CUP

Crushed garlic or spearmint to taste
1 cup plain yogurt

Mix garlic or spearmint into yogurt, to taste.

Approx. 160 calories per 1 cup
9g protein, 8g fat, 4g saturated fat, 0 trans fat,
13g carbohydrates, 0 cholesterol, 160mg sodium, 0 fiber

LEMON DRESSING
MAKES ABOUT ½ CUP OF DRESSING

¼ cup extra-virgin olive oil
¼ cup fresh-squeezed lemon juice
1 medium clove fresh garlic, crushed to a paste
Scant pinch of salt
Freshly ground pepper to taste

Combine all ingredients in a bowl and mix well.

Approx. 61 calories per tablespoon
<0.1g protein, 7g total fat, 0.7g saturated fat, 0 trans fat,
1g carbohydrates, 0 cholesterol, 0.1mg sodium, 0 fiber

LEMON-PEPPER SALAD DRESSING

MAKES ½ CUP

½ cup extra-virgin olive oil
2 tablespoons vinegar
1 tablespoon non-caloric sweetener
2 teaspoons lemon pepper seasoning

Combine all ingredients in a salad dressing shaker and shake well to blend. Drizzle on salad.

Approx. 720 calories per ½ cup (roughly 90 calories per tablespoon)
0 protein, 84g total fat, 11g saturated fat, 0 trans fat,
0 carbohydrates, 0 cholesterol, 0 sodium, 0 fiber

A GREAT SALAD DRESSING

MAKES I CUP

¼ cup apple cider vinegar
1¼ teaspoons Dijon mustard
1¼ teaspoons minced shallot
1 teaspoon non-caloric sweetener
¾ cup extra-virgin olive oil
Salt and freshly ground pepper to taste

Whisk together vinegar, mustard, shallot, and sweetener in a small bowl. Add in olive oil and salt and pepper to taste and whisk again. Set aside for 15 minutes before using to blend flavors. Drizzle on salad.

Approx. 1,080 calories per cup (roughly 67 calories per tablespoon)
0 protein, 126g total fat, 16g saturated fat, 0 trans fat,
0 carbohydrates, 0 cholesterol, 0 sodium, 0 fiber

SICILIAN DRESSING
MAKES 1 CUP

¼ cup water
⅔ cup extra-virgin olive oil
Juice from 1 lemon
2 cloves fresh garlic, sliced
½ cup chopped fresh parsley
1 teaspoon oregano

Bring water to a boil and pour into a bowl. Add olive oil and beat. Add lemon juice, garlic, parsley, and oregano, and beat again until well mixed. Place mixture in a double boiler and cook for additional 5 minutes, stirring constantly. Use as fish topper or let cool and serve over salad.

Approx. 80 calories per tablespoon
0 protein, 9g total fat, 1.2g saturated fat, 0 trans fat,
0 carbohydrates, 0 cholesterol, 0 sodium, 0 fiber

FRESH FIG VINAIGRETTE
MAKES ROUGHLY ½ CUP

3 figs, quartered
3 tablespoons balsamic vinegar
1 tablespoon maple syrup
Salt and freshly ground pepper to taste
3 tablespoons extra-virgin olive oil

Combine figs, vinegar, syrup, and salt and pepper to taste in a blender or food processor. Process until smooth. Turn off processor and scrape down mixture from sides. Start processing again while slowly adding olive oil. When vinaigrette has thickened, drizzle on salad.

Approx. 450 calories based on entire amount dressing
1g protein, 42g total fat, 5g saturated fat, 0 trans fat,
25g carbohydrates, 0 cholesterol, 1mg sodium, 4g fiber

MINT VINAIGRETTE DRESSING

MAKES ROUGHLY ¼ CUP

1 teaspoon red wine vinegar
1 teaspoon freshly squeezed lemon juice
1 tablespoon finely minced shallot
¼ cup extra-virgin olive oil
¼ cup chopped fresh mint

Whisk together vinegar, lemon juice, and shallot in a bowl. Add olive oil slowly while continuing to whisk ingredients. Stir in mint and allow dressing to sit to infuse for 10 minutes before using on salad.

Approx. 340 calories per entire amount of dressing
0 protein, 42g total fat, 5g saturated fat, 0 trans fat,
0 carbohydrates, 0 cholesterol, 0 sodium, 0 fiber

CHIVE VINAIGRETTE

MAKES ROUGHLY 1½ CUPS

6 tablespoons aged white wine vinegar
6 tablespoons extra-virgin olive oil
2 packages fresh chives (roughly ¾ ounce)
6 tablespoons Dijon mustard
6 tablespoons pure honey
Salt and freshly ground pepper to taste

Combine all ingredients in a blender and puree. Pour into salad cruet to store and shake well before serving over salad.

Approx. 60 calories per serving
0 protein, 7g total fat, 0 saturated fat, 0 trans fat,
8g carbohydrates, 0 cholesterol, 0 sodium, 0 fiber

SHALLOT-BALSAMIC VINAIGRETTE

MAKES ROUGHLY ⅔ CUP

4 tablespoons balsamic vinegar

4 tablespoons extra-virgin olive oil

2 tablespoons minced shallot

2 teaspoons pure maple syrup

1 teaspoon Dijon mustard

Salt and freshly ground pepper to taste

Combine all ingredients in a small bowl and briskly whisk to blend. Serve drizzled over salad.

Approx. 80 calories per serving

0 protein, 9g total fat, 1g saturated fat, 0 trans fat,

0 carbohydrates, 0 cholesterol, 0 sodium, 0 fiber

APPENDICES

The Atherogenic Metabolic Stew

If you ask most people what the cause of heart disease is, they'll say cholesterol. However, there are many other risk factors that increase your likelihood of developing heart disease that you can measure with a blood test.

First of all, cholesterol may be good or bad. Good (HDL) cholesterol helps to remove bad (LDL) cholesterol from our arteries. Triglycerides are another lipid, or fat, that can contribute to plaque buildup in our arteries.

Other metabolic risk factors that increase our risk of cardiovascular disease include:

- *Homocysteine*: a protein in the blood that has been linked to cardiovascular disease because of the damage it does to the lining of the blood vessels. It also leads to enhanced clotting. Although homocysteine predicts an increased risk of cardiovascular disease, it has not been demonstrated that lowering homocysteine levels with medication or vitamins will also lower the risk.
- *Fibrinogen*: another protein that, when elevated, can lead to an increased risk of clotting.
- *Infectious agents (such as viruses and bacteria)*: chronic infection leads to chronic inflammation, which increases the risk of heart attack and stroke.
- *Lipoprotein (a) (LPa)*: a "bad" cholesterol particle that increases the risk of heart attack and stroke. LPa contributes to atherosclerotic plaque formation and also increases the risk of blood clotting.
- *High sensitivity C-reactive protein (hs-CRP)*: a marker of inflammation that is linked to an increased risk of cardiovascular disease. Several studies have shown that hs-CRP is a better predictor of heart attack than total cholesterol or bad (LDL) cholesterol.

- *Particle size*: the size of the particles that carry cholesterol. This can be more important in predicting heart attack risk than the cholesterol level itself. Small bad (LDL) cholesterol particles are more dangerous than large bad cholesterol particles. Likewise, small good (HDL) cholesterol particles are less effective in removing bad (LDL) cholesterol particles from the blood vessel wall than large good (HDL) cholesterol particles.

Collectively, all of the risk factors mentioned above, along with other emerging risk factors, are termed "the atherogenic metabolic stew." These metabolic risk factors can be measured by most commercial labs. The task of the preventive cardiologist is to treat all of the known risk factors, thereby decreasing this deadly stew. This will result in a decrease in atherosclerotic plaque buildup as well as a decrease in the risk of heart attack, stroke, and peripheral vascular disease.

Important Medications for Cardiovascular Disease Prevention

Cardiovascular disease prevention begins with lifestyle modification. A proper diet and exercise program, along with stress management and smoking cessation, form the foundation of our heart disease prevention guidelines. There are people who nevertheless develop heart disease, even though they follow these guidelines. These individuals have a genetic basis for their heart disease and require medications along with a healthy lifestyle.

Many types of medications are used in the treatment of cardiovascular disease. The most commonly used medications for cardiovascular disease prevention are listed below.

- *HMG-CoA reductase inhibitors (also known as statins)*: medications that reduce cholesterol levels by decreasing the production of cholesterol in the body. Clinical trials that have evaluated the impact of statins on heart disease prevention have demonstrated a significant lowering of heart attack risk and death from coronary heart disease.
- *Niacin, fibrates, resins, and cholesterol absorption inhibitors*: medications that can also lower cholesterol and triglyceride levels.
- *ACE inhibitors*: medications that lower blood pressure and help stabilize the blood vessel wall. They have been shown to lower heart attack risk in patients with heart disease risk factors.
- *Beta blockers*: medications that decrease blood pressure and heart rate by blocking adrenaline. These drugs are especially useful in patients who have high blood pressure and cardiac arrhythmias (heart rhythm disorder). In addition, beta blockers have been shown to reduce the risk of sudden death

in certain high-risk patients. Finally, beta blockers have also been shown to be useful in the treatment of congestive heart failure.

• *Aspirin*: a medication that decreases the risk of heart attack and stroke by blocking the effects of platelets, which are cells that contribute to thrombus (clot formation). Low-dose aspirin appears to be as effective as high-dose aspirin for cardiovascular protection. Unless there is a good reason not to, most physicians advise all patients with cardiovascular disease to take aspirin on a regular basis. In men and women without cardiovascular disease, low-dose aspirin has been shown to reduce the risk of heart attack in men over the age of fifty and reduce the risk of stroke in women over the age of sixty-five. As always, you should discuss the risks and benefits of aspirin therapy with your physician.

Many other medications are used in cardiovascular disease prevention. Calcium channel blockers and angiotensin receptor blockers, for instance, are blood pressure medications used to treat patients with cardiovascular disease. New medications are constantly being developed to battle heart disease. A more efficient good (HDL) cholesterol, developed through genetic engineering, could help to reverse heart disease by decreasing plaque buildup in our arteries.

It is very important to become knowledgeable about all the medications used to treat cardiovascular disease, and it is equally important to understand all of their potential side effects. There is no substitute for regular medical follow-up and discussion between you and your doctor about the medications that are best for your cardiovascular health.

Tips on Purchasing, Preparing, and Eating Foods in the Mediterranean Diet

Olive Oil

People who live in the Mediterranean grow up with the taste of their local olive oil ingrained in their senses. When you consume a local olive oil, you can almost smell the soil and envision the tree that produced its fruit.

Buying olive oil can be both exciting and confusing because of the vast variety of oils available in supermarkets and specialty food markets. There are emerald green-colored oils and golden oils. There are virgin oils and pure oils. The oils come packaged in different shapes and sizes, from exquisite glass bottles to metal tins and even plastic containers. So how does one even start to make a selection?

Olive oils range from pale yellow to a deep, cloudy green. One can easily assume that the green oil is from green, barely ripe olives, but its color is often actually an indication that the oil has a wonderfully fresh, intensely fruity taste. The color yellow, however, does usually mean that the olives were picked late in the season, when black and ripe, often resulting in a sweeter, rounder flavor.

There are various grades of olive oil:

- *Extra-virgin olive oil*: obtained from the first pressing of the olive; has less than 1% acidity
- *Fine virgin olive oil*: obtained from the second pressing of the olives; usually made from slightly riper olives than extra-virgin olive oil; has a slightly higher level of acidity, about 1.5%

- *Refined olive oil*: created by using chemicals to extract the oil from the olives; a basically tasteless olive oil with an acidity level higher than 3.2%
- *Pure olive oil*: a blend of refined and virgin olive oils that is lighter in color and blander in taste than virgin olive oil; an all-purpose olive oil; the word "pure" simply refers to the fact that no oils other than olive oil have been added

Virgin olive oil has more antioxidant properties than refined olive oil and tends to raise good (HDL) cholesterol more effectively than refined olive oil. People with high cholesterol who replace the saturated fat in their diet with olive oil, particularly virgin olive oil, decrease their total cholesterol and bad (LDL) cholesterol.

Bulk oils are generally blends of olive oils from either a particular region or country, or sometimes even from different countries. They are blended together by manufacturing companies and sold in large-quantity tins, plastic bottles, even pails, that range in size from 1 gallon to as much as 55 gallons. This does not mean that they are inferior oils; however, these oils are not the special quality first, cold-pressed olive oils, which can be as expensive as very fine wines. All olive oils have the same amounts of monounsaturated and polyunsaturated fats (good fats); however, first cold-pressed olive oil will have more naturally occurring antioxidants than the regular-pressed olive oils. Blended bulk oils are sometimes a blend of first cold-pressed and regular-pressed oils. They still provide some of the health benefits of a pure first cold-pressed olive oil but can be sold at a cheaper price.

When you buy olive oil, consider how you will use it. If you want to make a pasta sizzle, a young, peppery Tuscan oil might be your best bet, whereas a good, cured, full-bodied oil would be appropriate for a traditional Greek salad made of the best quality tomatoes and finest feta available. However, if you want a hint of olive oil with a background flavor, then a light fruity olive oil, perhaps one from Liguria or Provence that adds a layer of flavor but does not stand out, would be the way to go.

A few other tips:

- Olive oil far exceeds the health benefits of other oils, butters, margarines, or lard; it should be used to replace these items, not in conjunction with them.
- If an oil smells or tastes rancid, that usually indicates that it has been exposed to sunlight or another source of light, which reduces olive oil's delicate aromatic qualities and vitamin E content.
- When selecting an oil, look for the harvest date on the bottle. No olive oil improves with age; it should be no more than eighteen months old.

- An excellent olive oil can range from thirty to forty dollars a bottle or as high as eighty dollars a bottle, much like an expensive bottle of wine of corresponding quality.
- Heating olive oil, especially at high temperatures as in deep frying, can decrease the levels of antioxidants in the oil.

Canola Oil

Canola oil is another heart-healthy oil. The word "canola" in "canola oil" comes from the words "Canada" and "oil"; it was developed in Canada during the late 1960s and early 1970s. It comes from a genetically engineered hybrid plant developed from different mustard seed plants and the turnip rapeseed.

Canola oil contains essential fatty acids that have been proven beneficial to health. Canola oil has zero trans fat and high levels of heart-healthy monounsaturated fats and omega-3 fat.

Beans

Humble bean dishes are a staple in the Mediterranean, made with grains and an abundance of vegetables. On wintry days, throughout the countryside you can smell the delicious aroma of hearty bean soups that have been simmering for days. Beans are served hot or cold, as a first course or as a main dish, as part of a stew or perhaps a dip, to be scooped up with bread or vegetables—there are so many delicious ways in which they can be served.

But the best thing about beans is how healthy they are. They're high in complex carbohydrates, amino acids, fiber, iron, and folic acid. They contain little to no fat and no cholesterol, but an abundance of soluble fiber, which benefits our hearts by lowering cholesterol levels. They are also an excellent low-fat source of protein.

A good rule of thumb for purchasing beans is to buy only beans that are smooth and bright in color; beans that appear cracked, dull, and/or wrinkled are old, and the older the bean, the longer the cooking time needed. One cup of dry beans equals 2 to 2½ cups of cooked beans. Most dried beans must be soaked before they are cooked; the only exception is lentils.

There are two methods you can use for soaking beans: the power-soak method and the long-soak method. In the power-soak method, dried beans are boiled in water for about three minutes, then covered and set aside for two to four hours. After four hours the water is drained off and discarded and the beans are rinsed under fresh running water. The beans are then returned to a heavy-bottomed pot, covered with fresh water, and cooked per package directions.

In the long-soak method, the beans are soaked for eight hours or more. After the required soaking time, the water covering the beans is also discarded. As in the power-soak method, the beans are rinsed under fresh water then returned to a heavy-bottomed pot with fresh water and cooked per package directions.

With either method of soaking, you can test that a bean has been adequately soaked simply by cutting the bean in half to check its color. If the center is opaque, the beans need to be soaked longer. A bean is fully cooked when it can be mashed with a fork.

Below are a few major beans used in the Mediterranean region. Note that the following soaking instructions are for beans cooked in a pressure cooker; cooking beans in a pressure cooker requires less soaking time than conventional stovetop cooking.

Cannellini Bean: one of the most popular beans used in cuisines of central Italy. The cannellini bean is a small white kidney-shaped bean that is high in protein. These beans are great in soups and salads as well as by themselves with just a little olive oil drizzled over them. Soaking time is about 1½ hours (use a ratio of 1 cup of beans to 3 cups of water). One half (½) cup of cooked cannellini beans is roughly 100 calories.

Fava Bean (white or brown; also called the "broad bean"): a bean that goes back almost to the beginning of Mediterranean agriculture. Fava beans have tough outer skins (which are usually discarded after soaking) and a sweet, nutty-flavored inner taste. They are great in soups and salads and are often used for dips and pâté. Soaking time is about 3 hours (use a ratio of 1 cup of beans to 4 cups of water). One half (½) cup of fava beans is roughly 93 calories.

Chickpea or Garbanzo Bean: another Old World bean with a long history in Mediterranean agriculture. Chickpeas are an excellent source of protein and iron. In North African regions they are used to make hummus. Soaking time is about 3 hours (use a ratio of 1 cup of beans to 4 cups of water). One half (½) cup of cooked chickpeas is roughly 130 calories.

Navy Bean: a member of the white bean family. These beans are great in soups and salads and also stand alone well just in an oil-and-vinegar marinade. Soaking time is about 2½ hours (use a ratio of 1 cup of beans to 4 cups of water). One half (½) cup of cooked navy beans is roughly 130 calories.

Great Northern Bean: also a member of the white bean family, similar in flavor to the navy bean but larger in size. These beans do well in many dishes, as well as in an oil-and-vinegar marinade. Soaking time is about 2 hours (use a ratio of 1 cup of beans to 3 cups of water). One half (½) cup of cooked great northern is roughly 100 calories.

Lentil (brown, red, or green): a staple in many Mediterranean cuisines. Brown and green lentils do well in salads, whereas red ones are better suited for pâté and soups. NOTE: Never substitute Indian lentils in a Mediterranean dish. Indian lentils are meant to disintegrate into a thick sauce upon cooking, and in Mediterranean cuisine, the lentils are meant to remain intact. No soaking is required. One half (½) cup of cooked red or brown lentils is roughly 120 calories. One half (½) cup of cooked green lentils is roughly 110 calories.

Some favorite spices used in France and Italy to flavor beans include rosemary, fennel, sage, caraway, tarragon, and marjoram. Lighter spices often include bay leaves, garlic, oregano, parsley, thyme, and dill. In the Middle Eastern countries stronger spices such as cumin, cinnamon, mint, and coriander prevail; on the lighter end, garlic, ginger, nutmeg, fresh pepper, marjoram, parsley, cilantro, saffron, paprika, and turmeric are often used.

A few hints for basic bean seasoning: When using chopped onions, garlic cloves, bay leaves, and cumin, cook them with the beans from the start. Wait until the beans are almost done before adding major seasonings. Adding spices too soon can cause them to break down and disappear before the meal is served.

Bean-related flatulence can be a major problem for some people. Many beans contain a sugar molecule called oligosaccharides. When bacteria breaks down this sugar molecule in the large intestine, it causes flatulence as a by-product. To reduce the occurrence of flatulence, never use the same water that the beans have been soaking in to also cook the beans, always discard soaking water, rinse beans, and cook in fresh water. By soaking the beans for several hours and then discarding the water, you soak off and get rid of some of the offending sugars, reducing the problem of flatulence and possibly eliminating it completely.

Grains

Grains, which make up the foundation of the Mediterranean diet, appear at almost every meal in one form or another. They provide the bulk of the Mediterranean diet's protein and many of its calories, and in the form of complex carbohydrates are the perfect energy source.

Grains can be divided into two groups: whole grains (the grains commonly used in a traditional Mediterranean diet) and refined grains. Whole grains include the entire grain kernel, consisting of the bran, the germ, and the endosperm. Refined grains are whole grains that have been milled, a process that destroys the bran and germ of the kernel, removing dietary fiber, iron, and B-vitamins. Refining gives grains a smoother texture and makes them last longer on the shelf, which is why it has become a common practice in the United States. Many refined grains have been "enriched," meaning that iron and some vitamins have been put back into the product, but the fiber cannot be replaced.

The following are some of the most commonly used grains.

Wheat

Wheat is one of the cornerstones of the Mediterranean diet, in the form of bread, pasta, couscous, and bulgur. There are many types of wheat ranging from very soft wheat (*Triticum aestivum*) to very hard wheat (*Triticum durum*). The terms "soft" and "hard" do not refer to the texture of the wheat but to the protein content of the wheat: hard wheat is generally higher both in protein and in the gluten needed for bread making (gluten is responsible for the stretchiness of dough). Soft wheat is most often used for commercial pizza dough and pastries.

Durum hard grain is the hardest wheat grown. Although it is a soft creamy yellow in color, its texture is coarser than regular wheat flour. When durum wheat is milled—when the outer portions of the wheat are stripped away, leaving only its heart—the result is called semolina flour. Golden in color, semolina flour has an even higher proportion of protein and gluten content than whole durum and is used almost exclusively for pasta production; in Morocco, it is also used to make couscous and homemade breads.

Bread

Semolina flour is often used to make bread, sometimes alone but usually combined with unbleached or all-purpose flour. The best all-purpose flour is a blend of hard and soft wheat that is unbleached and unbromated. ("Unbleached" means that the flour has not been treated with chemicals such as chlorine or peroxide to make it whiter; "unbromated" means the flour has not been enriched using chemicals like potassium bromate.) Most health food stores carry at least one unbleached and unbromated type of all-purpose flour.

Whole wheat flour, another great flour for bread making, is flour that contains the whole wheat kernel, or berry. The amount of husk and wheat germ retained by the flour varies depending on how it is milled; a flour's performance, flavor, and nutrition are greatly affected by the type of mill that grinds the grain. Whole wheat flour for instance, is stone-ground. Stone-ground mills produce the best flour because they do not overheat it as in other milling methods, instead flaking layers off the grain. This results in more of the nutrients being retained in the flour.

Pasta

Pasta comes in many shapes, flavors, and textures, but shares the same basic ingredients: flour and water. The best industrial pasta is made from semolina flour because it absorbs much less water than other flours. That's why pastas imported from Italy are usually of such high quality—the pastas usually list durum wheat flour or semolina among their ingredients.

One pound of pasta generally feeds six people as an appetizer or four people as a main course. Two ounces of uncooked pasta generally equals one cup of cooked pasta. When pairing sauces with pastas, generally pureed, creamy, or clinging sauces are best served with thin strands of pasta like spaghetti, fettuccine, cappellini, or linguine because they will allow the sauce to flow evenly over the noodle. Thinner, runnier sauces are better held by pastas that have twisted or curled shapes because they trap the liquid, making sure the sauce coats the pasta rather than the plate, whereas chunky sauces go best with chunky pastas, particularly ones that contain an opening, like elbow macaroni or shell pastas. Tiny pastas like orzo are great with just a little olive oil and herbs; rich sauces tend to overwhelm them.

Tips for cooking pasta:

- Use three quarts of rapidly boiling water for ½ pound of pasta and four quarts for one pound of pasta.
- Make sure your pot is large and roomy.
- Salt the water before adding pasta, not after (generally one teaspoon of salt per ½ pound of pasta).
- Do not stir noodles that stick to the bottom of the pot; instead, gently lift them with a fork.
- Check pasta at two to four minutes for thin pasta and eight to ten minutes for denser pasta.
- Drain pasta once it's finished cooking but do not rinse; this keeps the pasta moist and helps the sauce stick.

- Add sauce immediately after draining and serve. If not serving immediately, toss pasta with one to two tablespoons of olive oil; this will prevent pasta from sticking.
- If you're making a pasta salad, put dressing on hot noodles immediately to let it sink in; the starchiness of the hot pasta helps the sauce cling to the noodles.
- If pasta is going to be cooked further, such as in a baked dish, undercook it slightly when boiling. This is called cooking it *al dente*.

Various sizes and shapes of pastas:

Shaped pasta: pastas in shapes such as shells, bow ties, spirals, wheels, and curly shapes. The smaller of these varieties do best with a simple, plain sauce; however, the larger ones can usually handle a thicker, chunkier sauce because they are sturdier. Some examples:

- Cavatelli shells (small, narrow shells)
- Conchigliette (medium-sized shells)
- Fusilli (short, twisted, curly pastas)
- Gnocchi shells (small shells made from potato dough)
- Ruotine (small wheels)
- Rotini (spirals)
- Farfalle (bow ties)

Tubular pastas: any pastas in the shape of a tube, from short and wide to long and narrow. The outside can be smooth or textured, and the ends can be cut off straight or at an angle. These pastas are hearty and can handle very chunky, thick sauces, which cling well to both the inside and outside of the pasta. The larger varieties of these tubular pastas are great for stuffing with meat and/or cheese. Some examples:

- Penne (two-inch-long smooth tubes)
- Rigatoni (thick tubes that can be two inches long or longer, often with outside grooves)
- Ziti (straight or slightly curved tubes, either smooth or grooved on the outside)
- Cannelloni (very large tubes; great for stuffing)

- Manicotti (very large tubes, slightly smaller than Cannelloni, that often come flat for rolling; also great for stuffing)

Strand pastas: long rods of pasta that come in a variety of thickness, from very long and thin to very short and thick. The thicker kinds do well with heavy sauces, whereas the very thin kinds require light, plain sauces. Some examples:

- Spaghetti (long rods of various medium thicknesses)
- Capellini, or angel hair (long, very thin rods)
- Vermicelli (long round rods somewhere in thickness between a thinner spaghetti and capellini)
- Linguine (long, flat, thin pasta)
- Tagliateline (long, flat, thin pasta slightly wider than linguine)
- Fettuccine (long, flat, thin pasta wider than both linguine and tagliateline)

Ribbon pastas: long flat pieces of pasta that come in a variety of lengths and widths; can be curled or straight on the sides. These pastas are generally used with a thick sauce. Some examples:

- Lasagna (long rectangular pieces roughly 2–3 inches wide and curly on both side edges)
- Tagliatelle (long rectangular pieces roughly 1 inch wide and curly on both side edges)
- Pappardelle (long rectangular pieces about 1–1½ inches wide and curly on both side edges)

Soup pastas: small to tiny pastas, most frequently used in soups, that come in a variety of shapes. The larger of the small size can be used with thicker soups while the tiny ones are better in a thinner broth. Shapes include flat pieces, balls, tubes, rings, stars, grain shapes, thin strands, and even letters or numbers. Some examples:

- Orzo (small rice-shaped pasta)
- Ditalini (tiny tubes less than ¼-inch long)
- Tubettini (very tiny tubes, smaller than ditalini)
- Alfabeto (alphabet-shaped pasta)
- Anchellini (thin, short, flat pieces of pasta)

Because pastas come in many shapes and flavors, their caloric value per cup varies greatly.

The key to keeping pasta a healthy low-fat food is to use whole grain pasta and to not top with a rich, fatty sauce.

Couscous

What pasta is to the Italians and rice is to the Chinese, couscous is to the inhabitants of Morocco, Algeria, and Tunisia; it's used to make appetizers, soups, salads, main course dishes, and even desserts. When entering a kitchen during mealtime, it's quite common to see a steaming platter of couscous topped with vegetables, meat, or fish. Couscous is often eaten with only vegetables and perhaps goat cheese and/or nuts. When meat is used, it is usually lamb, chicken, or pork.

Couscous is made from durum wheat. The wheat is milled into semolina, rolled into thin strands, crumbled into tiny pieces, steamed, and dried. (Unlike pasta, it is not kneaded during the semolina-water mixture stage.) The word "couscous" refers both to this dry semolina product and the popular prepared dish in which it is the principal ingredient.

The coarsest, largest size of couscous is used primarily for soups. Medium-sized couscous, which is mostly what we see here in the United States, is all-purpose. Tiny or ant-sized couscous is reserved for special dishes and desserts.

When convenience is needed, pre-steamed couscous is used. Pre-steamed couscous greatly reduces the final cooking time for a dish, since it needs only fifteen minutes in boiling liquid before it is ready to serve.

Bulgur

Bulgur is commonly used in salad preparations, but most often used to make tabbouleh. It is made by cracking parboiled whole wheat kernels (kernels boiled until they are partially cooked) and drying them. Bulgur wheat does not need to be cooked but should be soaked in warm water for twenty to thirty minutes (to soften it) before using. However, when making pilaf (another popular use for bulgur), you don't need to soak the bulgur before using it—you are cooking all the ingredients together at the same time, and the bulgur will soften during that process.

Rice

Worldwide, rice is the most consumed food, eaten by millions every day. In the Mediterranean diet, rice is as popular as wheat flour, and in some regions it's even preferred. In the regions of the western Mediterranean, it takes the form of dishes like risotto and paella. In Greece, Turkey, and the Levant, it shows up as long-grain rice, originally from India and Persia, and is used to make pilaf (long-grain rice makes a better paella because it cooks up dry and fluffy, whereas short-grain rice becomes tender and sticky when cooked). Brown rice, unquestionably a healthier product, is not often used in the Mediterranean except by people eating a macrobiotic diet.

To cook most rice, use a ratio of 1 cup of rice to 1½ or 2 cups of water. Put the rice in a heavy pot with water and salt and cover with a tight-fitting lid; bring to a boil, then reduce heat to medium-low and let simmer for 1 hour, or until water is completely absorbed. Finally, when the time is up, keep the pot covered tightly for another 10 minutes before serving.

Polenta

Polenta is a favorite dish in northern Italy, where it is cooked in water and then eaten with a drizzle of olive oil and a sprinkle of Parmesan cheese or with tomato sauce. It is a traditional dish and often replaces rice, pasta, or potatoes.

Polenta is made of gluten-free, coarsely ground cornmeal that is either white or yellow in color, rather like semolina in appearance. The best polenta is stone-ground cornmeal, where the whole grain, including the germ, is retained.

Fish

In the past decade one of the single most important health recommendations has been to increase our dietary intake of omega-3 fatty acids. Numerous scientific studies tout their health benefits: they have been shown to reduce blood pressure and systemic and vascular inflammation and decrease triglyceride levels and heart rhythm disturbances. Consequently, omega-3 fatty acids may be helpful in treating or improving a wide variety of diseases, such as rheumatoid arthritis, inflammatory bowel diseases, periodontal diseases, depression, acne, asthma, and other disorders.

Cold water fish is rich in EPA and DHA, two omega-3 fatty acids that have been proven beneficial to heart health. But that's not all fish has to offer. Fish is an excellent source of protein and lower in calories than other meat sources. Fish is also lower in fat, particularly cholesterol and saturated fat.

The American Heart Association states that "eating a variety of fish is beneficial to fetal development in pregnant women." However, pregnant women (and children) should avoid certain species of fish (swordfish, shark, tilefish, and king mackerel) as these large predatory fish may contain higher levels of environmental contaminants like mercury. Because of the mercury content of some fish, it is recommended that the skin of the fish be removed before cooking—higher levels of mercury may be concentrated in the skin.

The chart below provides a general overview of the omega-3 content of some popular varieties of finfish (fish with a bony skeleton) and shellfish, based on a 3-ounce raw edible portion for finfish and a 3½-ounce raw edible portion for shellfish.

Fish Omega-3/mg

Catfish, channel or farmed 373
Cod, Atlantic...........................184
Cod, Pacific............................215
Dolphin; Mahi-mahi.............108
Flounder; Sole 199
Grouper, mixed species..........248
Haddock 185
Hake 225
Halibut, Atlantic and Pacific....495
Herring, Atlantic.................1,571
Herring, Pacific 1,658
Mackerel, Atlantic 2,299
Mackerel, Pacific 1,442
Ocean Perch 289
Perch 253
Pollack, Atlanta 421
Pompano, Florida.................568
Sablefish...............................1,395
Salmon, Atlantic.................1,435
Salmon, King Chinook 1,355
Salmon, Sockeye.................1,200
Sea bass, mixed species 590
Sea trout, mixed species.........373
Shark, mixed species..............845

Snapper, mixed species 311
Swordfish 639
Trout, Rainbow 568
Tuna, Blue Fin....................1,173
Tuna, Skipjack......................256
Tuna, Yellow Fin..................218
Turbot, Greenland................920
Whitefish, mixed species 1,258

Shellfish Omega-3/mg

Clams, mixed species.............142
Crab, Alaska King 400
Crab, Blue.............................320
Crab, Dungeness 400
Crab, Queen 375
Crawfish, mixed species.........175
Lobster..................................373
Mussels..................................440
Octopus 150
Oysters..................................678
Scallops, mixed species 198
Shrimp, mixed species 480
Squid, mixed species.............488

Nuts

Nut consumption has been shown to be beneficial for cardiovascular health and to reduce the risk of heart attack. Several landmark studies have revealed the importance of regular nut consumption:

- The Adventist Health Study of 31,000 men and women in 1992 at Loma Linda University in California showed that those who consumed nuts more than five times a week had up to 60 percent fewer heart attacks than those who ate nuts less than once monthly.
- Harvard Men's Health Watch showed that healthy men and men who have suffered a heart attack can actually decrease their cardiovascular risk by eating nuts on a regular basis.
- Iowa Women's Healthy Study in 1996, involving more than 34,000 postmenopausal women, found that those who ate nuts more than four times a week were 40% less likely to die of heart disease.
- Physician's Health Study in 2002 found that men who consumed nuts two or more times per week had reduced risk of sudden cardiac death.

Nuts are a great source of protein and are rich in fiber. In addition, they contain phytonutrients and antioxidants such as vitamin E and selenium. They are high in plant sterol, but mostly contain healthy monounsaturated and polyunsaturated fats like omega-3 that have been shown to lower bad (LDL) cholesterol. As little as two ounces of nuts a week may help lower heart disease risk.

If you are afraid the caloric content of nuts will make you gain weight (an ounce of nuts can contain more than 200 calories, after all), instead of simply adding nuts to your diet, eat them as a replacement for foods that are high in saturated fats and limit your intake to one or two ounces a day. For instance, don't add chocolate chips or icing to cookies; instead, sprinkle on some nuts. Or instead of making a meat or cheese sandwich, try a nut-butter sandwich. In most markets today you can find several varieties of nut butters, from almond nut butter to cashew and even macadamia nut butter.

Peanut butter, of course, is another healthy choice; however, peanuts are not actually nuts—they're legumes. They are, however, as healthy a snack as nuts since they also contain fiber, micronutrients, and antioxidants that are essential for good health. Several studies involving peanuts, such as the ground-breaking Harvard School of Public Health Study, report that eating an ounce of nuts or one tablespoon of peanut butter five times or more a week reduced the risk of developing type II diabetes by 21–27 percent.

Purdue University conducted a study that found that peanuts and peanut butter produced greater feelings of satiety and fullness than other high-carbohydrate snacks. Peanuts kept the participants satisfied for as much as 2–2½ hours longer than other snacks. Furthermore, the participants self-adjusted their caloric intake after eating peanuts: they did not add extra calories to their daily intake. The Purdue University Study showed that nut- and peanut-eaters tend to have lower body mass index

(BMI) than non-nut-eaters. It also showed that when people ate peanuts, they naturally decreased what they ate at other times of the day, resulting in improved weight control.

Eating Out on the Mediterranean Diet (The Restaurant Survival Guide)

It's easy to follow the Mediterranean diet at home, but what do you do when you're faced with a restaurant menu? Relax. You can take the Mediterranean diet on the road and still have a great time. Just use these easy-to-follow guidelines:

- Don't go to a restaurant when you're starving. Drink a glass of water and enjoy a handful of almonds before you go. That way, you won't be tempted to devour the breadbasket while you're waiting for your meal.
- Speaking of that breadbasket, avoid it. Instead, ask to exchange it for whole grain bread and a small dish of olive oil (to be used sparingly on bread instead of margarine or butter). But remember, if you're watching your calories, a tablespoon of olive oil has 120 calories; be sure to use it in moderation.
- Choose fish or skinless poultry over red meat.
- Avoid foods that are fried; opt for grilled, baked, or broiled instead.
- Steer clear of processed or frozen food. Fresh food is healthier and tastes much better.
- Be certain that food isn't cooked with trans fats (hydrogenated oils). Ask to be sure!
- When ordering pasta, ask for whole grain.
- Order a salad with fresh vegetables and balsamic or olive oil dressing.
- Select brown rice instead of white rice.
- Avoid fruit drinks and sodas.

- Eat half your portion and take the rest home—in fact, ask for half of it to be wrapped up ahead of time, before it is even brought to the table!
- Order fresh fruit for dessert.
- Consider hot green tea after your meal.

Glossary

Al dente: Italian for pasta cooked until it is slightly resistant to the bite.

All-purpose flour: a blend of soft and hard wheat; the best type is unbleached.

Antioxidants: compounds that may have the potential to prevent numerous diseases by interfering with the cellular destruction caused by free radicals.

Basil: a very aromatic herb with a sweet, mildly pungent flavor that is widely used in Italy.

Bay leaf: another aromatic herb, with a slightly bitter taste; the greener the leaf, the more flavor it has. When fresh, the leaf is dark green on one side and lighter on the other. Properly dried bay leaf should be olive green in color.

Bruschetta: crusty slices of bread drenched with extra-virgin olive oil, rubbed with generous amounts of garlic, and grilled or toasted on both sides.

Bulgur: whole wheat kernels that are steamed, dried, and crushed. Bulgur has a tender, chewy consistency and comes in three grades: coarse, medium, and fine. The coarser size is best for pilaf, while the medium size is good for tabbouleh.

Calorie: a unit of heat energy that expresses the energy exchanges of the body and the potential energy values of food.

Canola/olive oil spread: trans fat–free, plant-based buttery spreads that can be used to replace butter and other buttery products, which often contain saturated fat and even trans fats. Examples of plant-based spreads include Smart Balance and Promise.

Carbohydrates: the source of energy gained from food; they can be either complex or simple.

Cayenne: the dried, powdered fruit of the red hot pepper. It is much like paprika in appearance and is used in small amounts to give a fiery kick to many dishes.

Cholesterol: a type of fat derived from animal sources. Cholesterol is transported through the body by carriers called lipoproteins. Excessive amounts of cholesterol circulating in the blood can build up on artery walls and eventually lead to heart attack and stroke.

Cilantro: a very pungent herb; part of the parsley family and often used instead of parsley in dishes where a stronger accent is desired.

Complex carbohydrates: energy-yielding nutrients that provide the most efficient fuel source for the body. Complex carbohydrates metabolize more slowly than simple carbohydrates, providing the body with energy over a longer period of time. Examples of complex carbohydrates are legumes, vegetables, and whole grains.

Cornmeal: a white or yellow grain (though yellow is more typical) that has a grainy texture and a sweet taste. In Italy cornmeal is called polenta.

Couscous: a type of pasta made from semolina and water. What rice is in China, couscous is in Morocco, Algeria, and Tunisia. Couscous is now available in an instant form, which just needs to be covered with boiling water.

Crostini: thin slices of crusty bread baked in an oven at 350 degrees until golden in color, rubbed with garlic, and drenched in extra-virgin olive oil.

Cumin: a dried, slightly bitter fruit that is part of the parsley family. It has a strong scent and flavor.

Dietary fiber: the parts of fruits and vegetables and whole grains that are not digested or absorbed by the body. There are two types of dietary fiber: soluble and insoluble. Soluble fiber forms a jell-like mass around food parts and helps to prevent the absorption of cholesterol by promoting its excretion. Insoluble fibers add bulk to stools and help you feel satiated.

Durum flour: flour ground from durum wheat. Durum flour is very fine flour that is very high in gluten.

Fat: one of three main classes of nutrients that provide energy to the body. Fats are either saturated or unsaturated.

Feta cheese: cheese made from pasteurized sheep's or goat's milk.

Focaccia: an Italian oven-baked round or rectangular bread filled with herbs, onions, spices, and often an array of vegetables.

Free radicals: unstable products of metabolism that have a destructive effect on cells' DNA. The damaged DNA not only suppresses the immune system but has also been implicated in the development of many diseases, such as heart disease, cancer, and other chronic illnesses.

Garlic: a member of the onion family with a distinctively rich, hot flavor (though the flavor can be mild or strong, depending on how it is sliced or chopped and how long it is cooked). Garlic has been shown to have beneficial effects on blood pressure, cholesterol, and other risk factors.

Gluten: a protein substance (especially of wheat flour) that gives cohesiveness to dough.

Harissa, hareesa, or hreesa: a fiery hot paste made by pounding together red chili peppers, spices, and olive oil. It is used to season couscous and many North African dishes.

Italian frittatas: savory omelets cooked into a thick cake brimming with potatoes and onions or other vegetables. It is most delicious when served warm from the oven.

Kesra: a dense round loaf of bread predominately seen in the Northwestern African regions, largely Morocco, Algeria, and Tunisia. Kesra is flavored with whole aniseeds or sesame seeds and is great for dipping in soups or eating with stews.

Khubz: Arab pita bread used to scoop up sauces, dips, yogurts, and liquids, or cut in half and filled with shish kabobs, falafel, or salads. Arabs eat bread with every meal and consider bread to be a divine gift from God.

Lavosh: a very crispy flat Egyptian bread.

Lipoproteins: combinations of fat and protein that transport lipids (fats) in the blood.

Low-calorie baking sweeteners: refined sugar substitutes that do well in recipes when the recipe calls for heat, such as in baking and cooking. These products usually have half or less than half the calories of refined sugar.

Mediterranean crusty country bread: a favorite, hearty, slightly sour crusty bread consumed throughout France, Italy, Spain, and Portugal.

Mint: an herb with a strong sweet aroma that is available fresh or dried. Also great as a garnish.

Monounsaturated fat: a naturally occurring heart-healthy fat found in plant foods. Research has found that monounsaturated fats actually play an important role in helping prevent heart disease and cancer. It is believed that it generally helps to maintain or raise good (HDL) cholesterol while decreasing bad (LDL) cholesterol. A few examples of foods high in monounsaturated fats are nuts, olives, and avocados.

Mozzarella: a soft spongy white cheese with a slightly sour flavor.

Non-caloric sweeteners: replacements for refined sugar that have no caloric value such as Splenda, Equal, Stevia, and Sweet'N Low.

Obesity: a condition in which a person exceeds the healthy weight for his or her height and body composition by 20% or more. The BMI, or body mass index, is used to define obesity. The BMI categories are

< 18.5	*underweight*
18.5–24.9	*normal weight*
25–29.9	*overweight*
> 30	*obese*

Oregano: a very popular Italian herb closely related to marjoram.

Paella: a variable Spanish rice dish often containing chicken, mussels, whitefish, peas, and rice, flavored with saffron, salt, pepper, and pimiento.

Parmesan cheese: a hard cheese made from semi-skim unpasteurized cow's milk.

Parsley: one of the most commonly used herbs. It adds both flavor and color to many dishes.

Pecorino: a sheep's milk cheese that has recently become more available in finer cheese shops here in the United States.

Pesto: a paste made from basil, olive oil, and pine nuts. The word comes from the Italian verb *pestare*, which means "to pound." It was often handmade using a mortar and pestle to grind the herbs, lending a wonderful coarseness in texture. It was said that this assertive green sauce was a traditional favorite of Genoese sailors. In Italy, cooks are discreet with their pesto use; a little of this rich, highly flavored sauce goes a long way. Today, pre-made pesto sauces are available in most markets. The fresh pesto in tubs usually has more flavor than the jar varieties; however, nothing is as good as homemade.

Pistou: a pounded pesto-like sauce made of nuts, olive oil, garlic, and basil. It is unique to the Mediterranean region in France and adds both body and herbaceous flavor to soups and stews.

Pita bread: a flat, round, hollow bread common to the cuisines of Africa and the Middle East.

Polenta: coarse-textured cornmeal. Pre-cooked instant polenta is now available in most markets but does not taste as good as homemade polenta.

Polyunsaturated fat: highly unsaturated fats obtained from plants like corn, sunflower, and safflower oils that help reduce bad (LDL) cholesterol levels. They are also present in food such as oily fish, walnuts, and certain types of seeds.

Ratatouille: a vegetable casserole of tomatoes, eggplant, green peppers, zucchini, onions, and seasonings.

Risotto: an Italian rice dish made with butter, chopped onion, stock or wine, and Parmesan cheese. Meats or seafood and vegetables may also be added.

Saffron: a rather expensive dried yellow crocus native to the Mediterranean with a strong yellow color and a delicate flavor that is used in many Mediterranean dishes.

Saturated fat: a type of fat found in animal foods such as red meat and poultry, and dairy products, such as butter and whole milk. Other foods high in saturated fats include tropical cooking oils such as palm and coconut oils. High intakes of saturated fats have been linked to cardiovascular disease and cancer.

Semolina: roughly ground durum wheat used to make pasta and bread. It is technically not a grain but a nutritive tissue of durum wheat, the hardest of all wheat, and it is traditionally used to make pasta.

Simple carbohydrates: sugars that are quickly absorbed into the bloodstream, providing an immediate source of energy. Food sources like candy and soda are good examples of simple carbohydrates.

Sodium-free salt substitute: salt substitutes that contain either no sodium or reduced sodium content. Examples include No Salt and Salt Sense.

Soft and hard (wheat): this refers not just to the texture of the wheat but also to the protein content. Most hard wheat is higher in protein as well as in the gluten necessary for bread making than soft wheat.

Tahini: a paste made from crushed sesame seeds.

Tapas: Spanish appetizers, often called the "little dishes of Spain."

Trans fat: a type of fat found in stick margarine, vegetable shortening, and any food product that lists hydrogenated oils as one of its ingredients. The consumption of food products containing trans fats has been linked with the development of heart disease, diabetes, obesity, and cancer.

Turmeric: a relatively inexpensive rich yellow spice with flavoring similar to saffron that is used as a replacement for saffron in many dishes. It is a member of the ginger family.

Whole wheat flour: dark whole grain flour that has not had the bran and germ milled out of it. Some whole wheats are coarser than others. The best stoneground whole wheat has a nutty wholesome flavor.

Whole wheat pastry flour: flour made from softer wheat that is more finely milled than whole wheat flour. In Italy it is used to make pizza and other pastries.

Recipe Index

A

Acorn Squash
Baked 335
Roasted................................ 334
Alfalfa Sprouts, Hummus and 454
Almonds
Broccoli with Olives and....................... 323
Toasted, Lime Sauce with 480
Anchovy
Dressing 94
Dressing, Escarole with........................... 94
and Garlic Sauce.............................. 490
and Garlic Sauce, Whole Wheat Spaghetti
with 203
Pizza, Sundried Tomato and 146
Sauce, Tomato and, with Pasta.............. 225
Angel Food Cupcakes, Orange 437
Angel Hair (Pasta)
with Fresh Marinara 304
Spicy Shrimp with 183
Antipasti 451
Appetizers
Antipasti.................................... 451
Apple, Gorgonzola, and Walnut Crostini.... 454
Avocado and Mango Salsa 455
Avocado Spread with Crusty
Garlic Toast 452
Avocado Toasts 461
Baby Shrimp on Toasted Rye 453
Bay Scallops with Smoked Paprika......... 455

Cheesy Crab Bites 458
Crispy Chicken Parmesan Tenders......... 459
Crispy Polenta Topped with a Spicy
Marinara.......................... 462
Crostini with Pesto, Prosciutto,
Mozzarella, and Sundried Tomatoes 456
Hummus and Alfalfa Sprouts 454
Italian Crostini 449
Mushroom Crostini............................ 450
Pizza Zucchini Boats 460
Roasted Garlic 445
Roasted Tomato Boats 457
Stuffed Grape Leaves (Dolmas)............. 446
Tomato and Fresh Parmesan Cheese
Bruschetta.......................... 448
Tomato and Garlic Bruschetta 447
Yogurt Sauce............................ 447
Apple(s)
Baked, Crème de Banana...................... 403
Braised, Scallops with 267
Crostini, Gorgonzola, Walnut, and........ 454
Omelet, Cheesy Apple Raisin Cinnamon ...155
Pancakes, Multigrain Nut and 168
Pie, Homestyle 423
Spiced............................ 419
-Walnut Raisin Wrap 379
Apple Sauce, Chunky 417
Apricot(s)
Drunken............................ 407
Sorbet............................417

Arborio Rice, Swiss Chard and 351
Artichoke(s)
    Baby, Spinach Fettuccine with 296
    Risotto 362
    Roasted Baby, and Parmesan Cheese 328
    Salad, Broiled 91
    Steamed 358
Arugula and Asian Pear Salad 89
Asparagus
    with Fresh Garden Herbs 317
    Gnocchi with Shrimp and 245
    Lemon Garlic 343
    Salad, Tangy Orange Roasted 71
Assorted Mushroom and Swiss
    Cheese Pizza 141
Avocado
    and Crab Stuffed Pita Pockets 366
    Dip, Chilled 463
    Halves, Broiled, and Cheddar Cheese 323
    and Mango Salsa 455
    Salad 75
    Soup, Chilled 111
    Spread, with Crusty Garlic Toast 452
    Toasts 461
    Wrap, Shrimp and 381

B

Baby Shrimp and Mozzarella
    Cheese Pizza 142
Baby Shrimp on Toasted Rye 453
Baked Acorn Squash 335
Baked Chilean Sea Bass 271
Baked Eggplant with Garlic and Basil ... 353
Baked Flounder with Capers and
    Baby Shrimp 222
Baked Meatballs 279
Baked or Grilled Mussels 238
Baked Parsnip Fries with Rosemary 341
Baked Potato Fingers with Shallots
    and Fresh Herbs 321
Baked Stuffed Trout 172
Baked Sweet Potato Fries with
    Basil Pesto 360
Baked Tilapia 195

Banana
    Buttermilk Pancakes 166
    Muffins, Healthy Banana-Nut 433
    Smoothie, Banana Peach Vanilla
       Soy Milk 443
    Toasted Sautéed, and Strawberry
       Crêpes 425
    -Walnut Loaf 386
Barley
    Broiled Chicken with Vegetables and 266
    Salad, Mushroom and 98
Basic Lentil Soup 122
Basic Rice Pilaf 352
Basil Pesto
    Baked Sweet Potato Fries with 360
    Easy 481
    Fettuccine with Smoked Salmon and 230
    Sauce 488
    Snap Peas with 336
    Bay Scallops with Smoked Paprika 455
Bean(s). *See also specific types of beans*
    Beans and More Beans 291
    Dip, Greek 468
    Mixed, Feta and 345
    Pasta e Fagioli Soup 135
    Salad, Corn and 100
    Soup, Hearty 129
Beet and Tomato Salad 104
Beets, Boiled Fresh Red 326
Black Bean(s)
    and Brown Rice 301
    Couscous, Tomatoes, and 316
    Seafood Burgers 228
Blackened Swordfish 198
Blackened Tuna Steaks with Mustard
    Ginger Sauce 217
Blackening Seasoning Mix 477
Black Olive(s)
    Bow Tie Pasta with Eggplant and 200
    Lamb and 198
    Paste 480
    Paste, Fettuccini with Provolone
       Cheese and 241
Blueberry Burst Whey Smoothie 439

Blueberry Pancakes, Multigrain Nutty
    Blueberry......................................167
Boiled Fresh Red Beets..........................326
Boneless Chicken Cutlets.......................270
Bouillabaisse.....................................174
Bow Tie Pasta with Eggplant and
    Black Olives....................................200
Branzino, Whole Roasted, with Buttery
    Lemon Sauce...................................285
Bread
    Banana-Walnut Loaf.............................386
    Cranberry Nut Whole Wheat.................389
    Egyptian Khubz (Pita Bread).................385
    Focaccia..383
    Honey Whole Wheat.............................388
    Lavosh..385
    Mixed Fruit and Nut Whole Wheat......390
    Nutty Pomegranate Whole Wheat.........391
    Nutty Whole Wheat.............................392
    Sesame (Kersa).................................387
    Sundried Tomato Basil White Wheat.....393
Bread Machine Whole Grain Thin
    Crust Pizza Dough...........................153
Broccoli
    with Almonds and Olives......................323
    Flatbread Pizzas, Pecorino and...............140
    Florets, Orzo with Feta Cheese and.......310
    with Fresh Garlic..............................317
    Frittata, Cheese and............................159
    Italian...329
    -Potato Soup with Greens.....................112
    Roasted..339
    Whole Wheat Penne with Shrimp
        and...221
Broccolini, Crispy Tender.....................330
Broccoli Rabe, Spicy, with Penne Pasta..175
Broiled Artichoke Salad..........................91
Broiled Avocado Halves and Cheddar
    Cheese..323
Broiled Chicken and Barley with
    Vegetables.....................................266
Broiled Garlic Lamb Chops...................224
Broiled Halibut Steaks with
    Tomato Pesto..................................231

Broiled Mango Chicken Breast Fillets ...219
Broiled Red Snapper with Garlic...........181
Broiled Scallops with Orange
    Ginger Sauce..................................234
Broiled Spicy Rainbow Trout................265
Broiled Spicy Turkey Burgers................220
Broiled Tuna and Tomato.....................208
Broth, Fresh Chicken..........................108
Brownies...429
Brown Rice
    Black Beans and................................301
    Mom's...359
Bruschetta
    Tomato and Fresh Parmesan Cheese......448
    Tomato and Garlic.............................447
    Brussels Sprouts, Caramelized,
        with Garlic and Red Chili Peppers....337

C

Cabbage Soup, Chunky Chicken and 127
Caesar Salad, Light................................78
Cake(s)
    Lemon...414
    Spice..398
Calamari in Spicy Red Sauce.................300
Cannellini Beans, Garlicky....................355
Cannelloni, Mushroom and Ricotta.......242
Cantaloupe Sorbet...............................404
Caramelized Brussels Sprouts with Garlic
    and Red Chili Peppers.......................337
Caramelized Onions and Roasted Kale..338
Caramelized Pears...............................434
Caramelized Pineapple and
    Pistachios......................................418
Carrot(s)
    Mashed Parsnips and..........................344
    Salad, Tunisian.................................76
Cauliflower
    Garlic Roasted..................................361
    Soup..119
Cheddar Cheese
    Broiled Avocado Halves and.................323
    Grilled Polenta with Sundried
        Tomatoes and.............................324

Cheese. *See also specific types of cheese*
Frittata, Broccoli and 159
Medallions, Greens with 74
Pizza, Assorted Mushroom and Swiss.....141
Pizza, Baby Shrimp and Mozzarella 142
Pizza, Fresh Basil and Mozzarella 141
Pizza, Smoked Salmon and Mozzarella....139
Quiche, Spinach and Swiss 272
Twice-Baked Sweet Potatoes with Fresh
    Sage and 333
Cheesy Apple Raisin Cinnamon
    Omelet 155
Cheesy Crab Bites 458
Cherries, Honey-Sweetened, Phyllo
    Tartlets with 408
Chicken
Baked, Mustard and Smoked Paprika 257
Breast Fillets, Broiled Mango 219
Breasts, Crusted.....................................241
Breasts, Rosemary Roasted.....................297
Breasts, Stuffed Sesame 218
Broiled, and Barley with Vegetables 266
Broth, Fresh...108
Cacciatore 255
Crunchy, and Fruit Salad........................96
Cutlets, Boneless 270
and Eggplant 179
and Feta...239
Great Northern Beans and.....................173
Grilled, Pomodora Sauce and 274
Lemony, Vegetables and..........................210
Parmesan Tenders, Crispy 459
and Penne Pasta in a Garlic Sauce..........247
Pesto Wrap 380
Piccata...207
with Pomegranate Sauce 206
Soup, Chicken Escarole 132
Soup, Chunky Chicken and Cabbage 127
Soup, Lemony Chicken and Orzo 110
Soup, Mom's..136
Spanish Paella with Saffron Rice,
    Seafood, and.....................................170
Spicy, with Couscous 190
and Spicy Hummus.................................298

White Beans and Wild Mushrooms
    with 259
and Wild Rice with Garden Vegetables ...248
Yummy Marinade for 494
Chicken Rub 477
Spicy 478
Chickpea(s)
with Couscous..347
and Garden Vegetables............................91
Pita Pockets 370
Sandwich, Fresh Spinach and 372
Soup, Savory Mediterranean..................123
Chilean Sea Bass, Baked 271
Chilled Avocado Dip 463
Chilled Avocado Soup 111
Chilled Cucumber Soup 133
Chilled Stuffed Pasta Shells 313
Chilly Tomato Soup 125
Chive
Sauce, Grilled Whole Rainbow
    Trout and...216
Vinaigrette...498
Chocolate
Bites 471
Cupcakes, Healthy.................................432
Mousse Whey Smoothie 442
Pudding, Dark Double 436
Smoothie, Chocolate Raspberry
    Soy Milk...444
Sweet Treats...438
Chowder
Chunky Fish, with Saffron......................131
Red Clam 117
Chunky Apple Sauce 417
Chunky Chicken and Cabbage Soup 127
Chunky Fish Chowder with Saffron 131
Chutney, Mango 466
Cinnamon
Couscous..350
and Flaxseed Wafers...............................472
Honey Dip, Fresh Fruit Kabobs and......401
Citrus Scallops and Shrimp 191
Clam(s)
Bouillabaisse..174

Chowder, Red.................................117
Pasta with Wine, Red Hot Peppers,
   and..202
   Red Clam Sauce 489
   Red Clam Sauce, Pasta with......201
Classic Greek Salad 77
Classic Spinach and Pine Nuts 312
Classic Tabbouleh 69
Cod(fish)
   Bouillabaisse..............................174
   Grilled.....................................254
   in Sundried Tomato Pesto Sauce 232
Cole Slaw, Spicy...........................106
Compote
   Peach Marsala...........................399
   Sweet Plum...............................430
   Vanilla-Rhubarb 415
Cookies
   Meringue..................................427
   Orange Macaroons 430
   Raspberry Meringues...................428
   Sour Cream and Walnut...............421
   Cooler, Summer Rhubarb.............440
Cool Refreshing Orange Pops 415
Corn and Bean Salad.........................100
Cornish Hens, Roasted........................273
Corn on the Cob, Great 320
Cornstarch Paste 483
Couscous
   Chickpeas with.........................347
   Cinnamon.................................350
   Fruit-Glazed Salmon with 184
   Garlic, Sautéed Mixed Fish over 244
   Lemon-Almond..........................335
   Mushroom, Sautéed Shrimp and 278
   and Parsley Salad, Easy 83
   Spicy 348
   Spicy Chicken with 190
   Tomatoes, Black Beans, and............316
   with Turnips and Greens................325
Crab
   and Avocado Stuffed Pita Pockets 366
   Bites, Cheesy 458
   Cakes......................................243

   Pasta Fresca with Lemon and.........260
   Patty Burgers 235
   Steamed Dungeness....................215
Cranberry Nut Whole Wheat Bread 389
Creamy Green Garden Soup................109
Crème de Banana Baked Apples 403
Crêpes, Toasted Sautéed Banana and
   Strawberry...........................425
Crispy Chicken Parmesan Tenders 459
Crispy Polenta Topped with a Spicy
   Marinara 462
Crispy Tender Broccolini 330
Crispy Tender Ratatouille 318
Crispy Thin Whole Wheat Pizza
   Dough 150
Crostini
   Apple, Gorgonzola, and Walnut 454
   Italian.....................................449
   Mushroom 450
   with Pesto, Prosciutto, Mozzarella,
      and Sundried Tomatoes 456
Crunchy Chicken and Fruit Salad 96
Crusted Chicken Breasts 241
Cucumber
   Salad.......................................100
   Salsa.......................................465
   Soup, Chilled 133
   Yogurt Dip, Herb 469
   and Yogurt Salad, Syrian...............68
Cupcakes
   Healthy Chocolate......................432
   Orange Angel Food 437

D

Dark Double Chocolate Pudding 436
Dates, Stuffed.................................402
Deliciously Sweetened Yogurt...............412
Desserts
   Apricot Sorbet 417
   Brownies..................................429
   Cantaloupe Sorbet......................404
   Caramelized Pears.......................434
   Caramelized Pineapple and Pistachios.....418
   Chocolate Sweet Treats 438

Chunky Apple Sauce 417
Cool Refreshing Orange Pops...............415
Crème de Banana Baked Apples 403
Dark Double Chocolate Pudding 436
Deliciously Sweetened Yogurt 412
Drunken Apricots...................................407
Drunken Peaches....................................406
Drunken Strawberries............................412
Easy Peach Cobbler 413
Figs in Plain Yogurt 396
Fresh Fruit and Nut Platter...................395
Fresh Fruit in Yogurt with Rum.............401
Fresh Fruit Kabobs and Cinnamon
    Honey Dip 401
Fresh Pineapple in Spicy Rum Syrup 431
Fruited Nutty Pastry Rolls 426
Healthy Banana-Nut Muffins 433
Healthy Chocolate Cupcakes.................432
Homestyle Apple Pie 423
Honeydew Sorbet...................................405
Honey Mousse Delight...........................397
Honey Nests 410
Lemon Cakes..414
Lemon Sherbet 420
Meringue Cookies 427
Meringue Key Lime Dessert Cups 422
Moroccan Sweet Oranges 409
Orange Angel Food Cupcakes 437
Orange Macaroons 430
Peach Marsala Compote 399
Phyllo Tartlets with Honey-Sweetened
    Cherries..408
Plum Sorbet 435
Pumpkin Pudding 409
Raspberry Meringues.............................428
Sautéed Peaches or Nectarines
    with Maple Syrup 399
Sour Cream and Walnut Cookies 421
Spice Cake..398
Spiced Apples 419
Strawberries Amaretto 419
Strawberries and Balsamic Syrup 405
Strawberry and Poached Pears...............395
Strawberry-Rhubarb Quinoa Pudding.....411

Strawberry Sauce 395
Strawberry-Walnut Trifle.......................416
Stuffed Dates...402
Sweet Italian Rice Pudding 402
Sweet Mango Mousse 400
Sweet Plum Compote.............................430
Toasted Crêpe Cups with Fresh
    Berries in a Lemon Yogurt Sauce.......424
Toasted Sautéed Banana and Strawberry
    Crêpes 425
Vanilla-Rhubarb Compote 415

Dill Sauce
Encrusted Red Snapper and..................213
Lightly Pan-Fried Crusted Trout with....284

Dip
Chilled Avocado 463
Cinnamon Honey, Fresh Fruit
    Kabobs and......................................401
Cucumber Salsa.....................................465
Greek Bean..468
Greek Feta and Walnut..........................467
Herb Cucumber Yogurt 469
Hummus...467
Hummus with Tahini 470
Mango Chutney 466
Mediterranean Salsa...............................465
Remoulade Dipping Sauce 466
Roasted Pepper 470
Smoked Trout..464

Dipping Sauce, Remoulade 466
Dolmas 446
Dressing
Anchovy 94
Chive Vinaigrette...................................498
Fresh Fig Vinaigrette.............................497
A Great Salad Dressing 496
Lemon...495
Lemon-Pepper.......................................496
Mint Vinaigrette....................................498
Orange-Mustard, Kale with 322
Shallot-Balsamic Vinaigrette..................499
Sicilian 497
Walnut 81
Yogurt 495

Drunken Apricots....................................407
Drunken Peaches....................................406
Drunken Strawberries 412

E

Easy Baked Eggplant Parmesan 275
Easy Basil Pesto.....................................481
Easy Couscous Parsley Salad....................83
Easy Peach Cobbler 413
Easy Pizza Sauce....................................149
Easy Turkey Meatloaf.............................252
Egg(s)
    Cheesy Apple Raisin Cinnamon
        Omelet 155
    -Lemon Pasta Soup...............................107
    Poached, in a Garden............................156
    Spanish Omelet.....................................158
    Vegetable Omelet with Pesto 163
Eggplant
    Baked, with Garlic and Basil..................354
    Bow Tie Pasta with Black Olives and 200
    Chicken and...179
    Crispy Tender Ratatouille......................318
    Grilled...356
    Parmesan, Easy Baked 275
    Pizza, Tomato, Basil, and 143
    Salad, Moroccan.....................................79
    Sauce, Hardy...481
    Sicilian-Style Linguine with Roasted
        Peppers and 177
    Soup...115
    Soup, with Dry Sherry and Feta Cheese..134
    Spicy...308
Egyptian Khubz (Pita Bread).................385
Encrusted Red Snapper and Dill Sauce.....213
Endive Spinach Salad 88
Escarole Chicken Soup 132
Escarole with Anchovy Dressing...............94
Exotic Pear Salad...................................101

F

Fava Bean(s)
    and More Beans.....................................291
    with Pesto Sauce...................................344

    Salad, Savory Greek 70
    White, Salad, Savory Greek 70
Fennel
    Salad...75
    Tuscan Braised.....................................346
Feta (Cheese)
    Chicken and...239
    Eggplant Soup with Dry Sherry and......134
    Greek Dip, Walnut and 467
    and Mixed Beans...................................345
    Orzo with Broccoli Florets and..............310
    Pasta, Greek Olive and 67
    Soup, Spinach and.................................130
Fettuccine (Fettuccini)
    with Provolone Cheese and Black
        Olive Paste.............................241
    with Smoked Salmon and Basil Pesto.....230
    with Sundried Tomatoes and Goat
        Cheese....................................204
Fiery Tomato and Basil Pizza Sauce........148
Fig(s)
    in Plain Yogurt 396
    Salad, Prosciutto and 90
    Vinaigrette, Fresh Fig............................497
Fish. *See also specific types of fish*
    Bouillabaisse..174
    Branzino, Whole Roasted, with
        Buttery Lemon Sauce..............285
    Chowder, with Saffron, Chunky............131
    Great Marinade for 493
    Parmesan-Crusted 289
    Sautéed Mixed, over Garlic Couscous....244
    Smoked, and Roasted Pepper
        Sandwich................................373
Flaxseed and Cinnamon Wafers.............472
Florentine Roasted Pork 205
Flounder
    Baked, with Capers and Baby Shrimp....222
    Tahini Baked 189
Focaccia...383
French Pistou Soup 128
Fresh Basil and Mozzarella
    Cheese Pizza 141
Fresh Chicken Broth 108

Fresh Chopped Garden Salad 99
Fresh Fig Vinaigrette 497
Fresh Fruit
    Kabobs, and Cinnamon Honey Dip......401
    and Nut Platter...................................395
    in Yogurt with Rum.............................401
Fresh Garden Gazpacho.........................124
Fresh Herb Sauce, Rigatoni in a 287
Freshly Chopped Salad with Walnut
    Dressing 81
Fresh Pineapple in Spicy Rum Syrup.....431
Fresh Spinach with Roasted
    Mushrooms 340
Fresh Stewed Tomatoes 332
Frittata
    Broccoli and Cheese 159
    Ham and Zucchini 160
    Mixed Vegetable 157
    Zucchini..162
Fruit. *See also Fresh Fruit*
    -Glazed Salmon with Couscous 184
    Salad, Crunchy Chicken and 96
Fruited Nutty Pastry Rolls.....................426
Fusilli and Fresh Tomato.......................283

G

Garden Vegetables
    Chicken and Wild Rice with 248
    Chickpeas and 91
    Fresh Chopped Garden Salad 99
    Soup, Creamy Green Garden.................109
Garlic
    Pasta..189
    Rice..315
    Roasted..445
    Roasted Cauliflower.............................361
    Salmon Linguini.................................269
Garlicky Cannellini Beans 355
Garlicky Swiss Chard 319
Gazpacho, Fresh Garden........................124
Gingered Green Beans and Pea Pods 357
Ginger Garlic Marinade 493
Glaze, Sweet and Spicy 479
Gnocchi with Shrimp and Asparagus.....245

Goat Cheese
    Fettuccine with Sundried
        Tomatoes and 204
    Lemony Pasta with Spinach and 249
    and Pesto Sandwich 377
    -Stuffed Tomatoes...................................68
Gorgonzola Crostini, Apple,
    Walnut, and....................................454
Grape Leaves, Stuffed 446
Great Corn on the Cob 320
Great Fish Marinade...............................493
A Great Marinade...................................494
Great Northern Beans and Chicken.......173
A Great Salad Dressing...........................496
Great Tuna Salad on Whole Grain
    Toast...375
Greek Bean Dip.....................................468
Greek Feta and Walnut Dip 467
Greek Olive and Feta Cheese Pasta..........67
Greek Rice...314
Greek Salad, Classic 77
Green Beans
    and Baby Portobellos 360
    Gingered, Pea Pods and 357
Greens. *See also specific types of greens*
    with Cheese Medallions..........................74
    Couscous with Turnips and 325
    Mediterranean Mixed 72
    Potato-Broccoli Soup with.....................112
Grilled Blackened Salmon 303
Grilled Chili Tuna Sandwich.................378
Grilled Citrus Salmon with
    Garlic Greens.................................176
Grilled Cod 254
Grilled Eggplant....................................356
Grilled Grouper.....................................240
Grilled Jumbo Portobello Mushrooms....346
Grilled Jumbo Portobello Mushroom
    Sandwich 367
Grilled Polenta with Cheddar
    Cheese and Sundried Tomatoes 324
Grilled Tilapia.......................................223
Grilled Whole Rainbow Trout a
    nd Chive Sauce 216

Grilled Whole Sea Bass............................306
Grouper
    Grilled...240
    Lightly Breaded Grilled 193

H

Halibut
    Pan-Seared, with Lemon-Caper Sauce.....293
    Steaks, Broiled, with Tomato Pesto 231
Ham and Zucchini Frittata....................160
Hardy Eggplant Sauce 481
Harissa (Red Pepper Spice).....................476
Healthy Banana-Nut Muffins 433
Healthy Chocolate Cupcakes.................432
Hearty Bean Soup 129
Herb Cucumber Yogurt Dip..................469
Herbed Potato Salad................................92
Homestyle Apple Pie..............................423
Honeydew Sorbet...................................405
Honey Mousse Delight 397
Honey Mustard Sauce 486
Honey Mustard Shrimp 263
Honey Nests...410
Honey Whole Wheat Bread....................388
Horseradish Encrusted Salmon 211
Hummus
    and Alfalfa Sprouts 454
    Dip...467
    Spicy, Chicken and 298
    Spicy, in Toasted Pita Loaves..................369
    with Tahini Dip.....................................470

I

Italian Broccoli.....................................329
Italian Crostini......................................449
Italian Egg Drop Soup...........................121
Italian Minestrone Soup with Pesto.......126
Italian Poached Scallops 192

K

Kale
    with Orange-Mustard Dressing..............322
    Orecchiette with Spinach, Toasted Bread
       Crumbs, Pine Nuts, and, in a Red Sauce.268

    Roasted, Caramelized Onions and.........338
    Sautéed..336
    Sautéed, and Spinach with Mushrooms
       and Tomato 327
Kersa...387
Key Lime Dessert Cups, Meringue.........422
Khubz (Pita Bread)
    Egyptian...385
    Stuffed Whole Wheat 368

L

Lamb
    and Black Olives....................................198
    Chops, Broiled Garlic............................224
    Ground, Rigatoni with 199
    Skewered Mediterranean Grilled, and
       Vegetables 171
    Wrap 364
Lasagna
    Made Easy 280
    Meatless..227
Lavosh...385
Leek Potato Soup with Smoked Salmon...137
Lemon
    -Almond Couscous................................335
    Cakes..414
    -Caper Sauce, Pan-Seared Halibut with 293
    Dressing 495
    -Egg Pasta Soup....................................107
    Garlic Asparagus...................................343
    -Pepper Salad Dressing 496
    -Pepper Salmon 282
    -Pepper Tilapia, Pan-Seared 294
    Sherbet...420
    Shrimp Pasta 305
    Yogurt Sauce, Toasted Crêpe Cups
       with Fresh Berries in 424
Lemony Chicken and Orzo Soup 110
Lemony Chicken and Vegetables 210
Lemony Pasta with Goat Cheese and
    Spinach..249
Lentil Soup, Basic 122
Lentil Stew..302
Light Caesar Salad..................................78

Lightly Breaded Grilled Grouper...........193
Lightly Pan-Fried Crusted Trout
   with Dill Sauce...................................284
Lime Sauce with Toasted Almonds........480
Linguine (Linguini)
   Garlic Salmon.......................................269
   and Mixed Seafood...............................197
   Sicilian-Style, with Eggplant and
      Roasted Peppers...........................177
Lobster, Bouillabaisse...........................174

M

Macaroons, Orange...............................430
Main dishes
   Angel Hair with Fresh Marinara............304
   Baked Chilean Sea Bass........................271
   Baked Flounder with Capers and Baby
      Shrimp..222
   Baked Meatballs....................................279
   Baked or Grilled Mussels......................238
   Baked Stuffed Trout.............................172
   Baked Tilapia..195
   Beans and More Beans..........................291
   Black Beans and Brown Rice.................301
   Black Bean Seafood Burgers..................228
   Blackened Swordfish.............................198
   Blackened Tuna Steaks with Mustard
      Ginger Sauce................................217
   Boneless Chicken Cutlets......................270
   Bouillabaisse...174
   Bow Tie Pasta with Eggplant and Black
      Olives..200
   Broiled Chicken and Barley with
      Vegetables....................................266
   Broiled Garlic Lamb Chops...................224
   Broiled Halibut Steaks with Tomato
      Pesto..231
   Broiled Mango Chicken Breast Fillets....219
   Broiled Red Snapper with Garlic...........181
   Broiled Scallops with Orange Ginger
      Sauce...234
   Broiled Spicy Rainbow Trout.................265
   Broiled Spicy Turkey Burgers.................220
   Broiled Tuna and Tomato......................208

Calamari in Spicy Red Sauce.................300
Chicken and Eggplant...........................179
Chicken and Feta..................................239
Chicken and Penne Pasta in a Garlic
   Sauce...247
Chicken and Spicy Hummus..................298
Chicken and Wild Rice with Garden
   Vegetables..248
Chicken Cacciatore...............................255
Chicken Piccata....................................207
Chicken with Pomegranate Sauce..........206
Citrus Scallops and Shrimp...................191
Codfish in Sundried Tomato Pesto
   Sauce...232
Crab Cakes...243
Crab Patty Burgers...............................235
Crusted Chicken Breasts.......................241
Easy Baked Eggplant Parmesan.............275
Easy Turkey Meatloaf............................252
Encrusted Red Snapper and Dill Sauce.....213
Fettuccine with Smoked Salmon
   and Basil Pesto....................................230
Fettuccine with Sundried Tomatoes
   and Goat Cheese..................................204
Fettuccini with Provolone Cheese
   and Black Olive Paste..........................241
Florentine Roasted Pork........................205
Fruit-Glazed Salmon with Couscous......184
Fusilli and Fresh Tomato.......................283
Garlic Pasta..189
Garlic Salmon Linguini.........................269
Gnocchi with Shrimp and Asparagus.....245
Great Northern Beans and Chicken.......173
Grilled Blackened Salmon.....................303
Grilled Citrus Salmon with Garlic
   Greens...176
Grilled Cod..254
Grilled Grouper....................................240
Grilled Tilapia......................................223
Grilled Whole Rainbow Trout and
   Chive Sauce...216
Grilled Whole Sea Bass.........................306
Honey Mustard Shrimp.........................263
Horseradish-Encrusted Salmon.............211

Italian Poached Scallops............................192
Lamb and Black Olives............................198
Lasagna Made Easy.................................280
Lemon-Pepper Salmon 282
Lemon Shrimp Pasta 305
Lemony Chicken and Vegetables 210
Lemony Pasta with Goat Cheese and
    Spinach...249
Lentil Stew 302
Lightly Breaded Grilled Grouper 193
Lightly Pan-Fried Crusted Trout
    with Dill Sauce 284
Linguine and Mixed Seafood 197
Meatless Lasagna 227
Mom's Turkey Burgers 229
Mushroom and Ricotta Cannelloni 242
Mussels in Spicy Red Sauce 237
Mustard and Smoked Paprika Baked
    Chicken..257
Orange Horseradish-Encrusted Scallops....214
Orecchiette Pasta and Roasted
    Tomatoes 292
Orecchiette with Spinach, Kale, Toasted
    Bread Crumbs, and Pine Nuts in
    a Red Sauce 268
Pan-Grilled Ground Pork Burgers..........236
Pan Roasted Salmon Fillets....................271
Pan-Seared Halibut with Lemon-Caper
    Sauce 293
Pan-Seared Lemon-Pepper Tilapia 294
Pan-Seared Parmesan Cheese Scallops
    with Rice Pilaf 281
Parmesan-Crusted Fish 289
Pasta and White Beans............................288
Pasta Fresca with Fresh Crab
    and Lemon 260
Pasta Primavera with Shrimp 185
Pasta with Clams, Wine, and Red Hot
    Peppers 202
Pasta with Pine Nuts and Scallops 182
Pasta with Red Clam Sauce.....................201
Pasta with Salmon Sauce.........................256
Pasta with Tofu in a Spicy Marinara
    Sauce 295

Penne with Pancetta and Mushrooms 258
Penne with Rosemary and Balsamic
    Vinegar...178
Peppered Fillet of Sole 264
Pesto Stuffed Shells.................................187
Pomodora Sauce 274
Pomodora Sauce and Grilled Chicken 274
Pork Chops and Sage...............................251
Pork Marsala..246
Rigatoni in a Fresh Herb Sauce..............287
Rigatoni with Ground Lamb 199
Roasted Cornish Hens.............................273
Roasted Salmon with Wilted Spinach 261
Roasted Seafood Medley..........................250
Rosemary Roasted Chicken Breasts 297
Salmon Cakes with Sour Cream
    Dill Sauce 212
Salmon with Smoked Paprika.................290
Sardines Pasta with Lemon and Garlic ...286
Sautéed Mixed Fish over Garlic
    Couscous...244
Sautéed Shrimp and Mushroom
    Couscous...278
Scallops with Braised Apples...................267
Seared Golden Sea Scallops.....................282
Shrimp in Spicy Black Bean Sauce.........209
Sicilian-Style Linguine with Eggplant
    and Roasted Peppers 177
Skewered Mediterranean Grilled
    Lamb and Vegetables 171
Spanish Paella with Saffron Rice,
    Seafood, and Chicken 170
Spicy Broccoli Rabe with Penne Pasta....175
Spicy Chicken with Couscous 190
Spicy Eggplant..308
Spicy Mediterranean Pasta 276
Spicy Rigatoni with Mussels 196
Spicy Shrimp with Angel Hair Pasta 183
Spicy Sole 169
Spicy Stuffed Tilapia...............................194
Spicy Whole Wheat Capellini
    with Garlic 180
Spinach and Swiss Cheese Quiche 272
Spinach Fettuccine with Baby Artichokes......296

Steamed Dungeness Crab 215

Steamed Mussels with Garlic and Dry
    Vermouth 226

Steamed Sea Bass 188

Stuffed Sesame Chicken Breasts............218

Stuffed Zucchini with Vegetables
    and Sweet Italian Sausage................262

Tahini Baked Flounder 189

Tomato and Anchovy Sauce with Pasta.....225

Trout Almandine 233

Turkey Meatballs with Whole Grain
    Pasta and Tomato Sauce...................299

Turkey Tetrazzini 253

Turkish Mussel Stew 186

Veal Scaloppine 307

White Beans and Smoked Paprika
    Shrimp 277

White Beans and Wild Mushrooms
    with Chicken..................................259

Whole Roasted Branzino with Buttery
    Lemon Sauce 285

Whole Wheat Penne with Shrimp
    and Broccoli 221

Whole Wheat Spaghetti with
    Anchovy and Garlic Sauce 203

Mango
    Chutney 466
    Mousse, Sweet 400
    Salsa, Avocado and 455

Marinade
    Ginger Garlic 493
    Great Fish......................................493
    A Great Marinade...........................494
    Yummy, for Chicken 494

Marinara Sauce, Simply Great 491

Mashed Parsnips and Carrots 344

Meatless Lasagna...............................227

Meatless Sloppy Joe............................376

Meatloaf, Easy Turkey.........................252

Mediterranean Mixed Greens 72

Mediterranean Salsa 465

Melon Madness Whey Smoothie...........444

Meringue(s)
    Cookies 427

Key Lime Dessert Cups 422
    Raspberry 428

Minestrone Soup with Pesto, Italian......126

Mint Vinaigrette Dressing....................498

Mixed Fruit and Nut Whole Wheat
    Bread 390

Mixed Spices 475

Mixed Vegetable Frittata 157

Mom's Brown Rice 359

Mom's Chicken Soup 136

Mom's Turkey Burgers 229

Moroccan Eggplant Salad......................79

Moroccan Sweet Oranges 409

Mousse, Sweet Mango...........................400

Muffins, Healthy Banana-Nut...............433

Multigrain Apple and Nut Pancakes......168

Multigrain Nutty Blueberry Pancakes.....167

Mushroom(s). *See also* **Portobello**
    Mushroom(s)
    and Barley Salad 98
    Cannelloni, Ricotta and.........................242
    Couscous, Sautéed Shrimp and..............278
    Crostini 450
    Penne with Pancetta and.....................258
    Pizza, Swiss Cheese and 141
    Pizza, Wild Mushroom.......................145
    Polenta with Garlic and 355
    and Ricotta Cannelloni........................242
    Roasted, Fresh Spinach with 340
    Sautéed Kale and Spinach with Tomato and
        327
    -Shallot Sauce 482
    Wild, White Beans with Chicken and 259
    Wrap, Spicy 371

Mussel(s)
    Baked or Grilled 238
    in Spicy Red Sauce 237
    Spicy Rigatoni with 196
    Steamed, with Garlic and Dry Vermouth ...226
    Stew, Turkish 186

Mustard and Smoked Paprika Baked
    Chicken 257

Mustard Ginger Sauce Blackened Tuna
    Steaks with 217

N

Nectarines, Sautéed, with Maple Syrup 399
North African Zucchini Salad.................73
Nut(s). See also specific types of nuts
    Fresh Fruit and Nut Platter...................395
    Fruited Nutty Pastry Rolls......................426
    Muffins, Healthy Banana Nut..............433
    Multigrain Apple and Nut Pancakes......168
    Multigrain Nutty Blueberry Pancakes....167
Nutty Pomegranate Whole Wheat
    Bread 391
Nutty Whole Wheat Bread....................392

O

Old-Fashioned Oyster Stew...................114
Olive(s)
    Black, Bow Tie Pasta with Eggplant
        and 200
    Black, Lamb and...................................198
    Black Olive Paste...................................480
    Black Olive Paste, Fettuccini with
        Provolone Cheese and....................241
    Broccoli with Almonds and 323
    Greek Olive and Feta Cheese Pasta 67
Omelet
    Cheesy Apple Raisin Cinnamon 155
    Spanish...158
    Vegetable, with Pesto 163
Onions, Caramelized, and Roasted
    Kale 338
Orange(s)
    Angel Food Cupcakes...........................437
    Ginger Sauce 478
    Ginger Sauce, Broiled Scallops with.......234
    Horseradish-Encrusted Scallops.............214
    Macaroons..430
    Moroccan Sweet 409
    -Mustard Dressing, Kale with 322
    Pops, Cool Refreshing 415
Orecchiette
    and Roasted Tomatoes 292
    with Spinach, Kale, Toasted Bread
        Crumbs, and Pine Nuts in a Red
        Sauce 268

Orzo
    with Feta Cheese and Broccoli Florets....310
    Soup, Lemony Chicken and 110
Oven-Roasted Potato Wedges................326
Oyster Stew, Old-Fashioned..................114

P

Paella, Spanish, with Saffron Rice,
    Seafood, and Chicken 170
Pancakes
    Banana Buttermilk 166
    Multigrain Apple and Nut.....................168
    Multigrain Nutty Blueberry...................167
    Strawberry Buttermilk 165
Pancetta, Penne with Mushrooms and 258
Pan-Grilled Ground Pork Burgers 236
Pan Roasted Salmon Fillets 271
Pan-Seared Halibut with
    Lemon-Caper Sauce...........................293
Pan-Seared Lemon-Pepper Tilapia 294
Pan-Seared Parmesan Cheese Scallops
    with Rice Pilaf 281
Parmesan-Crusted Fish...........................289
Parsnip(s)
    Fries, Baked, with Rosemary.................341
    Mashed, and Carrots 344
Pass the Peas, Please 320
Pasta. See also specific types and shapes
    of pasta
    with Clams, Wine, and Red Hot
        Peppers 202
    Fresca, with Fresh Crab and Lemon.......260
    Garlic 189
    Gnocchi with Shrimp and Asparagus.....245
    Greek Olive and Feta Cheese.................67
    Lemon Shrimp 305
    Lemony, with Goat Cheese and
        Spinach......................................249
    with Pine Nuts and Scallops 182
    Primavera, with Shrimp.........................185
    with Red Clam Sauce 201
    with Salmon Sauce 256
    Sardines, with Lemon and Garlic...........286
    and Shrimp Salad 85

Soup, Egg-Lemon.................................107
Spicy Mediterranean............................276
with Tofu in a Spicy Marinara Sauce......295
Tomato and Anchovy Sauce with...........225
and Tomato Sauce, Turkey Meatballs
    with 299
and White Beans 288
Pasta e Fagioli Soup............................ 135
Pasta Salad
Shrimp and 85
Summer...93
Tomato..102
Pasta Sauce, Sardine 487
Paste
Black Olive...480
Cornstarch 483
Pastry Rolls, Fruited Nutty....................426
Pea(s)
Pass the Peas, Please.............................320
Pods, Gingered Green Beans and...........357
Snap, with Basil Pesto...........................336
Snow, Spicy 334
Snow Pea Salad 104
Peach(es)
Cobbler, Easy 413
Drunken...406
Marsala, Compote 399
Sautéed, with Maple Syrup.....................399
Smoothie, Banana Peach Vanilla Soy
    Milk 443
Pea Pods, Gingered Green Beans and 357
Pear(s)
Caramelized...434
Poached, Strawberry and 395
Salad, Asian Pear and Arugula 89
Salad, Exotic..101
Salad, Walnut and 95
Salad, Watercress and.............................97
Sandwich, Cream Cheese, Red Onion,
    and 377
Penne
Chicken in a Garlic Sauce with..............247
with Pancetta and Mushrooms 258
with Rosemary and Balsamic Vinegar 178

Whole Wheat, with Shrimp
    and Broccoli 221
Pepper(s)
Crispy Tender Ratatouille 318
Dip, Roasted Pepper 470
Pizza, Spicy Sweet................................144
Red Hot, Pasta with Clams, Wine,
    and 202
Roasted..311
Roasted, Sandwich, Smoked Fish and....373
Roasted, Sicilian-Style Linguine with
    Eggplant and 177
Sandwich, Smoked Fish and Roasted
    Pepper 373
Sicilian-Style Linguine with Eggplant
    and 177
Peppered Fillet of Sole............................264
Peppery Watercress Salad.........................92
Pesto
Basil 488
Basil, Baked Sweet Potato Fries with 360
Basil, Fettuccine with Smoked
    Salmon and 230
Basil, Snap Peas with 336
Chicken Pesto Wrap 380
Crostini with Prosciutto, Mozzarella,
    Sundried Tomatoes, and 456
Easy Basil 481
and Goat Cheese Sandwich 377
Italian Minestrone Soup with 126
Spicy Pistachio....................................486
-Stuffed Shells.....................................187
Sundried Tomato 485
Tomato, Broiled Halibut Steaks with.....231
Vegetable Omelet with 163
Pesto Sauce
Fava Beans with...................................344
Red...479
Spicy Garlicky 484
Sundried Tomato, Codfish in,................232
Phyllo Tartlets with Honey-Sweetened
    Cherries.....................................408
Pie, Homestyle Apple..........................423
Pineapple

Caramelized, and Pistachios....................418
Fresh, in Spicy Rum Syrup 431
Smoothie, Pineapple Delight Whey.......443

Pine Nuts
Orecchiette with Spinach, Kale, Toasted
   Bread Crumbs, and, in a Red Sauce 268
Pasta with Scallops and..........................182
Spinach and, Classic 312

Pistachio(s)
Caramelized Pineapple and....................418
Pesto, Spicy 486
Pistou Soup, French...............................128

Pita Loaves
Spicy Hummus in Toasted......................369
Stuffed Whole Wheat Khubz.................368
Pita Pockets. See also Khubz
   (Pita Bread)
Chickpea 370
Crab and Avocado Stuffed 366

Pizza
Assorted Mushroom and Swiss Cheese....141
Baby Shrimp and Mozzarella Cheese 142
Broccoli and Pecorino Flatbread 140
Fresh Basil and Mozzarella Cheese.........141
Margherita...142
Smoked Salmon and Mozzarella
   Cheese 139
Spicy Sweet Pepper 144
Sundried Tomato and Anchovy 146
Tomato, Eggplant, and Basil..................143
Wild Mushroom....................................145

Pizza Dough
Bread Machine Whole Grain Thin
   Crust 153
Crispy Thin Whole Wheat.....................150
Thin Crust...152
Whole Wheat 151

Pizza Sauce
Easy...149
Fiery Tomato and Basil 148
Spicy Garlic, Olive Oil, and Sundried
   Tomato 148
Traditional...147
Pizza Zucchini Boats 460

Plum
Compote, Sweet 430
Sorbet..435
Poached Eggs in a Garden 156
Polenta..354
Crispy, Topped with a Spicy Marinara.......462
Grilled, with Cheddar Cheese
   and Sundried Tomatoes 324
with Mushrooms and Garlic..................355
Pomegranate Molasses, Thick................484
Pomegranate Sauce, Chicken with.........206
Pomodora Sauce....................................274
   and Grilled Chicken 274
Pork
Burgers, Pan-Grilled 236
Chops, and Sage....................................251
Chops, Sage and....................................251
Florentine Roasted.................................205
Marsala..246
Porridge, Quinoa and Raisins................161
Portobello Mushroom(s)
Baby, Green Beans and 360
Burger, with Caramelized Onions..........374
Grilled Jumbo..346
Sandwich, Grilled Jumbo.......................367
Sautéed, with Garlic and Parsley............354
Potato(es)
-Broccoli Soup with Greens...................112
Fingers, Baked, with Shallots and
   Fresh Herbs 321
Salad, Herbed..92
Soup, Potato Leek, with Smoked
   Salmon 137
Wedges, Oven Roasted..........................326
Prosciutto
Crostini with Pesto, Mozzarella,
   Sundried Tomatoes, and 456
Salad, Fig and..90
Pudding
Chocolate, Dark Double 436
Pumpkin 409
Quinoa, Strawberry-Rhubarb 411
Rice, Sweet Italian 402
Pumpkin Pudding...................................409

Q

Quiche, Spinach and Swiss Cheese 272
Quinoa and Raisins Porridge 161
Quinoa Pudding, Strawberry-Rhubarb 411

R

Raspberry Meringues 428
Ratatouille, Crispy Tender 318
Red Cabbage Salad, Sweet 103
Red Clam Chowder 117
Red Clam Sauce 489
    Pasta with 201
Red Pepper
    Roasted, Sandwich 363
    Spice (Harissa) 476
Red Pesto Sauce 479
Red Sauce, Spicy, Mussels in 237
Red Snapper
    Broiled with Garlic 181
    Encrusted, and Dill Sauce 213
Remoulade Dipping Sauce 466
Rhubarb
    Cooler, Summer 440
    -Strawberry Quinoa Pudding 411
    -Vanilla Compote 415
Rice
    Arborio, Swiss Chard and 351
    Brown, Black Beans and 301
    Brown, Mom's 359
    Garlic 315
    Greek 314
    Pilaf, Basic 352
    Pilaf, Pan-Seared Parmesan Cheese
        Scallops with 281
    Risotto, Artichoke 362
    Saffron 309
    Saffron, Spanish Paella with Seafood,
        Chicken, and 170
    Wild, Chicken and, with Garden
        Vegetables 248
Rice Pudding, Sweet Italian 402
Ricotta and Mushroom Cannelloni 242
Rigatoni
    in a Fresh Herb Sauce 287
    with Ground Lamb 199
    Spicy, with Mussels 196
Risotto, Artichoke 362
Roasted Acorn Squash 334
Roasted Baby Artichokes and Parmesan
    Cheese 328
Roasted Broccoli 339
Roasted Caesar Parmesan Romaine 342
Roasted Cornish Hens 273
Roasted Garlic 445
Roasted Pepper Dip 470
Roasted Peppers 311
Sicilian-Style Linguine with Eggplant
    and 177
Roasted Red Pepper Sandwich 363
Roasted Salmon with Wilted Spinach 261
Roasted Seafood Medley 250
Roasted Tomato Boats 457
Romaine, Roasted Caesar Parmesan 342
Rosemary Roasted Chicken Breasts 297

S

Saffron Rice 309
    Spanish Paella with Seafood,
        Chicken, and 170
Salad
    Arugula and Asian Pear 89
    Avocado 75
    Beet and Tomato 104
    Broiled Artichoke 91
    Chickpeas and Garden Vegetables 91
    Classic Greek 77
    Classic Tabbouleh 69
    Corn and Bean 100
    Crunchy Chicken and Fruit 96
    Cucumber 100
    Easy Couscous Parsley 83
    Endive Spinach 88
    Escarole with Anchovy Dressing 94
    Exotic Pear 101
    Fennel 75
    Fig and Prosciutto 90
    Fresh Chopped Garden 99
    Freshly Chopped, with Walnut Dressing 81

Goat Cheese Stuffed Tomatoes 68
Greek Olive and Feta Cheese Pasta 67
Greens with Cheese Medallions 74
Herbed Potato 92
Light Caesar 78
Mediterranean Mixed Greens 72
Moroccan Eggplant 79
Mushroom and Barley 98
North African Zucchini 73
Pasta and Shrimp.................................85
Pear and Walnut 95
Pear and Watercress 97
Peppery Watercress 92
Sardine 84
Savory Greek White Fava Bean 70
Simple Spanish 82
Snow Pea 104
Spicy Cole Slaw 106
Spinach 103
Summer Pasta......................................93
Sweet Red Cabbage 103
Syrian Cucumber and Yogurt.................68
Tangy Orange Roasted Asparagus 71
Tangy Tangerine Cress 86
Toasted Capri 87
Tomato, with Basil, Capers, and
    Vinaigrette....................................105
Tomato Pasta.....................................102
Tunisian Carrot 76
Tunisian Tuna......................................80
Watermelon...93

Salad dressing. See Dressing

Salmon
Cakes, with Sour Cream Dill Sauce 212
Fillets, Pan Roasted.............................271
Fruit-Glazed, with Couscous 184
Garlic Salmon Linguini 269
Grilled Blackened 303
Grilled Citrus, with Garlic Greens 176
Horseradish-Encrusted 211
Lemon-Pepper....................................282
Roasted, with Wilted Spinach 261
Sauce, Pasta with 256
Smoked, Fettuccine with Basil Pesto and 230

Smoked, Potato Leek Soup with 137
with Smoked Paprika............................290

Salsa
Avocado and Mango.............................455
Cucumber 465
Mediterranean 465

Sandwich. *See also* **Pita Pockets; Wrap**
Chickpea and Fresh Spinach..................372
Goat Cheese and Pesto 377
Grilled Chili Tuna 378
Pear, Cream Cheese, and Red Onion 377
Roasted Red Pepper..............................363
Smoked Fish and Roasted Pepper 373

Sardine(s)
Pasta, with Lemon and Garlic...............286
Pasta Sauce 487
Salad..84

Sauce(s)
Anchovy and Garlic..............................490
Anchovy and Garlic, Whole Wheat
    Spaghetti with...............................203
Basil Pesto 488
Black Olive Paste 480
Chive, Grilled Whole Rainbow Trout
    and, ...216
Cornstarch Paste..................................483
Dill, Encrusted Red Snapper and...........213
Dill, Lightly Pan-Fried Crusted Trout
    with 284
Easy Basil Pesto 481
Fresh Herb, Rigatoni in 287
Hardy Eggplant 481
Honey Mustard 486
Lemon Caper, Pan Seared Halibut
    with 293
Lemon Yogurt, Toasted Crêpe Cups
    with Fresh Berries in a 424
Lime, with Toasted Almonds 480
Mushroom-Shallot 482
Mustard Ginger, Blackened Tuna
    Steaks with 217
Orange Ginger 478
Orange Ginger, Broiled Scallops with 234
Pesto, Fava Beans with.........................344

Pomegranate, Chicken with...................206
Pomodora..274
Pomodora, and Grilled Chicken............274
Red Clam..489
Red Clam, Pasta with 201
Red Pesto..479
Remoulade Dipping Sauce 466
Salmon Pasta with 256
Sardine Pasta 487
Simple Quick Tomato 483
Simple Tomato Pasta 492
Simply Great Marinara 491
Sour Cream Dill, Salmon Cakes with 212
Spicy Black Bean, Shrimp in.................209
Spicy Garlicky Pesto 484
Spicy Pistachio Pesto.............................486
Spicy Red, Calamari in 300
Spicy Red, Mussels in 237
Strawberry..395
Sundried Tomato Pesto..........................485
Sweet and Spicy Glaze 479
Thick Pomegranate Molasses 484
Tomato and Anchovy, with Pasta...........225
Tomato-Basil 485
White Wine...482
Yogurt 447

Sausage, Sweet Italian, Stuffed Zucchini
with Vegetables and 262
Sautéed Garlic Spinach.......................361
Sautéed Kale..336
Sautéed Kale and Spinach with
Mushrooms and Tomato..................327
Sautéed Mixed Fish over Garlic Couscous ...
244
Sautéed Peaches or Nectarines
with Maple Syrup 399
Sautéed Portobellos with Garlic
and Parsley 354
Sautéed Shrimp and Mushroom
Couscous 278
Sautéed Vegetables with Fresh Thyme....349
Savory Greek White Fava Bean Salad.......70
Savory Mediterranean Chickpea
Soup 123

Scallops
Bay, with Smoked Paprika 455
with Braised Apples 267
Broiled, with Orange Ginger Sauce 234
Orange Horseradish-Encrusted..............214
Pan-Seared Parmesan Cheese,
with Rice Pilaf 281
Pasta with Pine Nuts and 182
Poached, Italian 192
Sea, Seared Golden 282
and Shrimp, Citrus 191
Sea Bass
Chilean, Baked 271
Grilled Whole...306
Steamed..188
Seafood. *See also* **Fish;** *specific types*
of seafood
Black Bean Seafood Burgers..................228
Bouillabaisse..174
Mixed, Linguine and 197
Roasted Seafood Medley........................250
Spanish Paella with Saffron Rice,
Chicken, and 170
Seared Golden Sea Scallops 282
Seasoning Mix, Blackening.................477
Sesame Bread (Kersa) 387
Shallot-Balsamic Vinaigrette.................499
Shells, Pesto Stuffed 187
Sherbet, Lemon.....................................420
Shrimp
and Avocado Wrap 381
Baby, and Mozzarella Cheese Pizza 142
Baby, Baked Flounder with Capers and 222
Baby, on Toasted Rye.............................453
Gnocchi with Asparagus and 245
Honey Mustard 263
Lemon Shrimp Pasta 305
Pasta Primavera with..............................185
Salad, Pasta and 85
Sautéed, and Mushroom Couscous........278
Scallops and, Citrus 191
Smoked Paprika, White Beans and 277
Spicy, with Angel Hair Pasta.................183
in Spicy Black Bean Sauce 209

Whole Wheat Penne with Broccoli and.....221

Sicilian Dressing.....................................497

**Sicilian-Style Linguine with Eggplant
and Roasted Peppers.........................177**

Side dishes

Artichoke Risotto 362

Asparagus with Fresh Garden Herbs 317

Baked Acorn Squash.................................335

Baked Eggplant with Garlic and Basil....353

Baked Parsnip Fries with Rosemary 341

Baked Potato Fingers with Shallots
and Fresh Herbs...............................321

Baked Sweet Potato Fries with Basil
Pesto 360

Basic Rice Pilaf..352

Boiled Fresh Red Beets 326

Broccoli with Almonds and Olives.........323

Broccoli with Fresh Garlic 317

Broiled Avocado Halves and Cheddar
Cheese..323

Caramelized Brussels Sprouts with
Garlic and Red Chili Peppers............337

Caramelized Onions and Roasted Kale 338

Chickpeas with Couscous.......................347

Chilled Stuffed Pasta Shells....................313

Cinnamon Couscous 350

Classic Spinach and Pine Nuts...............312

Couscous, Tomatoes, and Black Beans 316

Couscous with Turnips and Greens........325

Crispy Tender Broccolini 330

Crispy Tender Ratatouille 318

Fava Beans with Pesto Sauce 344

Feta and Mixed Beans.............................345

Fresh Spinach with Roasted
Mushrooms 340

Fresh Stewed Tomatoes...........................332

Garlicky Cannellini Beans 355

Garlicky Swiss Chard...............................319

Garlic Rice 315

Garlic Roasted Cauliflower 361

Gingered Green Beans and Pea Pods......357

Great Corn on the Cob 320

Greek Rice..314

Green Beans and Baby Portobellos.........360

Grilled Eggplant.......................................356

Grilled Jumbo Portobello Mushrooms 346

Grilled Polenta with Cheddar Cheese
and Sundried Tomatoes 324

Italian Broccoli 329

Kale with Orange-Mustard Dressing......322

Lemon-Almond Couscous.......................335

Lemon Garlic Asparagus..........................343

Mashed Parsnips and Carrots.................344

Mom's Brown Rice 359

Orzo with Feta Cheese and Broccoli
Florets..310

Oven-Roasted Potato Wedges 326

Pass the Peas, Please 320

Polenta 354

Polenta with Mushrooms and Garlic......355

Roasted Acorn Squash 334

Roasted Baby Artichokes and Parmesan
Cheese..328

Roasted Broccoli......................................339

Roasted Caesar Parmesan Romaine........342

Roasted Peppers..311

Saffron Rice..309

Sautéed Garlic Spinach 361

Sautéed Kale...336

Sautéed Kale and Spinach with
Mushrooms and Tomato...................327

Sautéed Portobellos with Garlic
and Parsley...354

Sautéed Vegetables with Fresh Thyme....349

Snap Peas with Basil Pesto 336

Spicy Couscous..348

Spicy Julienned Sweet Potato Fries.........331

Spicy Snow Peas.......................................334

Steamed Artichokes 358

Swiss Chard and Arborio Rice 351

Tuscan Braised Fennel 346

Twice-Baked Sweet Potatoes with
Cheese and Fresh Sage 333

Zesty Lemon Swiss Chard.......................310

Simple Quick Tomato Sauce 483

Simple Spanish Salad...............................82

Simple Tomato Pasta Sauce...................492

Simply Great Marinara Sauce 491

Skewered Mediterranean Grilled
    Lamb and Vegetables 171
Sloppy Joe, Meatless............................... 376
Smoked Fish and Roasted Pepper
    Sandwich 373
Smoked Salmon
    Fettuccine with Basil Pesto and.............. 230
    and Mozzarella Cheese Pizza................. 139
    Potato Leek Soup with......................... 137
Smoked Trout Dip 464
Smoothie
    Soy Milk, Banana Peach Vanilla............. 443
    Soy Milk, Chocolate Raspberry 444
    Whey, Blueberry Burst......................... 439
    Whey, Chocolate Mousse 442
    Whey, Melon Madness 444
    Whey, Pineapple Delight....................... 443
    Whey, Strawberry Sundae...................... 441
Snack foods
    Chocolate Bites 471
    Cinnamon and Flaxseed Wafers............. 472
Snap Peas, with Basil Pesto..................... 336
Snow Peas, Spicy 334
Snow Pea Salad 104
Sole
    Peppered Fillet of................................ 264
    Spicy 169
Sorbet
    Apricot 417
    Cantaloupe.. 404
    Honeydew 405
    Plum 435
Soup
    Basic Lentil....................................... 122
    Cauliflower.. 119
    Chicken Escarole................................ 132
    Chilled Avocado 111
    Chilled Cucumber............................... 133
    Chilly Tomato 125
    Chunky Chicken and Cabbage.............. 127
    Chunky Fish Chowder with Saffron 131
    Creamy Green Garden.......................... 109
    Egg-Lemon Pasta 107
    Eggplant.. 115

    Eggplant, with Dry Sherry and
        Feta Cheese...................................... 134
    French Pistou 128
    Fresh Chicken Broth............................ 108
    Fresh Garden Gazpacho........................ 124
    Hearty Bean 129
    Italian Minestrone, with Pesto 126
    Lemony Chicken and Orzo 110
    Mom's Chicken 136
    Old-Fashioned Oyster Stew................... 114
    Pasta e Fagioli 135
    Potato-Broccoli, with Greens 112
    Potato Leek, with Smoked Salmon 137
    Red Clam Chowder.............................. 117
    Savory Mediterranean Chickpea 123
    Spicy Vegetable Stew............................ 118
    Spinach Feta Cheese 130
    Spinach Tortellini 116
    Stracciatella (Italian Egg Drop)............. 121
    Tomato Tortellini 120
    Vegetable and Tortellini....................... 113
Sour Cream and Walnut Cookies 421
Sour Cream Dill Sauce, Salmon
    Cakes with.. 212
Spaghetti, Whole Wheat, with
    Anchovy and Garlic Sauce................. 203
Spanish Omelet.................................... 158
Spanish Paella with Saffron Rice,
    Seafood, and Chicken 170
Spanish Salad, Simple............................ 82
Spice Cake... 398
Spiced Apples 419
Spice Rub.. 476
    Chicken.. 477
    Spicy Chicken 478
Spices
    Harissa (Red Pepper Spice) 476
    Mixed... 475
Spicy Black Bean Sauce, Shrimp in........ 209
Spicy Broccoli Rabe with Penne Pasta..... 175
Spicy Chicken Rub............................... 478
Spicy Chicken with Couscous 190
Spicy Cole Slaw................................... 106
Spicy Couscous 348

Spicy Eggplant 308
Spicy Garlic, Olive Oil, and Sundried
   Tomato Pizza Sauce 148
Spicy Garlicky Pesto Sauce 484
Spicy Hummus in Toasted Pita Loaves 369
Spicy Julienned Sweet Potato Fries 331
Spicy Mediterranean Pasta 276
Spicy Mushroom Wrap 371
Spicy Pistachio Pesto 486
Spicy Red Sauce, Calamari in 300
Spicy Rigatoni with Mussels 196
Spicy Shrimp with Angel Hair Pasta...... 183
Spicy Snow Peas 334
Spicy Sole.. 169
Spicy Stuffed Tilapia 194
Spicy Sweet Pepper Pizza........................ 144
Spicy Vegetable Stew 118
Spicy Whole Wheat Capellini with
   Garlic... 180
Spinach
   and Chickpea Fresh Spinach Sandwich.....372
   Fettuccine, with Baby Artichokes...........296
   Fresh, with Roasted Mushrooms............340
   Lemony Pasta with Goat Cheese and.....249
   Orecchiette with Kale, Toasted Bread
      Crumbs, Pine Nuts, and, in a Red
      Sauce 268
   and Pine Nuts, Classic...........................312
   Quiche, Swiss Cheese and......................272
   Salad..103
   Salad, Endive and 88
   Sautéed Garlic 361
   Sautéed Kale and, with Mushrooms
      and Tomato 327
   Soup, Spinach Feta Cheese 130
   Soup, Tortellini....................................116
   and Swiss Cheese Quiche......................272
   Wilted, Roasted Salmon with 261
Steamed Artichokes................................ 358
Steamed Dungeness Crab........................ 215
Steamed Mussels with Garlic and
   Dry Vermouth 226
Steamed Sea Bass.................................... 188
Stew

Lentil..302
Old-Fashioned Oyster 114
Spicy Vegetable.................................... 118
Turkish Mussel 186
Stewed Tomatoes, Fresh.......................... 332
Stracciatella (Italian Egg Drop Soup)..... 121
Strawberry(-ies)
   Amaretto 419
   and Balsamic Syrup 405
   Buttermilk Pancakes 165
   Crêpes, Toasted Sautéed Banana and 425
   Drunken...412
   and Poached Pears 395
   -Rhubarb Quinoa Pudding...................411
   Sauce...395
   Sundae Whey Smoothie........................441
   -Walnut Trifle 416
Stuffed Dates.. 402
Stuffed Grape Leaves (Dolmas) 446
Stuffed Sesame Chicken Breasts 218
Stuffed Whole Wheat Khubz................. 368
Stuffed Zucchini with Vegetables
   and Sweet Italian Sausage 262
Summer Pasta Salad 93
Summer Rhubarb Cooler 440
Sundried Tomato(es)
   and Anchovy Pizza................................146
   Basil White Wheat Bread......................393
   Crostini with Pesto, Mozzarella,
      Prosciutto, and 456
   Fettuccine with Goat Cheese and 204
   Grilled Polenta with Cheddar Cheese
      and 324
   Pesto...485
   Pesto Sauce, Codfish in........................232
   Pizza, Anchovy and..............................146
   Pizza Sauce, Spicy Garlic, Olive Oil,
      and 148
Sweet and Spicy Glaze 479
Sweet Italian Rice Pudding.................... 402
Sweet Italian Sausage, Stuffed
   Zucchini with Vegetables and........... 262
Sweet Mango Mousse.............................. 400
Sweet Pepper Pizza, Spicy....................... 144

Sweet Plum Compote...........................430
Sweet Potato(es)
    Fries, Baked, with Basil Pesto.................360
    Fries, Spicy Julienned...........................331
    Twice-Baked, with Cheese and Fresh
        Sage...333
Sweet Red Cabbage Salad.....................103
Swiss Chard
    and Arborio Rice..................................351
    Garlicky..319
    Zesty Lemon..310
Swiss Cheese and Spinach Quiche.........272
Swordfish, Blackened 198
Syrian Cucumber and Yogurt Salad.........68

T

Tahini
    -Baked Flounder...................................189
    Dip, Hummus with...............................470
Tangerine Cress Salad, Tangy.................86
Tangy Orange Roasted Asparagus
    Salad...71
Tangy Tangerine Cress Salad...................86
Tartlets, Phyllo, with Honey-Sweetened
    Cherries...408
Thick Pomegranate Molasses.................484
Thin Crust Pizza Dough.......................152
Tilapia
    Baked...195
    Grilled..223
    Pan-Seared Lemon-Pepper....................294
    Spicy Stuffed 194
Toasted Capri Salad...............................87
Toasted Crêpe Cups with Fresh Berries
    in a Lemon Yogurt Sauce 424
Toasted Sautéed Banana and
    Strawberry Crêpes.............................425
Tofu, Pasta with, in a Spicy Marinara
    Sauce...295
Tomato(es). *See also* Sundried Tomato(es)
    and Anchovy Sauce with Pasta..............225
    -Basil Sauce..485
    Boats, Roasted.....................................457
    Broiled Tuna and..................................208

    Bruschetta, Fresh Parmesan Cheese
        and 448
    Bruschetta, Garlic and 447
    Couscous, Black Beans, and...................316
    Fresh Stewed.......................................332
    Fusilli and..283
    Goat Cheese Stuffed 68
    Pasta Salad...102
    Pasta Sauce, Simple..............................492
    Pesto, Broiled Halibut Steaks with........231
    Pizza, Eggplant, Basil, and....................143
    Pizza, Eggplant, Basil and.....................143
    Pizza, Sauce, Spicy Garlic, Olive Oil,
        and 148
    Pizza Sauce, Basil and 148
    Roasted, Orecchiette Pasta and.............292
    Salad, Beet and....................................104
    Salad, with Basil, Capers, and
        Vinaigrette..............................105
    Sauce, Simple Quick.............................483
    Sautéed Kale and Spinach with
        Mushrooms and.......................327
    Soup, Chilly 125
    Soup, Tortellini...................................120
    Sundried, Fettuccine with Goat
        Cheese and 204
    Sundried, Grilled Polenta with
        Cheddar Cheese and.................324
    Sundried, Pesto Sauce, Codfish in..........232
Tortellini
    Soup, Spinach Tortellini 116
    Soup, Tomato Tortellini........................120
    Soup, Vegetable and.............................113
Traditional Pizza Sauce........................147
Trifle, Strawberry-Walnut.....................416
Trout
    Almandine...233
    Baked Stuffed......................................172
    Dip, Smoked Trout...............................464
    Lightly Pan-Fried Crusted, with
        Dill Sauce 284
    Rainbow, Grilled Whole, and
        Chive Sauce............................216
Tuna

Broiled, Tomato and 208
Grilled Chili Tuna Sandwich 378
Salad, Great, on Whole Grain Toast.......375
Salad, Tunisian 80
Steaks, Blackened, with Mustard
  Ginger Sauce 217
Tunisian Carrot Salad...............................76
Tunisian Tuna Salad.................................80
Turkey
Burgers, Broiled Spicy 220
Burgers, Mom's.....................................229
Meatballs, with Whole Grain Pasta
  and Tomato Sauce.............................299
Meatloaf, Easy 252
Tetrazzini..253
Turkish Mussel Stew 186
Turnips, Couscous with Greens and 325
Tuscan Braised Fennel 346
**Twice-Baked Sweet Potatoes with
  Cheese and Fresh Sage 333**

V

Vanilla-Rhubarb Compote 415
Veal Scaloppine 307
**Vegetable(s). *See also* Garden
  Vegetables**
Broiled Chicken with Barley and 266
Lemony Chicken and 210
Mixed Vegetable Frittata.......................157
Omelet, with Pesto 163
Sautéed, with Fresh Thyme...................349
Skewered Mediterranean Grilled
  Lamb and 171
Soup, Tortellini and..............................113
Stew, Spicy 118
Stuffed Zucchini with Sweet Italian
  Sausage and 262
Veggie Wrap 365
Vinaigrette
Chive...498
Fresh Fig..497
Mint..498
Shallot-Balsamic....................................499

W

Walnut
Cookies, Sour Cream and......................421
Crostini, Apple, Gorgonzola, and 454
Dressing 81
and Greek Feta Dip 467
and Pear Salad 95
Watercress
Salad, Pear and 97
Salad, Peppery 92
Tangy Tangerine 86
Watermelon Salad 93
White Beans
Fava Bean Salad, Savory Greek 70
Pasta and 288
and Smoked Paprika Shrimp 277
and Wild Mushrooms with Chicken......259
White Wine Sauce...................................482
**Whole Roasted Branzino with Buttery
  Lemon Sauce 285**
Whole Wheat Khubz, Stuffed................368
**Whole Wheat Penne with Shrimp
  and Broccoli.......................................221**
Whole Wheat Pizza Dough 151
Crispy Thin 150
**Whole Wheat Spaghetti with
  Anchovy and Garlic Sauce.................203**
Wild Mushroom Pizza............................145
**Wild Rice, Chicken and, with Garden
  Vegetables 248**
Wrap
Apple-Walnut Raisin..............................379
Chicken Pesto..380
Lamb...364
Shrimp and Avocado 381
Spicy Mushroom 371
Veggie..365

Y

Yogurt
and Cucumber Salad, Syrian....................68
Deliciously Sweetened 412
Dip, Herb Cucumber Yogurt.................469
Dressing 495
Fresh Fruit in, with Rum 401

Plain, Figs in 396
Sauce 447
Yummy Marinade for Chicken 494

Z

Zesty Lemon Swiss Chard 310
Zucchini

Boats, Pizza 460
Frittata 162
Frittata, Ham and 160
Salad, North African 73
Stuffed, with Vegetables and Sweet
Italian Sausage 262

Index

A

abdominal fat
    and exercise, 25
    and whey consumption, 34
ACE inhibitors, 505
adrenaline, 15
Adventist Health Study, 519
aerobic exercise, 16
aging
    and free radicals, 35
    and hypertension, 24
AHA (American Heart
    Association), 517
AHA (American Heart
    Association) diet, 10, 19
alcohol
    drawbacks of consuming, 33
    and heart health, 33
    and hypertension, 24
almond milk, 34
Alzheimer's Disease Study, 10
American (Western) diet, 4
    fats in, 11
    free radicals from, 34–37
    omega-3 deficiency in, 28
    portion size in, 21–22
    saturated and trans fats in,
        28

American Heart Association
    (AHA), 517
American Heart Association
    Step 1 diet, 10, 19
American lifestyle, 4
    free radicals from, 34–37
    stress in, 14
American Society of
    Nephrology, 30
amino acids, 34
angiotensinogen, 25
angiotensin receptor blockers,
    506
antioxidants
    in coffee and tea, 32
    and free radicals, 35–37
    in fruit juices, 31
    in Mediterranean diet, 7,
        34–37
arthritis
    inflammation linked to, 7
    and olive oil consumption,
        13
aspirin, 506
asthma, olive oil consumption
    and, 13
atherogenic metabolic stew,
    503–504

atherosclerosis
    and free radicals, 35
    and pomegranate juice, 11
Atkins diet, 20

B

bad cholesterol. *See* LDL
    cholesterol
baking, 65
barley, 12
beans (legumes)
    canned, reducing sodium
        from, 45
    and free radical reduction,
        37
    in Mediterranean diet, 12
    soaking, 509–510
    tips for purchasing,
        preparing, and eating,
        509–511
beer, heart health and, 33
Benson, Herbert, 25
beta blockers, 505–506
beta-carotene, 37
beverages, 31–34
black tea, 32
blood clotting
    and alcohol consumption, 13

and chronic stress, 15
and free radicals, 35
and green tea
    consumption, 32
and trans fats, 28
blood glucose. *See* blood sugar
blood pressure
and chronic stress, 15
and exercise, 16, 25
and flavanols, 39
and fructose consumption,
    30
impact of Mediterranean
    diet on, 10, 23–24
normal reading, 23
and nutrients in
    Mediterranean diet, 25
and phytonutrients, 25
and pomegranate juice,
    11, 31
and salt intake, 39
and stress, 25
blood pressure medications,
    506
blood sugar (blood glucose)
and cinnamon
    consumption, 38
and flavanols, 39
impact of Mediterranean
    diet on, 10
boiling, 65
bone health, exercise and, 16
bread, 512–513
breathing techniques, 25
broad beans, 510
broiling, 65
bulgur, 516
bypass surgery, 5

C

caffeine
in coffee and teas, 32
and hypertension, 24
calcium channel blockers, 506
cancer
and bean consumption, 12
and fresh fruits and
    vegetables, 12

and green tea
    consumption, 32
and inflammation, 7, 11
and low-carb diets, 20
and olive oil consumption,
    13
reasons for Mediterranean
    diet's reduction of, 11
and saturated fats, 28
Seven Countries Study of,
    9–10
and tea consumption, 32
and trans fats, 28
and whole grain
    consumption, 11
cannellini beans, 510
canola oil, 509
carbohydrates. *See also specific
types of carbohydrates, e.g.:*
fruits
complex vs. simple, 22,
    29–30
in Mediterranean diet,
    29–30
cardiac arrhythmias
and low-carb diets, 20
and omega-3 consumption,
    12
cardiovascular disease, 4–7
and alcohol consumption,
    33
and choices we make, 41
medications for prevention
    of, 505–506
cardiovascular events
and chronic stress, 15
reduced with
    Mediterranean diet, 9
in Singh Indo-
    Mediterranean Diet
    Study, 10
cardiovascular health, 9–12
catecholamines, 25
cell death, 35
cheeses, 34
chickpeas, 510
chocolate, 39
cholesterol, 503. *See also* HDL

(good) cholesterol; LDL
(bad) cholesterol
and alcohol consumption,
    13
and cinnamon
    consumption, 38
and exercise, 23
and fish oil consumption,
    38
and flavanols, 39
impact of Mediterranean
    diet on, 10, 22–23
and low-carb diets, 20
and nut consumption, 12
and olive oil consumption,
    13
and omega-3 consumption,
    12
in Singh Indo-
    Mediterranean Diet
    Study, 10
and whole milk
    consumption, 33
cholesterol absorption
    inhibitors,
    505
chronic diseases, 7
chronic stress, 15
cinnamon, 38–39
coffee, 32
Columbia University Medical
    Center, 10
combination of foods, 7
complex carbohydrates, 22
cooking methods, 65
coronary artery spasm, free
    radicals and, 35
coronary heart disease, 4–7.
See also heart disease
and alcohol consumption,
    13
and cinnamon
    consumption, 38
and fatty fish
    consumption, 10
and nut consumption, 12
Seven Countries Study of,
    9–10

cortisol, 15
couscous, 516
cranberry juice, 31

D
dairy
    milk, 33–34
    whey, 34
    yogurt, 34
dark chocolate, 39
DART Study, 10
death due to cardiovascular
  problems, 41
    and AHA diet, 10, 19
    and exercise, 16
    and fatty fish
      consumption, 10
    and fish oil consumption,
      38
    impact of Mediterranean
      diet on, 9, 11
    and napping, 14
    and omega-3 consumption,
      12
    in Seven Countries Study,
      10
    in Singh Indo-
      Mediterranean Diet
      Study, 10
deep muscle relaxation, 25
dehydration, 32
dental plaque, 32
desserts, 39–40
diabetes
    and bean consumption, 12
    and cinnamon
      consumption, 38
    and coffee/tea
      consumption, 32
    and inflammation, 11
    and olive oil consumption,
      13
    and trans fats, 28
    and whole grain
      consumption, 11
diastolic blood pressure, 23, 24
diet(s). *See also* American
  (Western) diet;

Mediterranean diet
    fad/popular, 19–21
    and health, 3–5
    and heart disease
      prevention, 5–6
    low-carbohydrate, 20
    low-fat, 9, 19, 35
disease(s). *See also specific*
  diseases
    chronic, 7
    and free radicals, 35
    and inflammation, 7, 11
    linked to diet and lifestyle,
      4
    and milk consumption,
      33–34
    and red meat
      consumption, 36
    reduced by Mediterranean
      diet, 5, 9–12
durum hard grain, 512

E
eating out, 521–522
Eliot, Robert S., 25
environmental toxins, 35
Esposito, Katherine, 10
exercise
    for cholesterol control, 23
    in Mediterranean lifestyle,
      16, 25
    in stress management, 15,
      26
    for weight loss, 22

F
fad diets, 19–21
fat-free milk, 34
fats. *See also individual kinds*
  of fats
    in American (Western)
      diet, 11
    in chocolate, 39
    and free radicals, 35
    in Mediterranean diet,
      27–28
    monounsaturated, 12, 13,
      27

    in nuts, 12
    polyunsaturated, 27
    saturated, 11, 25, 28
    trans, 11, 22, 25, 28
    unsaturated, 27
    in whole milk, 33
fatty fish, 10
fava beans, 510
fiber, 7
fibrates, 505
fibrinogen, 503
fish
    and cardiovascular health,
      25
    contaminants in, 12–13
    fatty, 10
    and free radical reduction,
      37
    in Mediterranean diet,
      12–13
    tips for purchasing,
      preparing, and eating,
      517–518
fish oil, 38
flavanols, 39
food combinations, 7
free radicals, 34–37
fricasseeing, 65
fructose, 30
fruit drinks, 32
fruit juices, 31
fruits
    antioxidants from, 35, 37
    and cardiovascular health,
      25
    in Mediterranean diet, 7, 12
    nutrient depletion in, 28
frying, 65

G
gallstones, coffee/tea
  consumption and, 32
garbanzo beans, 510
garlic, cardiovascular health
  and, 25
glycemic index, 29–30
good cholesterol. *See* HDL
  cholesterol

grains. *See also* whole grains
refined, 12
    tips for purchasing,
        preparing, and eating,
        511–513
grapefruit juice, 31
grape juice (red or purple),
    13, 25, 31
Great Northern beans, 511
green tea, 32

H
Harvard Men's Health Watch,
    519
Harvard School of Public
    Health, 519
HDL (good) cholesterol, 503,
    504, 506
    and AHA diet, 19
    and alcohol consumption,
        13
    and exercise, 16, 23
    and Mediterranean diet, 22
    and olive oil consumption,
        13, 508
    trans fats, 28
    and whey consumption, 34
heart attack
    and AHA diet, 10, 19
    deaths from, 41
    and exercise, 16
    and fish oil consumption,
        38
    and grape juice, 13
    and high blood pressure, 23
    and nut consumption, 12
    and omega-3 consumption,
        12
    reduced with
        Mediterranean diet, 9
    and salt intake, 39
    in Seven Countries Study,
        10
    in Singh Indo-
        Mediterranean Diet
        Study, 10
heartbeat, chronic stress and,
    15

heart disease, 4–7. *See also*
    coronary heart disease
    and bean consumption, 12
    and fish oil consumption,
        38
    and fresh fruits and
        vegetables, 12
    and inflammation, 7, 11
    and low-carb diets, 20
    and napping, 14
    and olive oil consumption,
        13
    reasons for Mediterranean
        diet's reduction of, 11
    risk factors for, 503–504
    and saturated fats, 28
    and smoking, 26
    and tea consumption, 32
    and trans fats, 28
    and triglycerides, 30
    and whole grain
        consumption, 11
heart health
    Mediterranean diet for,
        9–12
    and monounsaturated fat,
        13
    and pomegranate juice, 31
    and whey consumption,
        34
herbal teas, 32
high-fat diets, 35
high-fructose corn syrup, 30
high sensitivity C-reactive
    protein
    (hs-CRP), 503
HMG-CoA reductase
    inhibitors (statins), 505
homocysteine, 503
hormones
    in milk, 33
    stress, 15
"hot reactors," 25
hs-CRP (high sensitivity
    C-reactive protein), 503
hydrogenated oils, 28
hypertension, 24, 25, 30. *See
    also* blood pressure

I
infectious agents, 503
inflammation
    and disease development,
        11
    impact of Mediterranean
        diet on, 7, 10
    and olive oil consumption,
        13
    and omega-3 consumption,
        12
    and trans fats, 28
Iowa Women's Healthy Study,
    519

J
juices, 31–32

K
kasha, 12
ketosis, 20
Keys, Ancel, 9
kidney disease, high blood
    pressure and, 23
kidney malfunction, low-carb
    diets and, 20
kidney stones, coffee/tea
    consumption and, 32

L
lactose, 34
LDL (bad) cholesterol, 503,
    504
    and alcohol consumption,
        13
    and exercise, 23
    and green tea
        consumption, 32
    and low-carb diets, 20
    and Mediterranean diet, 22
    and olive oil consumption,
        13, 508
    and saturated fats, 28
    and trans fats, 28
legumes. *See* beans (legumes)
lentils, 511
lifestyle. *See also*
    Mediterranean lifestyle

American, 4, 14, 34–37
and health, 3–4
and hypertension, 24
and prevention of heart
disease, 5–6
lipid peroxides, 35
lipids, 503
lipoprotein (a) (LPa), 503
Loma Linda University, 519
low-carbohydrate diets, 20
low-fat diets
comparison of
Mediterranean diet
and, 9
drawbacks of, 19
and lipid peroxide
production, 35
LPa (lipoprotein [a]), 503
lung function, exercise and,
16
Lyon Diet Heart Study, 10, 19

M

medications, for
cardiovascular disease
prevention, 505–506
meditation, 15, 25
Mediterranean diet, 9–14
adaptation of, 11
antioxidants for free radical
reduction in, 34–37
beans (legumes) in, 12
beverages in, 31–34
carbohydrates in, 29–30
chronic diseases reduced
by, 7
cinnamon in, 38–39
clinical trials
demonstrating impact
of, 9–12
dark chocolate in, 39
disease risks reduced by, 5
fats in, 27–28
fish in, 12–13
fresh fruits and vegetables
in, 12
health benefits of, 7
menu plan for, 45–63

nuts in, 12
olive oil in, 13
and omega-3 deficiency,
28–29
reasons for choosing, 21
red wine in, 13
restaurant survival guide,
521–522
ten commandments of, 17
tips for purchasing,
preparing, and eating
foods in, 507–520
and vitamin supplements,
37–38
water in, 31
whole grains in, 11–12
Mediterranean Diet Pyramid,
14
Mediterranean lifestyle, 14–16
benefits of, 21
exercise in, 16
stress reduction in, 14–16
ten commandments of, 17
menu plan, 45–63
metabolic syndrome, 10
Metabolic Syndrome Study, 10
micronutrients, 37
milk, 33–34
milk chocolate, 39
monounsaturated fats, 12,
13, 27
muscle growth, whey
consumption and, 34
muscle tone, 16

N

naps, 14
navy beans, 510
niacin, 37, 505
nutrition
with Mediterranean diet,
24–25
to protect from free
radicals, 37
and soil depletion, 28
nuts
and cardiovascular health,
25

and free radical reduction,
37
in Mediterranean diet, 12
tips for purchasing,
preparing, and eating,
518–520

O

oatmeal, 12
obesity
and exercise, 16
and high-fructose corn
syrup, 30
impact of Mediterranean
diet on, 10
and trans fats, 22
and whole milk
consumption, 33
olive oil
and cardiovascular health,
25
in Mediterranean diet, 13
tips for purchasing,
preparing, and eating,
507–509
types of, 507–508
omega-3 fatty acids, 12, 27,
517
and cardiovascular health,
25
deficiency of, 28–29
in fish, 518
from fish oils, 38
ratio of omega-6s and,
28–29
omega-6/omega-3 ratio, 28–
29
orange juice, 31
Ornish diet, 19
osteoporosis, exercise and, 16
oxidation, 34–35

P

pan broiling, 65
partially hydrogenated oils, 28
particle size (cholesterol), 504
pasta, 513–516
cooking, 513–514

size and shapes of, 514–515

peanut butter, 519

Physician's Health Study, 519

phytonutrients, 24–25, 37

phytosterols, 23

plant sterols, 23

plaques, 4–7

polenta, 517

polyunsaturated fats, 27

pomegranate juice, 11, 31

popular diets, 19–21

portion control, 21–22

potassium salt, 39

prayer, 15, 25

pre-hypertension, 23

preventive cardiology, 4–6, 41
  medications for, 505–506
  success of Mediterranean diet in, 11

Pritikin diet, 19

protein
  red meat, 36
  whey, 34

Purdue University, 519–520

Q

"quick fix" diets, 19–21

quinoa, 12

R

rapid heartbeat, chronic stress and, 15

red meat, 36

red wine
  and cardiovascular health, 25
  and heart health, 33
  in Mediterranean diet, 13

refined grains, 12, 512

The Relaxation Response (Herbert Benson), 25

relaxation response training, 15, 25–26

resins, 505

resistance training, 16

restaurant survival guide, 521–522

resveratrol, 13

rice, 516–517

roasting, 65

S

salt. *See also* sodium
  and hypertension, 24
  potassium, 39
  sodium in, 39

satiety, 22

saturated fats, 11, 25, 28

sautéing, 65

Scarmeas, Nikolaos, 10

secondary hypertension, 24

self-hypnosis, 15, 25

Seven Countries Study, 9–10

simmering, 65

simple carbohydrates, 22

Singh Indo-Mediterranean Diet Study, 10

smoking, 24, 26

sodium, 39. *See also* salt
  and blood pressure, 25
  from canned beans, 45
  and hypertension, 24
  in vegetable juices, 32

soft drinks, 30

spices, 511

statins, 38, 505

steaming, 65

stents, 5

stevia, 30

stewing, 65

stress hormones, 15

stress reduction
  exercise for, 25
  in Mediterranean lifestyle, 14–16
  techniques for, 25–26

stroke
  reduced with Mediterranean diet, 9
  and salt intake, 39
  and systolic pressure, 23

sugars
  high-fructose corn syrup, 30
  lactose, 34

from simple vs. complex carbohydrates, 29–30

surgery, 5, 24

sweeteners, 30

synergistic, Mediterranean diet as, 7

systolic blood pressure, 23, 24

T

tea, 32

The Ten Commandments of Mediterranean Diet and Lifestyle, 17

tomato juice, 31–32

toxins, 35

transcendental meditation, 25

trans fats, 11, 22, 25, 28

triglycerides, 503
  and exercise, 23
  and Mediterranean diet, 22
  and omega-3 consumption, 12
  and sugar intake, 30
  and whey consumption, 34

U

unsaturated fats, 27

V

vascular disease, high blood pressure and, 23

vascular inflammation, impact of Mediterranean diet on, 10

vegetable juices, 31–32

vegetable oils, 27, 28

vegetables
  antioxidants from, 35, 37
  and cardiovascular health, 25
  in Mediterranean diet, 7, 12
  nutrient depletion in, 28

vitamin A, 37

vitamin C, 37

vitamin E, 37

vitamin supplements, 37–38

V8 juice, 31–32

W

walking, and risk of heart
   attack/cardiovascular death,
   16
water, 31
weight control
   and exercise, 25
   fad/popular diets for,
      19–21
   and green tea
      consumption, 32
   and low-carb diets, 20

with Mediterranean diet,
   9–12, 21–22
and nut consumption, 12
and olive oil consumption,
   13
well-being, exercise and, 16
Western diet. *See* American
   diet
wheat, 512
whey, 34
whiskey, heart health and, 33
white tea, 32

whole grains, 512
   and free radical reduction, 37
   in Mediterranean diet, 7,
      11–12
whole wheat flour, 513
wine
   and heart health, 33
   red, 13, 25, 33

Y

yoga, 15, 25
yogurt, 34

About the Author

MICHAEL OZNER, MD, FACC, FAHA, is one of America's leading advocates for heart disease prevention. Dr. Ozner is a board-certified cardiologist, a Fellow of the American College of Cardiology and of the American Heart Association, medical director of Wellness & Prevention at Baptist Health South Florida, and a well-known regional and national speaker in the field of preventive cardiology. He is the medical director of the Cardiovascular Prevention Institute of South Florida and symposium director for "Cardiovascular Disease Prevention," an annual international meeting highlighting advances in preventive cardiology and dedicated to the prevention of heart attack and stroke. He was the recipient of the 2008 American Heart Association Humanitarian Award. Dr. Ozner is also the author of the BenBella Books titles *The Great American Heart Hoax*, *Heart Attack Proof*, and *The Mediterranean Diet*.

To contact Dr. Michael Ozner and for more information about the Mediterranean diet and instructional video cooking tutorials, please visit www.drozner.com.